Current Perspectives on the Treatment of Obstructive Sleep Apnea - Part I

Current Perspectives on the Treatment of Obstructive Sleep Apnea - Part I

Editor

Yüksel Peker

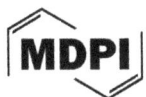

Basel • Beijing • Wuhan • Barcelona • Belgrade • Novi Sad • Cluj • Manchester

Editor
Yüksel Peker
Koc University
Istanbul, Turkey

Editorial Office
MDPI
St. Alban-Anlage 66
4052 Basel, Switzerland

This is a reprint of articles from the Special Issue published online in the open access journal *Journal of Clinical Medicine* (ISSN 2077-0383) (available at: https://www.mdpi.com/journal/jcm/special_issues/Obstructive_Apnea).

For citation purposes, cite each article independently as indicated on the article page online and as indicated below:

Lastname, A.A.; Lastname, B.B. Article Title. *Journal Name* **Year**, *Volume Number*, Page Range.

ISBN 978-3-0365-9742-3 (Hbk)
ISBN 978-3-0365-9743-0 (PDF)
doi.org/10.3390/books978-3-0365-9743-0

© 2023 by the authors. Articles in this book are Open Access and distributed under the Creative Commons Attribution (CC BY) license. The book as a whole is distributed by MDPI under the terms and conditions of the Creative Commons Attribution-NonCommercial-NoDerivs (CC BY-NC-ND) license.

Contents

Yüksel Peker, Henrik Holtstrand-Hjälm, Yeliz Celik, Helena Glantz and Erik Thunström
Postoperative Atrial Fibrillation in Adults with Obstructive Sleep Apnea Undergoing Coronary Artery Bypass Grafting in the RICCADSA Cohort
Reprinted from: *J. Clin. Med.* **2022**, *11*, 2459, doi:10.3390/jcm11092459 1

Peter M. Baptista, Natalia Diaz Zufiaurre, Octavio Garaycochea,
Juan Manuel Alcalde Navarrete, Antonio Moffa, Lucrezia Giorgi, et al.
TORS as Part of Multilevel Surgery in OSA: The Importance of Careful Patient Selection and Outcomes
Reprinted from: *J. Clin. Med.* **2022**, *11*, 990, doi:10.3390/jcm11040990 13

Baixin Chen, Miaolan Guo, Yüksel Peker, Neus Salord, Luciano F. Drager,
Geraldo Lorenzi-Filho, et al.
Effect of Continuous Positive Airway Pressure on Lipid Profiles in Obstructive Sleep Apnea: A Meta-Analysis
Reprinted from: *J. Clin. Med.* **2022**, *11*, 596, doi:10.3390/jcm11030596 23

Yeliz Celik, Baran Balcan and Yüksel Peker
CPAP Intervention as an Add-On Treatment to Lipid-Lowering Medication in Coronary Artery Disease Patients with Obstructive Sleep Apnea in the RICCADSA Trial
Reprinted from: *J. Clin. Med.* **2022**, *11*, 273, doi:10.3390/jcm11010273 33

Cheng-Yu Lin, Yi-Wen Wang, Febryan Setiawan, Nguyen Thi Hoang Trang and Che-Wei Lin
Sleep Apnea Classification Algorithm Development Using a Machine-Learning Framework and Bag-of-Features Derived from Electrocardiogram Spectrograms
Reprinted from: *J. Clin. Med.* **2022**, *11*, 192, doi:10.3390/jcm11010192 43

Maryam Maghsoudipour, Brandon Nokes, Naa-Oye Bosompra, Rachel Jen, Yanru Li,
Stacie Moore, et al.
A Pilot Randomized Controlled Trial of Effect of Genioglossus Muscle Strengthening on Obstructive Sleep Apnea Outcomes
Reprinted from: *J. Clin. Med.* **2021**, *10*, 4554, doi:10.3390/jcm10194554 63

Onintza Garmendia, Ramon Farré, Concepción Ruiz, Monique Suarez-Girón, Marta Torres,
Raisa Cebrian, et al.
Telemedicine Strategy to Rescue CPAP Therapy in Sleep Apnea Patients with Low Treatment Adherence: A Pilot Study
Reprinted from: *J. Clin. Med.* **2021**, *10*, 4123, doi:10.3390/jcm10184123 75

Ewa Olszewska, Piotr Fiedorczuk, Adam Stróżyński, Agnieszka Polecka, Ewa Roszkowska and B. Tucker Woodson
A Pharyngoplasty with a Dorsal Palatal Flap Expansion: The Evaluation of a Modified Surgical Treatment Method for Obstructive Sleep Apnea Syndrome—A Preliminary Report
Reprinted from: *J. Clin. Med.* **2021**, *10*, 3746, doi:10.3390/jcm10163746 85

Yung-An Tsou, Chun-Chieh Hsu, Liang-Chun Shih, Tze-Chieh Lin, Chien-Jen Chiu,
Vincent Hui-Chi Tien, et al.
Combined Transoral Robotic Tongue Base Surgery and Palate Surgery in Obstructive Sleep Apnea Syndrome: Modified Uvulopalatopharyngoplasty versus Barbed Reposition Pharyngoplasty
Reprinted from: *J. Clin. Med.* **2021**, *10*, 3169, doi:10.3390/jcm10143169 101

Clemens Heiser, Armin Steffen, Benedikt Hofauer, Reena Mehra, Patrick J. Strollo, Jr.,
Olivier M. Vanderveken and Joachim T. Maurer
Effect of Upper Airway Stimulation in Patients with Obstructive Sleep Apnea (EFFECT): A Randomized Controlled Crossover Trial
Reprinted from: *J. Clin. Med.* **2021**, *10*, 2880, doi:10.3390/jcm10132880 113

Hiroyuki Ishiyama, Masayuki Hideshima, Shusuke Inukai, Meiyo Tamaoka, Akira Nishiyama and Yasunari Miyazaki
Evaluation of Respiratory Resistance as a Predictor for Oral Appliance Treatment Response in Obstructive Sleep Apnea: A Pilot Study
Reprinted from: *J. Clin. Med.* **2021**, *10*, 1255, doi:10.3390/jcm10061255 . . . . **123**

Adam V. Benjafield, Liesl M. Oldstone, Leslee A. Willes, Colleen Kelly, Carlos M. Nunez, Atul Malhotra and on behalf of the medXcloud Group
Positive Airway Pressure Therapy Adherence with Mask Resupply: A Propensity-Matched Analysis
Reprinted from: *J. Clin. Med.* **2021**, *10*, 720, doi:10.3390/jcm10040720 . . . . **137**

Maria R. Bonsignore, Carolina Lombardi, Simone Lombardo and Francesco Fanfulla
Epidemiology, Physiology and Clinical Approach to Sleepiness at the Wheel in OSA Patients: A Narrative Review
Reprinted from: *J. Clin. Med.* **2022**, *11*, 3691, doi:10.3390/jcm11133691 . . . . **149**

Shahrokh Javaheri and Sogol Javaheri
Obstructive Sleep Apnea in Heart Failure: Current Knowledge and Future Directions
Reprinted from: *J. Clin. Med.* **2022**, *11*, 3458, doi:10.3390/jcm11123458 . . . . **161**

Catherine A. McCall and Nathaniel F. Watson
A Narrative Review of the Association between Post-Traumatic Stress Disorder and Obstructive Sleep Apnea
Reprinted from: *J. Clin. Med.* **2022**, *11*, 415, doi:10.3390/jcm11020415 . . . . **167**

Balint Laczay and Michael D. Faulx
Obstructive Sleep Apnea and Cardiac Arrhythmias: A Contemporary Review
Reprinted from: *J. Clin. Med.* **2021**, *10*, 3785, doi:10.3390/jcm10173785 . . . . **181**

Marta Stelmach-Mardas, Beata Brajer-Luftmann, Marta Kuśnierczak, Halina Batura-Gabryel, Tomasz Piorunek and Marcin Mardas
Body Mass Index Reduction and Selected Cardiometabolic Risk Factors in Obstructive Sleep Apnea: Meta-Analysis
Reprinted from: *J. Clin. Med.* **2021**, *10*, 1485, doi:10.3390/jcm10071485 . . . . **193**

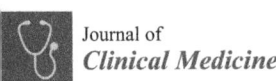

Article

Postoperative Atrial Fibrillation in Adults with Obstructive Sleep Apnea Undergoing Coronary Artery Bypass Grafting in the RICCADSA Cohort

Yüksel Peker [1,2,3,4,5,*], Henrik Holtstrand-Hjälm [3], Yeliz Celik [1], Helena Glantz [6] and Erik Thunström [3]

1. Department of Pulmonary Medicine, Koc University Research Center for Translational Medicine [KUTTAM], Istanbul 34450, Turkey; yecelik@ku.edu.tr
2. Division of Sleep and Circadian Disorders, Brigham and Women's Hospital and Harvard Medical School, Boston, MA 02115, USA
3. Department of Molecular and Clinical Medicine, Institute of Medicine, Sahlgrenska Academy, University of Gothenburg, 40530 Gothenburg, Sweden; henrik.holtstrand.hjalm@vgregion.se (H.H.-H.); erik.thunstrom@vgregion.se (E.T.)
4. Department of Clinical Sciences, Respiratory Medicine and Allergology, School of Medicine, Lund University, 22185 Lund, Sweden
5. Division of Pulmonary, Allergy, and Critical Care Medicine, University of Pittsburgh School of Medicine, Pittsburgh, PA 15213, USA
6. Department of Internal Medicine, Skaraborg Hospital, 53151 Lidköping, Sweden; helena.glantz@vgregion.se
* Correspondence: yuksel.peker@lungall.gu.se

Abstract: Postoperative atrial fibrillation (POAF) occurs in 20–50% of patients with coronary artery disease (CAD) after coronary artery bypass grafting (CABG). Obstructive sleep apnea (OSA) is also common in adults with CAD, and may contribute to POAF as well to the reoccurrence of AF in patients at long-term. In the current secondary analysis of the Randomized Intervention with Continuous Positive Airway Pressure (CPAP) in Coronary Artery Disease and Obstructive Sleep Apnea (RICCADSA) trial (Trial Registry: ClinicalTrials.gov; No: NCT 00519597), we included 147 patients with CABG, who underwent a home sleep apnea testing, in average 73 ± 30 days after the surgical intervention. POAF was defined as a new-onset AF occurring within the 30 days following the CABG. POAF was observed among 48 (32.7%) patients, occurring within the first week among 45 of those cases. The distribution of the apnea-hypopnea-index (AHI) categories < 5.0 events/h (no-OSA); 5.0–14.9 events/h (mild OSA); 15.0–29.9 events/h (moderate OSA); and ≥30 events/h (severe OSA), was 4.2%, 14.6%, 35.4%, and 45.8%, in the POAF group, and 16.2%, 17.2%, 39.4%, and 27.3%, respectively, in the no-POAF group. In a multivariate logistic regression model, there was a significant risk increase for POAF across the AHI categories, with the highest odds ratio (OR) for severe OSA (OR 6.82, 95% confidence interval 1.31–35.50; $p = 0.023$) vs. no-OSA, independent of age, sex, and body-mass-index. In the entire cohort, 90% were on β-blockers according to the clinical routines, they all had sinus rhythm on the electrocardiogram at baseline before the study start, and 28 out of 40 patients with moderate to severe OSA (70%) were allocated to CPAP. During a median follow-up period of 67 months, two patients (none with POAF) were hospitalized due to AF. To conclude, severe OSA was significantly associated with POAF in patients with CAD undergoing CABG. However, none of those individuals had an AF-reoccurrence at long term, and whether CPAP should be considered as an add-on treatment to β-blockers in secondary prevention models for OSA patients presenting POAF after CABG requires further studies in larger cohorts.

Keywords: coronary artery disease; coronary artery bypass grafting; atrial fibrillation; obstructive sleep apnea

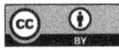

1. Introduction

Atrial fibrillation (AF) is the most common cardiac arrhythmia affecting up to 33% of general populations [1,2]. AF is associated with hypertension, coronary artery disease

(CAD), cardiomyopathies, and increases the risk for ischemic stroke and systemic embolism [2]. Moreover, the traditionally recognized risk factors for AF are also risk factors for ischemic stroke [3,4]. Many CAD patients require coronary artery bypass grafting (CABG) surgery, and postoperative atrial fibrillation (POAF) has been reported in 20–50% of those individuals [2,5–7]. Though many episodes of POAF are known to be self-terminating, there have been reports suggesting that POAF may increase the risk for recurrent AF in the next five years [8]. Moreover, it has been shown that POAF may be a risk factor for stroke, myocardial infarction, and mortality compared with non-POAF patients following cardiac and non-cardiac surgery [9–11]. Fatal embolic events have been proposed as the main contributing factor for the increased mortality risk in patients with POAF [12]. Other complications of POAF have been referred to prolonged hospital stay and increased health-care consumption [13,14].

Obstructive sleep apnea (OSA), being characterized by intermittent partial or complete collapse of the upper airways during sleep (hypopneas/apneas), leads to intermittent episodes of hypoxemia, hypercapnia, sympathetic activity, arousals, and intrathoracic pressure swings, altogether affecting normal physiology [15]. These changes are associated with increased inflammatory activity and endothelial dysfunction as well as remodeling of the left atrium, which in turn increases the risk of AF [16]. Unrecognized severe OSA has been related with new-onset AF in non-cardiac surgery [17]. It has also been shown that patients with OSA are at an increased risk for POAF [18,19], and readmission within 30 days following the CABG surgery [20]. In a questionnaire-based study, a high probability of OSA at baseline was found to be a significant predictor of POAF [21]. Moreover, obesity, closely linked with OSA, has also been related to the POAF [22].

To date, there is a lack of research evidence regarding a possible interaction between OSA and POAF, and whether it has influence on reoccurrence of AF and long-term adverse cardiovascular outcomes in patients undergoing CABG.

The Randomized Intervention with CPAP in CAD and OSA (RICCADSA) trial primarily addressed the impact of CPAP on the composite of repeat revascularization, myocardial infarction, stroke, and cardiovascular mortality in revascularized patients with CAD and OSA [23,24]. In the current study, we analyzed the prevalence of POAF in a subgroup of patients from the RICCADSA cohort, who had undergone CABG, and addressed the association between POAF and OSA, and its possible impact on the reoccurrence of AF and long-term adverse cardiovascular outcomes.

2. Materials and Methods

2.1. Study Population

The study design and methods of the RICCADSA trial have been published previously [23]. In brief, the RICCADSA cohort consisted of adults with CAD, who underwent revascularization (percutaneous coronary intervention (PCI) or CABG) in Skaraborg County, West Sweden, and investigated by a home sleep apnea test (HSAT) in a stable condition following the revascularization procedure. The patients were recruited between December 2005 and November 2010, and the final follow-up was in May 2013. In the parent trial, the CAD patients moderate to severe OSA (apnea –hypopnea-index (AHI) $\geq$ 15 events/h) who had no excessive daytime sleepiness (Epworth Sleepiness Scale (ESS) score < 10) were randomized to CPAP or no-CPAP, the ones with the excessive sleepiness (ESS score $\geq$ 10) were offered CPAP. The CAD patients without OSA (AHI < 5/h) were included in the observational arm and followed prospectively [21]. Patients with dominantly central sleep apnea/Cheyne–Stokes respiration (CSA/-CSR) were excluded. For the purpose of the current study, only patients with CABG at baseline and no history of AF before the CABG procedure (n = 147) were included in the cross-sectional analysis of the baseline cohort (Figure 1).

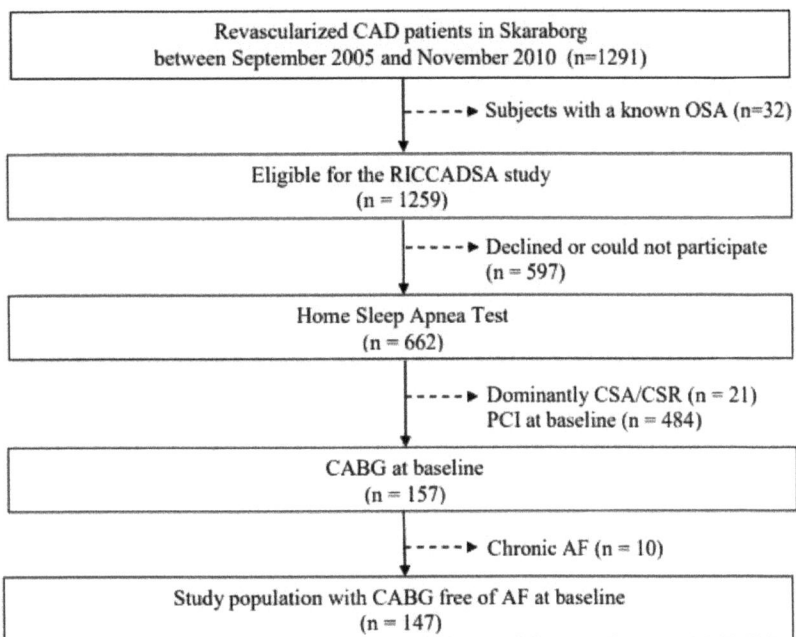

Figure 1. Consort flow chart of the analytic study sample. Definition of abbreviations: AF = atrial fibrillation; CAD = coronary artery disease; CABG = coronary artery bypass grafting; CSA/CSR = Central Sleep Apnea/Cheyne-Stokes Respiration; PCI = percutaneous coronary intervention; POAF = Postoperative atrial fibrillation; RICCADSA = Randomized Intervention with Continuous Positive Airway Pressure in Coronary Artery Disease and Obstructive Sleep Apnea.

2.2. Definition of Comorbidities

While the timeframe of POAF is not strictly defined in literature, it has been usually considered within a week after surgery with peak incidence between postoperative day 2 and 4 [2]. However, it has been shown that patients with OSA are at increased risk for readmission within 30 days following the CABG surgery [20], and we have therefore defined POAF as a new-onset AF within 30 days after the CABG for the current study. The POAF was detected by continuous electrocardiography telemetry during the initial postoperative care and by repeated electrocardiograms at the follow up visits. Body mass index (BMI) was calculated (body weight in kilograms divided my height in meters squared). Obesity was defined as BMI ≥ 30 kg/m^2 [25]. Current smoking was defined as current habitual smoking for at least 6 months at the time of the study start. Lung disease included chronic obstructive lung disease or asthma at baseline. Patients were labelled as hypertensive if they either had a hypertension diagnosis, and/or were receiving antihypertensive treatment. The ESS questionnaire was used to evaluate subjective excessive daytime sleepiness [26] and allocation of the patients to the randomized controlled arm or the observational arm of the main trial [23]. The ESS contains eight questions to evaluate the chance of dozing off under eight scenarios in the past month. Each item is scored from 0 to 3 (0 for would never doze, 1 for slight chance of dozing, 2 for moderate chance of dozing, and 3 for high chance of dozing). The ESS score ranges from 0 to 24. Excessive daytime sleepiness was defined as an ESS score of ≥ 10 as previously described [23]. Anthropometrics, smoking habits, medical history of the study population, as well as medications were obtained from the medical records.

2.3. Sleep Studies, Group Allocation

On average, the ambulatory HSAT was performed 73 ± 30 days after the CABG procedure. The portable, HSAT was conducted with the Embletta® Portable Digital System device (Embla, Broomfield, CO, USA), and consisted of the following tools: (1) nasal pressure detector using nasal cannula/pressure transducer system; (2) thoraco-abdominal movement detection through two XactTrace™ inductive belts with respiratory inductance plethysmography technology; (3) finger pulse oximeter detecting heart rate and oxyhemoglobin saturation (SpO_2); and (4) body position and movement detection. The sleep time was estimated on the basis of self-reporting as well as the pattern of body movement during the HSAT. Apneas were defined as an almost complete ($\geq$90%) cessation of airflow. Hypopneas were defined as a $\geq$50% reduction in thoraco-abdominal movement and/or a $\geq$50% decrease in the nasal pressure amplitude for $\geq$10 s [25]. In addition, the total number of significant oxyhemoglobin desaturations (decrease of $\geq$4% from the immediately preceding baseline) were scored, and the oxygen desaturation index (ODI) was calculated as the number of significant desaturations per hour of estimated sleep. Additionally, time spent below 90% saturation (T90%) was recorded. Events with a $\geq$30% reduction in thoraco-abdominal movement and/or a $\geq$30% decrease in the nasal pressure amplitude for $\geq$10 s were also scored as hypopneas when there was a significant desaturation ($\geq$4%) [27]. The reference group was the CAD patients with an AHI < 5.0 events/h, i.e., no-OSA. The widely used cut-offs for mild, moderate, and severe OSA are AHI 5.0 and 14.9 events/h; AHI 15.0–29.9 events/h, and AHI $\geq$ 30 events/h, respectively [28]. Mild OSA cases after screening with HSAT were included in the current protocol for baseline associations but not in the long-term follow-up as they were excluded from the main RICCADSA trial in order to avoid "overlapping" cases for OSA vs. no-OSA [23].

The 1:1 randomization of the participants with CAD and nonsleepy OSA in the main trial was scheduled with a block size of eight patients (four CPAP, four controls) stratified by sex and type of revascularization (PCI/CABG) [21,22]. The nonsleepy participants with OSA who were randomized to CPAP and the ones with sleepy OSA were fitted with an auto-adjusting device (S8® or S9®; ResMed, Sydney, Australia) by trained staff. Additional details of the follow-ups, including CPAP adherence, were published previously [24,29].

2.4. Blood Sampling

All blood samples were collected in EDTA and serum tubes on the morning following the baseline sleep recordings in the parent RICCADSA trial. As described previously [30], plasma N-terminal-prohormone of brain natriuretic peptide (p-NT-proBNP) levels were measured using the commercially available solid-phase 2-site chemiluminescent enzyme-labeled immunometric assay on an Elecsys system (Roche Diagnostics; Mannheim, Germany) on samples obtained from 2005 to 2007, and on an Immulite 2000 XPi (Siemens Healthcare Diagnostics, Cardiff, UK) from 2008 to 2010.

2.5. Transthoracic Echocardiography

As previously described in detail [30,31], cardiac function was assessed on the same day of the study following the collection of the blood samples. Echocardiographic examinations were conducted by experienced echocardiography technicians according to the study hospital's clinical practice on a commercially available cardiac ultrasound system (Vivid-7 General Electric Healthcare, Fairfield, CT, USA). Images were stored and evaluated with a commercially available software program (EchoPAC General Electric Healthcare). All examinations were evaluated by the same offline examiner (HG) who was unaware of the patients' clinical and sleep data. Left atrial diameter was measured on parasternal M-mode images as the linear distance between the trailing edge of the posterior aortic wall and the leading edge of the posterior wall. An overall evaluation of the left ventricular ejection fraction (LVEF) was performed by visual estimation, and when appropriate, by the Simpsons biplane method [30,31].

2.6. Statistical Analysis

For descriptive statistics, means and standard deviations were reported for continuous variables, and counts with percentages were given for categorical variables. Shapiro–Wilk test was used to test normality assumption of the current data for all variables. The baseline differences between the patients with POAF vs. no-POAF were tested by independent-sample T-test or Mann–Whitney U when appropriate for the continuous data, and by the Chi-square test for the categorical data. A binary logistic regression analysis was performed to determine the variables associated with POAF. Age, sex, obesity, and OSA severity were entered into the multivariate model with additional adjustments for the significant variables in the univariate analyses. All statistical tests were two-sided, odds ratios (ORs) with 95% confidence interval (CI) were reported, and a p-value < 0.05 was considered significant. Statistical analyses were performed using IBM Corp® Released 2019. IBM SPSS Statistics for Windows, Version 26.0 (IBM Corp, Armonk, NY, USA).

2.7. Outcomes and Sample Size

The main outcome of the current protocol was the occurrence of POAF in patients undergoing CABG, and its association with OSA as well as reoccurrence of AF and long-term outcomes in terms of hospitalization due to AF and/or cardiac failure. The clinical follow-up data were obtained from the patients' medical charts as well as from the Swedish Hospital Discharge Registry.

The sample size estimation for the main RICCADSA trial was based on the estimates for the primary endpoints, and no specific power estimate was established for the current post-hoc analysis.

3. Results

3.1. The Entire Study Population and Participants at Follow-Up

Among the 147 participants of the RICCADSA cohort who underwent CABG, 48 patients (32.7%) had POAF (Figure 2). HSAT was conducted in average 73 ± 30 days after the CABG surgery.

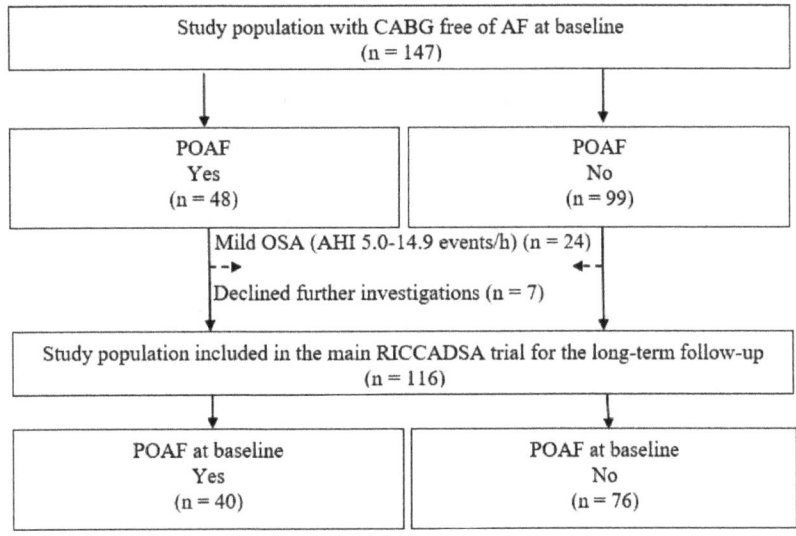

Figure 2. Consort flow chart for the follow-up sample. Definition of abbreviations: AF = atrial fibrillation; AHI = apnea hypopnea index; CABG = coronary artery bypass grafting; POAF = Postoperative atrial fibrillation; RICCADSA = Randomized Intervention with Continuous Positive Airway Pressure in Coronary Artery Disease and Obstructive Sleep Apnea.

As shown in Table 1, baseline demographic and clinical characteristics did not differ significantly between the patients with vs. without POAF. Almost all POAF cases were observed within seven days, except three cases occurring on days 9, 13, and 16, respectively (Figure 3). The β blocker use was similar in both groups. The proportion of patients without OSA was 4.2% in the POAF group vs. 14.1% in the no-POAF group, whereas severe OSA was observed among 45.8% of the patients with POAF compared to 27.3% in the no-POAF group ($p = 0.025$) (Table 1).

Table 1. Baseline characteristics of the entire study population ($n = 147$).

	POAF $n = 48$	No POAF $n = 99$
Age *, yrs	66.5 ± 7.5	63.1 ± 8.7
Male sex, %	89.6	84.8
BMI, kg/m^2	28.0 ± 4.5	27.7 ± 4.1
Obesity %	22.9	24.2
AHI categories *, %		
<5.0 events/h (no OSA)	4.2	16.2
5.0–14.9 events/h (mild)	14.6	17.2
15.0–29.9 events/h (moderate)	35.4	39.4
≥30.0 events/h (severe)	45.8	27.3
ESS ≥ 10, %	37.5	32.3
Current smoking, %	4.2	14.1
Hypertension, %	64.6	61.2
Diabetes, %	33.3	21.2
Stroke, %	4.2	11.2
Lung disease, %	8.3	8.1
Diuretic use, %	34.3	30.9
β blocker use, %	89.2	89.7
Aspirin use, %	80.0	95.8
Clopidogrel use, %	4.6	1.5
Warfarin use, %	13.7	1.5
CCB use, %	18.2	17.0
ACE inhibitor use, %	34.3	37.2
ARB use, %	11.4	7.8
Lipid-lowering agent use, %	93.7	97.5
Echocardiography [†]	$n = 39$	$n = 75$
LAD *, mm	45.6 ± 5.9	43.4 ± 5.7
LVEF %	54.8 ± 8.4	56.9 ± 5.0
p-NT-proBNP, ng/mL	705.2 ± 1164.5	419.3 ± 416.5

Continuous variables are expressed as median and boundaries of interquartile ranges. Definition of abbreviations: ACE = angiotensin-converting enzyme; AHI = apnea–hypopnea index, ARB = angiotensin II receptor blocker; BMI = body mass index; CABG = Coronary artery bypass grafting; CCB = calcium channel blocker; ESS = Epworth Sleepiness Scale; LAD = left atrium diameter; LVEF = left ventricular ejection fraction; p-NT-proBNP = plasma N-terminal-prohormone of brain natriuretic peptide; POAF = Postoperative atrial fibrillation; RICCADSA = Randomized Intervention with Continuous Positive Airway Pressure in Coronary Artery Disease and Obstructive Sleep Apnea. [†] No data from the mild OSA group. * $p < 0.05$.

3.2. Occurrence of POAF and Its Association with OSA

As illustrated in Figure 4, the distribution of the occurrence of POAF was 11.1%, 29.2%, 30.4%, and 44.9%, respectively, across the OSA severity categories.

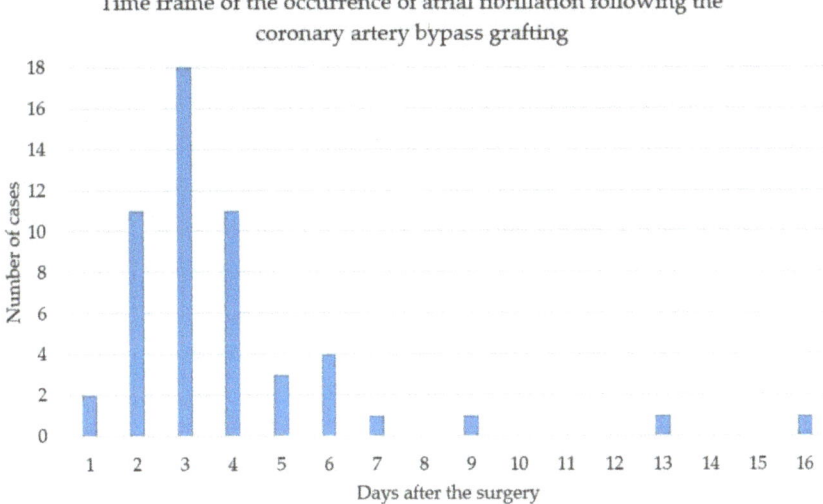

Figure 3. Time frame of the occurrence of POAF in 48 cases following the surgery.

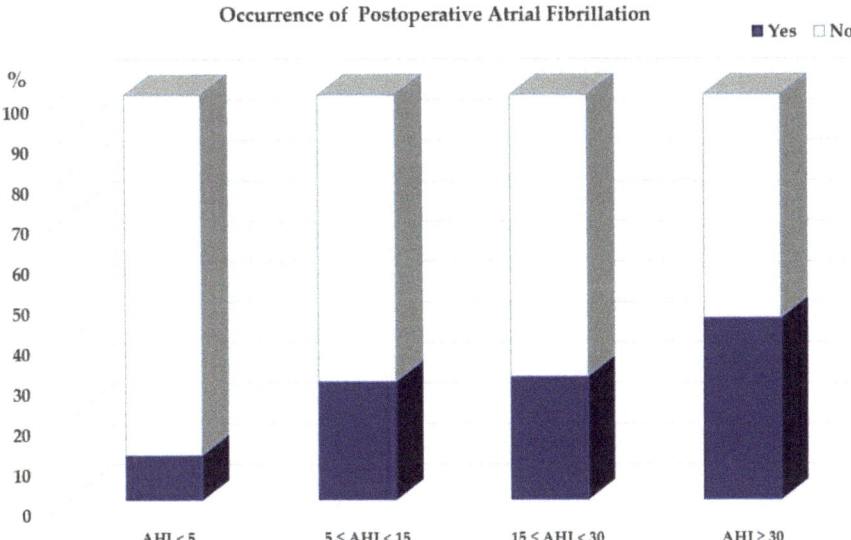

Figure 4. Proportion of occurrence of POAF across the AHI categories. Definition of abbreviations: AF = atrial fibrillation; AHI = apnea hypopnea index.

As shown in Table 2, age, AHI, ODI, and severe OSA were significantly associated with the occurrence of POAF in the univariate analyzes. There was a trend towards statistical significance for LAD and the circulating p-NT-proBNP values, but other demographic and clinical characteristics were not associated with the occurrence of POAF. In a multivariate logistic regression model, there was a significant risk increase for POAF across the AHI categories with the highest OR for severe OSA (OR 6.82, 95% CI 1.31–35.50; p = 0.023) vs. no-OSA, independent of age, sex, and body-mass-index.

Table 2. Unadjusted ORs (95% CIs) for variables associated with POAF.

	OR	Lower	Upper	p Value
Age, years	1.05	1.01	1.01	0.024
Male sex	1.54	0.52	4.51	0.435
BMI, kg/m^2	1.02	0.94	1.10	0.690
Obesity	0.93	0.41	2.10	0.860
Current smoking	0.26	0.06	1.21	0.087
Hypertension	1.16	0.56	2.37	0.694
Diabetes	1.86	0.86	4.01	0.115
Lung disease	1.03	0.30	3.62	0.958
AHI, events/h	1.03	1.01	1.05	0.003
ODI, events/h	1.04	1.01	1.06	0.007
T90%, %	1.01	0.99	1.02	0.545
AHI categories				
<5.0 events/h	1			
5.0–14.9 events/h	3.29	0.59	18.27	0.173
15.0–29.9 events/h	3.49	0.72	16.87	0.105
≥ 30 events/h	6.52	1.35	31.46	0.020
LAD, mm	1.07	0.99	1.14	0.068
LVEF %	1.05	0.98	1.11	0.157
p-NT-proBNP, pg/mL	1.00	1.00	1.00	0.090

Definition of abbreviations: AHI = apnea–hypopnea index, CI = confidence inetrval; LAD = left atrium diameter; LVEF = left ventricular ejection fraction; ODI = oxygen desaturation index; OR = odds ratio; p-NT-proBNP = plasma N-terminal-prohormone of brain natriuretic peptide; POAF = Postoperative atrial fibrillation; T90% = Time spent below 90% oxygen saturation.

3.3. Long-Term Outcomes

Among the 116 patients included in the main RICCADSA trial, 38 out of the 40 patients with POAF (95.2%) had moderate to severe OSA, of whom 28 (70%) were allocated to CPAP at baseline. At the one-year follow-up, 12 (42.9%) were using the device at least 4 h/night corresponding all nights. During a median follow-up of 67 months, only two patients (none with POAF at baseline) were hospitalized due to AF.

4. Discussion

The main findings of the current study included that almost one third of the patients undergoing CABG in the RICCADSA cohort demonstrated POAF, which is in line with the existing literature. We found that severe OSA, defined as an AHI of at least 30 events/h was independently associated with POAF. Notwithstanding, none of the patients with POAF at baseline had a new onset of AF, which required a hospital admission during a median follow-up of 67 months.

As aforementioned, AF is the most common cardiac arrhythmia affecting up to 33% of general populations [1,2]. AF is strongly related with hypertension, CAD, cardiomyopathies, ischemic stroke, and systemic embolism [3]. Moreover, POAF has been reported in 20–50% of CAD patients undergoing CABG [2,5,6]. In many cases, the episodes of POAF are self-terminating, but there have also been reports suggesting that POAF may increase the risk for recurrent AF in the next five years [8], and may be a risk factor for stroke, myocardial infarction, and mortality compared with non-POAF patients following cardiac and non-cardiac surgery [9–11]. Fatal embolic events [12] as well as prolonged hospital stay and increased health-care consumption [13,14] have also been reported.

It is widely known that obstructive events during sleep lead to intermittent episodes of hypoxemia, hypercapnia, sympathetic activity, arousals, and intrathoracic pressure swings, altogether affecting normal physiology [15]. These changes are also associated with increased inflammatory activity and endothelial dysfunction as well as remodeling of the left atrium, which in turn increases the risk of AF [16].

OSA has previously been found to be a risk factor of readmissions to hospital postoperatively [20,32]. In line with the previous studies, our results show that severe OSA is associated with AF, when compared to non-OSA patients, and with patients with no or mild to moderate OSA. In a meta-analysis by Qaddoura et al. [19], OSA patients had a two-fold risk increase in for POAF. Similar results were reported in a later meta-analysis by Nagappa et al. [33].

AF has been shown to be the most common of postoperative complications with associated sequelae [34]. In a study population consisting of almost 300,000 CABG patients, Jawitz et al. showed that new-onset AF was found in 30% during follow up, almost two and half times as common compared to the second most common complication (prolonged ventilatory support), and over six times as common as the third most common complication (renal failure) [35]. Similar results for POAF were reported in an earlier and smaller study conducted by Aranki et al. [36]. OSA is considered to lead to cardiac remodeling [37], and may therefore be involved in the development of AF. Thus, identifying and treating OSA may lead to reduce the adverse cardiovascular outcomes.

Interestingly, none of the patients who had POAF at baseline demonstrated reoccurrence during the follow-up period, which might be related with the fact that 90% of the entire cohort were on treatment with β-blockers at baseline before the start of the RICCADSA trial, and 70% of the OSA patients were allocated to CPAP.

Limitations of the Study

The small sample size of this post-hoc analysis of the CABG subgroup is the main limitation of the study, and the results should therefore be interpreted cautiously. We should also acknowledge that the patients were not screened for AF after discharge from the hospital. AF is often asymptomatic [1,38], and the reoccurrence of AF could therefore be missed during the follow-up period. Another limitation refers to the generalizability of the findings since the RICCADSA trial was a single-center, two-site study, and the results may not be valid for other geographic regions and races and other types of cardiac surgery.

5. Conclusions

Our results showed that severe OSA was significantly associated with POAF in patients with CAD undergoing CABG, of whom 90% were on β-blockers and 70% were allocated to CPAP treatment at the initiation of the study. None of the patients with the POAF history at baseline had reoccurrence of AF that required long-term hospitalization. Whether or not CPAP should be considered as an add-on treatment to β-blockers in secondary prevention models for OSA patients presenting POAF after CABG requires further studies in larger cohorts.

Author Contributions: Y.P. designed the main RICCADSA trial in 2005. Y.P., E.T. and H.G. performed the patient recruitment and clinical follow-ups. H.G. conducted the echocardiographic evaluations at baseline. Y.P., H.H.-H. and Y.C. performed the statistical analysis, prepared the manuscript, and drafted the article. All authors have read and agreed to the published version of the manuscript.

Funding: The main RICCADSA trial is supported by grants from the Swedish Research Council (521-2011-537 and 521-2013-3439); the Swedish Heart-Lung Foundation (20080592, 20090708 and 20100664); the "Agreement concerning research and education of doctors" of Västra Götalandsregionen (ALFGBG-11538 and ALFGBG-150801), Research fund at Skaraborg Hospital (VGSKAS-4731, VGSKAS-5908, VGSKAS-9134, VGSKAS-14781, VGSKAS-40271 and VGSKAS-116431); Skaraborg Research and Development Council (VGFOUSKB-46371); the Heart Foundation of Kärnsjukhuset; ResMed Foundation; and ResMed Ltd. ResMed Sweden provided some of the sleep recording devices and technical support. None of the funders had any direct influence on the design of the study, the analysis of the data, the data collection, drafting of the manuscript, or the decision to publish.

Institutional Review Board Statement: The study was conducted according to the guidelines of the Declaration of Helsinki and approved by the Regional Ethical Review Board in Gothenburg (approval nr 207-05; 13 September 2005; amendment T744-10; 26 November 2010; amendment T512-11; 16 June 2011). 2.2. The trial was registered with the ClinicalTrials.gov (NCT 00519597) as well as with the national researchweb.org (FoU i Sverige—Research and development in Sweden; nr VGSKAS-4731; 04.29.2005).

Informed Consent Statement: All patients provided written informed consent.

Data Availability Statement: Individual participant data that underlie the results reported in this article can be obtained by contacting the principal investigator of the RICCADSA trial; yuksel.peker@lungall.gu.se.

Conflicts of Interest: Yüksel Peker received institutional grants from ResMed for the main RICCADSA trial. Henrik Holtstrand-Hjälm, Erik Thunström, Helena Glantz and Yeliz Celik report no conflict of interest.

References

1. Dilaveris, P.E.; Kennedy, H.L. Silent atrial fibrillation: Epidemiology, diagnosis, and clinical impact. *Clin. Cardiol.* **2017**, *40*, 413–418. [CrossRef] [PubMed]
2. Hindricks, G.; Potpara, T.; Dagres, N.; Arbelo, E.; Bax, J.J.; Blomström-Lundqvist, C.; Boriani, G.; Castella, M.; Dan, G.-A.; Dilaveris, P.E. 2020 ESC Guidelines for the diagnosis and management of atrial fibrillation developed in collaboration with the European Association for Cardio-Thoracic Surgery (EACTS): The Task Force for the diagnosis and management of atrial fibrillation of the European Society of Cardiology (ESC) Developed with the special contribution of the European Heart Rhythm Association (EHRA) of the ESC. *Eur. Heart J.* **2021**, *42*, 373–498. [PubMed]
3. Wolf, P.A. Awareness of the Role of Atrial Fibrillation as a Cause of Ischemic Stroke. *Stroke* **2014**, *45*, e19–e21. [CrossRef] [PubMed]
4. Wańkowicz, P.; Nowacki, P.; Gołąb-Janowska, M. Atrial fibrillation risk factors in patients with ischemic stroke. *Arch. Med. Sci.* **2021**, *17*, 19–24. [CrossRef] [PubMed]
5. Echahidi, N.; Pibarot, P.; O'Hara, G.; Mathieu, P. Mechanisms, Prevention, and Treatment of Atrial Fibrillation after Cardiac Surgery. *J. Am. Coll. Cardiol.* **2008**, *51*, 793–801. [CrossRef] [PubMed]
6. Gillinov, A.M.; Bagiella, E.; Moskowitz, A.J.; Raiten, J.M.; Groh, M.A.; Bowdish, M.E.; Ailawadi, G.; Kirkwood, K.A.; Perrault, L.P.; Parides, M.K.; et al. Rate Control versus Rhythm Control for Atrial Fibrillation after Cardiac Surgery. *N. Engl. J. Med.* **2016**, *374*, 1911–1921. [CrossRef] [PubMed]
7. Lee, S.-H.; Kang, D.R.; Uhm, J.-S.; Shim, J.; Sung, J.-H.; Kim, J.-Y.; Pak, H.-N.; Lee, M.-H.; Joung, B. New-onset atrial fibrillation predicts long-term newly developed atrial fibrillation after coronary artery bypass graft. *Am. Heart J.* **2014**, *167*, 593–600.e1. [CrossRef]
8. Konstantino, Y.; Yovel, D.Z.; Friger, M.D.; Sahar, G.; Knyazer, B.; Amit, G. Postoperative Atrial Fibrillation Following Coronary Artery Bypass Graft Surgery Predicts Long-Term Atrial Fibrillation and Stroke. *Isr. Med. Assoc. J.* **2016**, *18*, 744–748.
9. Lin, M.-H.; Kamel, H.; Singer, D.E.; Wu, Y.-L.; Lee, M.; Ovbiagele, B. Perioperative/Postoperative Atrial Fibrillation and Risk of Subsequent Stroke and/or Mortality. *Stroke* **2019**, *50*, 1364–1371. [CrossRef]
10. AlTurki, A.; Marafi, M.; Proietti, R.; Cardinale, D.; Blackwell, R.; Dorian, P.; Bessissow, A.; Vieira, L.; Greiss, I.; Essebag, V.; et al. Major Adverse Cardiovascular Events Associated with Postoperative Atrial Fibrillation after Noncardiac Surgery: A Systematic Review and Meta-Analysis. *Circ. Arrhythm. Electrophysiol.* **2020**, *13*, e007437. [CrossRef]
11. Villareal, R.P.; Hariharan, R.; Liu, B.C.; Kar, B.; Lee, V.V.; Elayda, M.; Lopez, J.A.; Rasekh, A.; Wilson, J.M.; Massumi, A. Postoperative atrial fibrillation and mortality after coronary artery bypass surgery. *J. Am. Coll. Cardiol.* **2004**, *43*, 742–748. [CrossRef] [PubMed]
12. Mariscalco, G.; Klersy, C.; Zanobini, M.; Banach, M.; Ferrarese, S.; Borsani, P.; Cantore, C.; Biglioli, P.; Sala, A. Atrial Fibrillation After Isolated Coronary Surgery Affects Late Survival. *Circulation* **2008**, *118*, 1612–1618. [CrossRef] [PubMed]
13. Dobrev, D.; Aguilar, M.; Heijman, J.; Guichard, J.-B.; Nattel, S. Postoperative atrial fibrillation: Mechanisms, manifestations and management. *Nat. Rev. Cardiol.* **2019**, *16*, 417–436. [CrossRef]
14. Mathew, J.P.; Fontes, M.L.; Tudor, I.C.; Ramsay, J.; Duke, P.; Mazer, C.D.; Barash, P.G.; Hsu, P.H.; Mangano, D.T.; for the Investigators of the Ischemia Research and Education Foundation and the Multicenter Study of Perioperative Ischemia Research Group. A Multicenter Risk Index for Atrial Fibrillation after Cardiac Surgery. *JAMA J. Am. Med. Assoc.* **2004**, *291*, 1720–1729. [CrossRef] [PubMed]
15. Javaheri, S.; Barbe, F.; Campos-Rodriguez, F.; Dempsey, J.A.; Khayat, R.; Javaheri, S.; Malhotra, A.; Martinez-Garcia, M.A.; Mehra, R.; Pack, A.I.; et al. Sleep Apnea: Types, Mechanisms, and Clinical Cardiovascular Consequences. *J. Am. Coll. Cardiol.* **2017**, *69*, 841–858. [CrossRef]
16. Goyal, S.K.; Sharma, A. Atrial fibrillation in obstructive sleep apnea. *World J. Cardiol.* **2013**, *5*, 157–163. [CrossRef]
17. Chan, M.T.V.; Wang, C.Y.; Seet, E.; Tam, S.; Lai, H.Y.; Chew, E.F.F.; Wu, W.K.K.; Cheng, B.C.P.; Lam, C.K.M.; Short, T.G.; et al. Association of Unrecognized Obstructive Sleep Apnea with Postoperative Cardiovascular Events in Patients Undergoing Major Noncardiac Surgery. *JAMA J. Am. Med. Assoc.* **2019**, *321*, 1788–1798. [CrossRef]
18. Mooe, T.; Gullsby, S.; Rabben, T.; Eriksson, P. Sleep-disordered breathing: A novel predictor of atrial fibrillation after coronary artery bypass surgery. *Coron. Artery Dis.* **1996**, *7*, 475–478. [CrossRef]
19. Qaddoura, A.; Kabali, C.; Drew, D.; van Oosten, E.M.; Michael, K.A.; Redfearn, D.P.; Simpson, C.S.; Baranchuk, A. Obstructive Sleep Apnea as a Predictor of Atrial Fibrillation after Coronary Artery Bypass Grafting: A Systematic Review and Meta-analysis. *Can. J. Cardiol.* **2014**, *30*, 1516–1522. [CrossRef]

20. Feng, T.R.; White, R.S.; Ma, X.; Askin, G.; Pryor, K.O. The effect of obstructive sleep apnea on readmissions and atrial fibrillation after cardiac surgery. *J. Clin. Anesth.* **2019**, *56*, 17–23. [CrossRef]
21. Van Oosten, E.M.; Hamilton, A.; Petsikas, D.; Payne, D.; Redfearn, D.P.; Zhang, S.; Hopman, W.M.; Baranchuk, A. Effect of preoperative obstructive sleep apnea on the frequency of atrial fibrillation after coronary artery bypass grafting. *Am. J. Cardiol.* **2014**, *113*, 919–923. [CrossRef] [PubMed]
22. Sun, X.; Boyce, S.W.; Hill, P.C.; Bafi, A.S.; Xue, Z.; Lindsay, J.; Corso, P.J. Association of Body Mass Index with New-Onset Atrial Fibrillation after Coronary Artery Bypass Grafting Operations. *Ann. Thorac. Surg.* **2011**, *91*, 1852–1858. [CrossRef] [PubMed]
23. Peker, Y.; Glantz, H.; Thunström, E.; Kallryd, A.; Herlitz, J.; Ejdebäck, J. Rationale and design of the Randomized Intervention with CPAP in Coronary Artery Disease and Sleep Apnoea—RICCADSA trial. *Scand. Cardiovasc. J.* **2009**, *43*, 24–31. [CrossRef] [PubMed]
24. Peker, Y.; Glantz, H.; Eulenburg, C.; Wegscheider, K.; Herlitz, J.; Thunström, E. Effect of Positive Airway Pressure on Cardiovascular Outcomes in Coronary Artery Disease Patients with Nonsleepy Obstructive Sleep Apnea. The RICCADSA Randomized Controlled Trial. *Am. J. Respir. Crit. Care Med.* **2016**, *194*, 613–620. [CrossRef] [PubMed]
25. WHO. *Obesity: Preventing and Managing the Global Epidemic*; Report of a WHO Consultation; WHO Technical Report Series 894; WHO: Geneva, Switzerland, 2000.
26. Johns, M.W. A New Method for Measuring Daytime Sleepiness: The Epworth Sleepiness Scale. *Sleep* **1991**, *14*, 540–545. [CrossRef] [PubMed]
27. American Academy of Sleep Medicine Task Force. Sleep-related breathing disorders in adults: Recommendations for syndrome definition and measurement techniques in clinical research. The Report of an American Academy of Sleep Medicine Task Force. *Sleep* **1999**, *22*, 667–689. [CrossRef]
28. American Academy of Sleep Medicine. *International Classification of Sleep Disorders*, 3rd ed.; Darien, I., Ed.; American Academy of Sleep Medicine: Darien, IO, USA, 2014.
29. Peker, Y.; Thunström, E.; Glantz, H.; Wegscheider, K.; Zu Eulenburg, C. Outcomes in coronary artery disease patients with sleepy obstructive sleep apnoea on CPAP. *Eur. Respir. J.* **2017**, *50*, 1700749. [CrossRef]
30. Glantz, H.; Thunström, E.; Johansson, M.C.; Guron, C.W.; Uzel, H.; Ejdebäck, J.; Nasic, S.; Peker, Y. Obstructive sleep apnea is independently associated with worse diastolic function in coronary artery disease. *Sleep Med.* **2015**, *16*, 160–167. [CrossRef]
31. Glantz, H.; Johansson, M.C.; Thunström, E.; Guron, C.W.; Uzel, H.; Saygin, M.; Herlitz, J.; Peker, Y. Effect of CPAP on diastolic function in coronary artery disease patients with nonsleepy obstructive sleep apnea: A randomized controlled trial. *Int. J. Cardiol.* **2017**, *241*, 12–18. [CrossRef]
32. Zhao, L.-P.; Kofidis, T.; Chan, S.-P.; Ong, T.-H.; Yeo, T.-C.; Tan, H.-C.; Lee, C.-H. Sleep apnoea and unscheduled re-admission in patients undergoing coronary artery bypass surgery. *Atherosclerosis* **2015**, *242*, 128–134. [CrossRef]
33. Nagappa, M.; Ho, G.; Patra, J.; Wong, J.; Singh, M.; Kaw, R.; Cheng, D.; Chung, F. Postoperative Outcomes in Obstructive Sleep Apnea Patients Undergoing Cardiac Surgery: A Systematic Review and Meta-analysis of Comparative Studies. *Anesth. Analg.* **2017**, *125*, 2030–2037. [CrossRef] [PubMed]
34. Ahlsson, A.; Fengsrud, E.; Bodin, L.; Englund, A. Postoperative atrial fibrillation in patients undergoing aortocoronary bypass surgery carries an eightfold risk of future atrial fibrillation and a doubled cardiovascular mortality. *Eur. J. Cardio Thorac. Surg.* **2010**, *37*, 1353–1359. [CrossRef] [PubMed]
35. Jawitz, O.K.; Gulack, B.C.; Brennan, J.M.; Thibault, D.P.; Wang, A.; O'Brien, S.M.; Schroder, J.N.; Gaca, J.G.; Smith, P.K. Association of postoperative complications and outcomes following coronary artery bypass grafting. *Am. Heart J.* **2020**, *222*, 220–228. [CrossRef] [PubMed]
36. Aranki, S.F.; Shaw, D.P.; Adams, D.H.; Rizzo, R.J.; Couper, G.S.; VanderVliet, M.; Collins, J.J.; Cohn, L.H.; Burstin, H.R. Predictors of Atrial Fibrillation after Coronary Artery Surgery: Current trends and impact on hospital resources. *Circulation* **1996**, *94*, 390–397. [CrossRef]
37. Daubert, M.A.; Whellan, D.J.; Woehrle, H.; Tasissa, G.; Anstrom, K.J.; Lindenfeld, J.; Benjafield, A.; Blase, A.; Punjabi, N.; Fiuzat, M.; et al. Treatment of sleep-disordered breathing in heart failure impacts cardiac remodeling: Insights from the CAT-HF Trial. *Am. Heart J.* **2018**, *201*, 40–48. [CrossRef]
38. Freeman, J.V.; Simon, D.N.; Go, A.S.; Spertus, J.; Fonarow, G.C.; Gersh, B.J.; Hylek, E.M.; Kowey, P.R.; Mahaffey, K.W.; Thomas, L.E.; et al. Association Between Atrial Fibrillation Symptoms, Quality of Life, and Patient Outcomes. *Circ. Cardiovasc. Qual. Outcomes* **2015**, *8*, 393–402. [CrossRef]

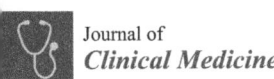

Journal of
Clinical Medicine

Article

TORS as Part of Multilevel Surgery in OSA: The Importance of Careful Patient Selection and Outcomes

Peter M. Baptista [1], Natalia Diaz Zufiaurre [1], Octavio Garaycochea [1], Juan Manuel Alcalde Navarrete [1], Antonio Moffa [2,3,*], Lucrezia Giorgi [2,3], Manuele Casale [2,3], Carlos O'Connor-Reina [4] and Guillermo Plaza [5]

1. Department of Otorhinolaryngology, Clinica Universidad de Navarra, Av. de Pío XII, 36, 31008 Pamplona, Spain; peterbaptista@gmail.com (P.M.B.); ndiazzu@unav.es (N.D.Z.); ogaraycoche@unav.es (O.G.); jalcalde@unav.es (J.M.A.N.)
2. School of Medicine, Campus Bio-Medico University, Via Alvaro del Portillo 21, 00128 Rome, Italy; l.giorgi@unicampus.it (L.G.); m.casale@unicampus.it (M.C.)
3. Integrated Therapies in Otolaryngology, Fondazione Policlinico Universitario Campus Bio-Medico, Via Alvaro del Portillo 200, 00128 Rome, Italy
4. Otolaryngology Head and Neck Surgery, USP Hospital, Av. Severo Ochoa, 20, 29603 Marbella, Spain; coconnor@us.es
5. Department of Otolaryngology, Hospital Universitario de Fuenlabrada, Cam. del Molino, 2, 28942 Fuenlabrada, Spain; guillermo.plaza@salud.madrid.org
* Correspondence: a.moffa@unicampus.it

Abstract: Transoral robotic surgery (TORS) for Obstructive Sleep Apnea (OSA) is a relatively young technique principally devised for managing apneas in the tongue base area. This study summarizes and presents our personal experience with TORS for OSA treatment, with the aim to provide information regarding its safety, efficacy, and postoperative complications. A retrospective study was conducted on patients undergoing TORS with lingual tonsillectomy through the Da Vinci robot. The effectiveness of the surgical procedure was assessed employing the Epworth Sleepiness Scale (ESS) and overnight polysomnography with the Apnea-Hypopnea Index (AHI). A total of 57 patients were included. Eighteen patients (31.6%) had undergone previous surgery. The mean time of TORS procedure was 30 min. Base of tongue (BOT) management was associated with other procedures in all patients: pharyngoplasty (94%), tonsillectomy (66%), and septoplasty (58%). At 6 months follow-up visit, there was a significant improvement in AHI values (from 38.62 ± 20.36 to 24.33 ± 19.68) and ESS values (from 14.25 ± 3.97 to 8.25 ± 3.3). The surgical success rate was achieved in 35.5% of patients. The most frequent major complication was bleeding, with the need for operative intervention in three cases (5.3%). The most common minor complications were mild dehydration and pain. TORS for OSA treatment appears to be an effective and safe procedure for adequately selected patients looking for an alternative therapy to CPAP.

Keywords: obstructive sleep apnea; robotic surgery; tongue base; multilevel collapse

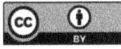

1. Introduction

Obstructive Sleep Apnea (OSA) is a prevalent disorder that affects up to 24% of adult men and 9% of adult women [1]. It is considered a severe social health problem that significantly increases cardiopulmonary and cerebrovascular morbidity, daytime sleepiness, poor work performance, and traffic accidents. OSA is an independent factor for hypertension, stroke, and myocardial infarction [2]. A multilevel collapse of the upper aerodigestive tract is the leading cause of OSA in most cases, causing repetitive partial and complete airway obstructions, intermittent hypoxemia, sympathetic nervous system output surges, and sleep arousals [3]. The retropalatal and retrolingual regions are the most frequent areas involved [4]. Continuous Positive Airway Pressure (CPAP) is considered the gold standard treatment for moderate to severe OSA. However, despite its proven effectiveness, a large percentage of patients are intolerant or reject its use [5]. Alternative therapeutic strategies are also available, including weight loss, positional therapy, oral appliances, myofunctional therapy, and surgical therapy. Several surgical procedures have been described for these situations. Since Vicini et al. [6] introduced the concept of Transoral Robotic Surgery (TORS) for the OSA treatment in 2010, many studies have been published regarding its efficacy [7]. In many ENT departments, TORS is nowadays considered a common surgical minimally approach for Base of Tongue (BOT) reduction in cases of OSA due to a lingual tonsil obstruction [8]. Furthermore, this procedure can be combined with other techniques, such as tonsillectomy, pharyngoplasty, genioglossal advancement, hyoid suspension, and many others in cases of a multilevel obstruction [9]. This study summarizes and presents our personal experience with TORS to manage OSA, whether as a standalone procedure or as a part of multilevel surgery. Our goal is to provide information regarding its safety, efficacy, and postoperative complications and to identify the outcome's predictive factors.

2. Materials and Methods

Patient Selection

A retrospective study was conducted at Department of Otorhinolaryngology at Clínica Universidad de Navarra (Pamplona, Navarra, Spain). From January 2011 to June 2021, 64 patients undergoing TORS with lingual tonsillectomy through the Da Vinci robot were included.

The procedure was either a standalone procedure or part of a multilevel operation, including pharyngeal, palatal, and/or nasal surgery. Nasal surgery included septoplasty and/or inferior turbinate reduction, endoscopic sinus surgery, and/or adenoidectomy. Palatal surgery included expansion sphincter pharyngoplasty or barbed reposition pharyngoplasty. Pharyngeal surgery included tonsillectomy. Tongue base surgery included lingual tonsillectomy, partial midline glossectomy, and epiglottoplasty. All procedures were performed by the same surgeon (PMB).

All patients underwent a complete ENT Physical exam, reporting awake BOT hypertrophy after Friedman's Lingual tonsil hypertrophy [10], Epworth sleepiness scale (ESS), type I polysomnogram, and detailed examination in supine and left/right decubitus positions with Drug-Induced Sleep Endoscopy (DISE) with propofol, administered through target infusion pump to determine the level of obstruction according to European position paper on drug-induced sleep endoscopy [11], following VOTE classification [12]. All patients were counseled on possible alternative treatments and gave their consent to the procedure.

The selection criteria used for the indication of TORS surgery were:
1. Presence of symptomatic OSA (Epworth Sleepiness Scale (ESS) score > 11) and/or moderate to severe OSA (Apnea-Hypopnea Index (AHI) > 15).
2. Low tolerability or drop-out from CPAP (CPAP use less than 3 h per night).
3. Lingual tonsil hypertrophy (Friedman Type 3 or 4).
4. Adequate BOT exposure assessed during sleep endoscopy. Patients must have a minimum distance of 1.5 cm between the superior and inferior incisor teeth.
5. No contraindications to surgery (ASA score < 3, absence of micrognathia).

Regarding TORS, in all the procedures, with the patient in the supine position, the tip of the tongue was fixed with a thick silk traction suture. A Storz Davis-Meyer mouth gag was used to obtain access and to visualize the lingual tonsil. BOT exposure was possible in all the cases. The robot was set up on the right side of the patient. Three Da Vinci robotic arms were used in the oral cavity, with the 30°-angled 3-dimensional endoscope in the center and the Maryland dissector in one arm. The second arm was the Monopolar cautery. The procedure began with a cut in the midline of the tongue base, from the foramen cecum to the vallecula. The incision was then extended laterally. In this way, it was possible to identify and preserve the neurovascular structures as the lingual artery and nerve. The right and left lingual tonsils were removed separately, with the right side followed by the left. An in-bloc resection of the lingual tonsil from superior to inferior and from medial to lateral was performed. We measured the volume of the tissue removed. Lingual tonsillectomy was always followed by epiglottoplasty. The epiglottis was held with the Maryland dissector and divided vertically along the midline 5 mm above the vallecula. A horizontal cut was then made in the right and the left portion to remove the upper one-third of the suprahyoid epiglottis (Figures 1 and 2; Supplementary Materials).

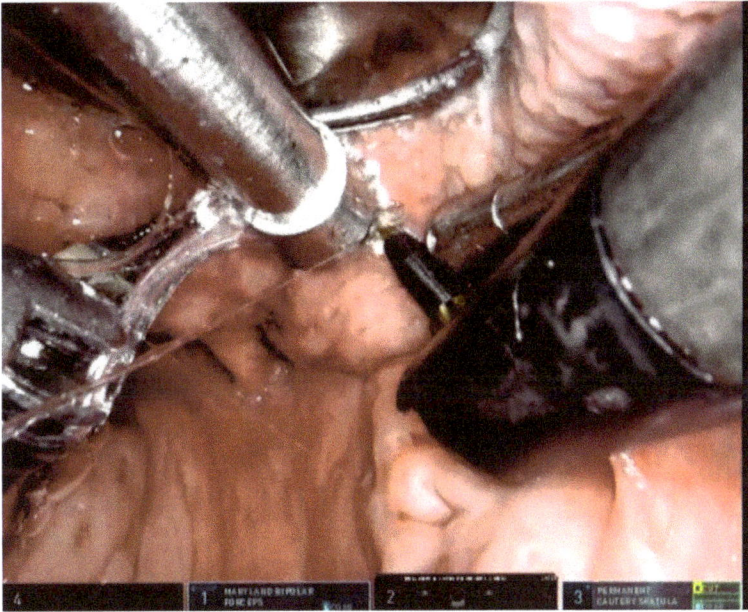

Figure 1. View of operative field before TORS: reduction of volume of tongue base and mouth aspirator, maryland dissector and bovie electrocautery.

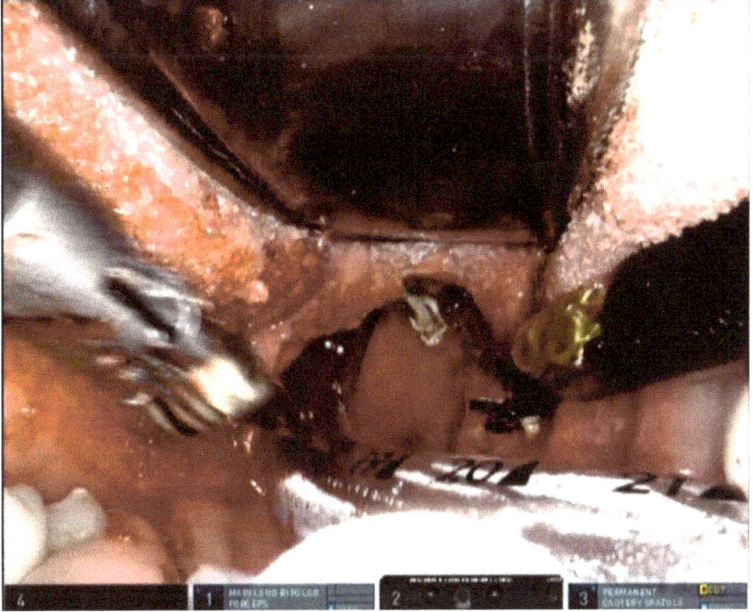

Figure 2. View of operative field after TORS: reduction of volume of tongue base and mouth aspirator, maryland dissector and bovie electrocautery.

The rate of immediate and delayed postoperative complications was also recorded. Complications were categorized as bleeding and other complications. Only patients with a minimum follow-up of 6 months were considered for surgical success assessment with ESS and a new type I polysomnogram. To report outcomes, Sher's criteria were used to define success (50% reduction in AHI and an AHI less than 20% after surgery) [13].

A t-test was used to determine the difference between the AHI index and ESS before and after the procedure. A chi-squared test was used to determine the association between age, BMI, and AHI index, with surgical success according to Sher's criteria. A value of $p < 0.001$ was regarded as being statistically significant. Quantitative data are shown as mean (SD), and qualitative data are represented as n (%). All statistical analyses were performed using IBM SPSS Statistics Visor.

3. Results

At the end of our selection process, 57 patients who satisfied the inclusion criteria were enrolled, 50 males (88%) and 7 females (12%). The mean age of the patients was 49.6 ± 12 years, and the mean BMI at the time of surgery was 28.8 ± 3.6 kg/m^2. Demographic characteristics, pre-treatment and post-treatment average, and median values of AHI and ESS are summarized in Table 1.

Table 1. Subject demographic characteristics.

	Mean	SD
Age	49.63	12.09
BMI	28.84	3.66
AHI Pre	38.62	20.36
ESS Pre	14.25	3.97
AHI Post	24.33	19.68
ESS Post	8.25	3.3

SD: Standart Deviation; BMI: Body Mass Index; EES: Epworth Sleepiness Scale; AHI: Apnea-hypopnea Index.

All the subjects included suffered from moderate to severe OSA except four. In these patients, the indication was due to the lack of adherence or failure of non-surgical treatments. Eighteen patients (31.6%) had undergone previous surgery (septoplasty, turbinoplasty, tonsillectomy, palate surgery, adenoidectomy, or endoscopic sinus surgery). During TORS, the mean volume of BOT removed was 10 cc (6–15 cc). The mean total surgical time was 133 min, including all the other procedures included. The mean time of TORS procedure was 30 min. BOT management was associated with other procedures in all patients. The most common secondary procedures were pharyngoplasty (94%), tonsillectomy (66%), and septoplasty (58%). Table 2 shows all procedures performed with their frequencies.

Table 2. Secondary procedures associated with TORS.

Intervention	n (%)
Septoplasty	33 (58%)
Turbinoplasty	32 (56%)
Adenoidectomy	3 (5%)
Tonsillectomy	38 (66%)
Pharingoplasty	54 (94%)
Epigotoplasty	28 (49%)
Nasal Endoscopic Surgery	2 (3%)

All patients were admitted to the surgical intensive care unit (ICU) postoperatively. The median number of days in the ICU and hospital was 1 and 3 days, respectively. None of our patients underwent tracheostomy.

At the 6-month follow-up visit, there was a significant improvement in AHI values (from 38.62 ± 20, 36 events/h to 24.33 ± 19.68 events/h) and ESS values (from 14.25 ± 3.97

to 8.25 ± 3.3); ($p < 0.001$) (Figure 3). The surgical success rate was achieved in 35.5% of patients. In particular, we recorded the following AHI results: four patients with AHI < 15 events/h, four patients with AHI < 10 events/h, and three patients with AHI < 5 events/h. In five patients, there was a worsening of the AHI, and in four cases, the improvement was minimal.

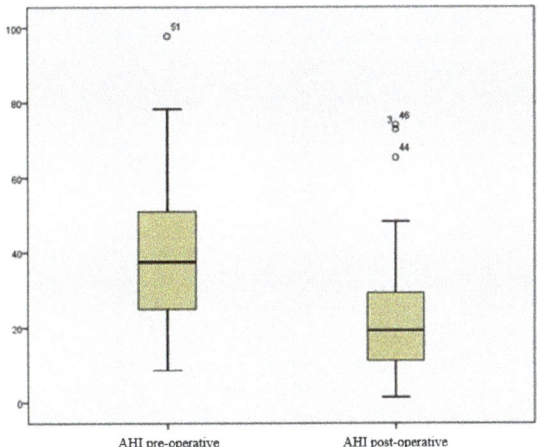

Figure 3. Pre-operative and post-operative AHI values. The central mark indicates the median, and the bottom and top edges of the box indicate the 25th and 75th percentiles, respectively. The whiskers extend to the most extreme data points not considered outliers, and the outliers are plotted individually using the 'o' marker symbol.

There were a total of 10 complications in 9 patients (15.8%). Complications were classified as bleeding (8.8%) and other complications (8.8%), including atrial fibrillation, pulmonary thromboembolism, flap dehiscence, or rehospitalization for pain control. Table 3 outlines the complications that occurred.

Table 3. Secondary procedures associated to TORS.

Complication	n (%)
No complications	48 (84%)
Bleeding	5 (8.8%)
Other Complications *	9 (16%)

* Atrial fibrillation, pulmonary thromboembolism, flap dehiscence, and rehospitalization for pain control.

The most frequent major complication was bleeding, with the need for operative intervention in three cases (5.3%). Bleeding was from the BOT in two cases and the tonsil in another case, and was controlled by transoral approach without the use of Da Vinci. The remaining two cases were self-limited bleeding, and the source could not be determined. Bleeding appeared in all cases between days 2 and 12 after the intervention.

The most common minor complications were mild dehydration and pain, although only two cases showed uncontrolled pain and required hospitalization for intravenous medications 5 and 10 days after the surgery. A few days later, the two patients were both discharged with no sequelae. No patient complained of impaired swallowing after the procedure after 2 weeks of surgery.

4. Discussion

OSA is an underestimated but severe health problem with a high social and economic impact. Since Vicini et al. described the application of TORS for BOT and epiglottis in

OSA patients in 2010, many authors have obtained satisfactory results in different series of patients [6]. TORS is nowadays considered a common surgical procedure in cases of OSA due to a lingual tonsil obstruction.

In 2012, Friedman et al. described a 66.7% surgical success rate in a series of 40 patients [13]. In 2014, Toh et al. described a cure rate of 35% (AHI < 5 events/h) [3]. The latest systematic reviews and meta-analyses have shown a success rate between 48.2% and 68.4%, respectively, with the essential conditioning factors being a BMI <30 kg/m^2 and its association with multilevel surgery as required [14]. Similarly, our study found a significant difference between pre- and post-operative AHI and the ESS values ($p < 0.001$). Moreover, more than one-third of the subjects (35.5%) achieved surgical success. Our study obtained a lower cure rate when compared to the results reported by Toh et al. [3], possibly because our sample was not homogeneous.

Our patients were subject to multilevel surgery. Therefore, our results are adequate as most patients had obstruction at diverse levels. In addition, some had poor prognostic features, such as BMI > 30 kg/m^2 or AHI > 60 events/h. Unlike previous studies, significantly worse results have been reported in patients with high BMI and preoperative high AHI values [10]. It should be noted that in our group, the mean BMI or AHI between patients with surgical success and those without it ($p = 0.8$ and $p = 0.18$, respectively) was not statistically significant. Nonetheless, in all patients whose surgical procedure was considered successful, the AHI score was <60 events/h, and the mean value was lower than in the non-cured group (44.41 and 33.56, respectively). In addition, the mean age between cured patients and non-cured ones ($p = 0.67$) was not significant.

Although we did not compare this surgical technique with others, previous studies have compared TORS surgery to other therapeutic options. Cammaroto at al. compared TORS with Coblation Tongue Base Resection (CTBR) and concluded that complications occurred in 21.3% of the patients treated with TORS and in 8.4% of the patients treated with Coblation surgery [15]. On one hand, TORS seems to give slightly better results, allowing a broader surgical view and a measurable, more consistent removal of lingual tissue. On the other hand, in a randomized controlled trial comparing TORS with CTBR, the AHI improved from 29.7 ± 9 events/h to 10.7 ± 3.9 events/h ($p < 0.001$) following TORS, and from 27.2 ± 6.4 events/h to 10.3 ± 4 events/h in the Coblation group [16,17].

In a meta-analysis comprising 18 studies on TORS (834 patients) and 11 studies on CTBR (294 patients), it was observed that TORS allows a greater resection of the tongue base tissue compared to CTBR. The mean differences of AHI, ESS, and lowest oxygen saturation for TORS were -23.92, -7.6, and 5.83% (all $p < 0.001$). However, it was observed that the surgical success of the two is similar (57.6% vs. 60.3%, $p = 0.4474$), with a lower postoperative bleeding rate with TORS (3.3% vs. 7.5%, $p = 0.0103$), a longer operative time with TORS compared to CTBR ($p > 0.0001$), and a similar hospitalization time ($p = 0.9047$) [18,19].

Post-surgical bleeding that requires surgical revision has been described in 2.5% of cases after TORS, which was slightly lower than that commented in our group (8.8%). All bleeding cases occurred in our first 15 cases. Therefore, we can attribute this to a learning curve. Bleeding appeared in all cases between day 2 and 12 after the intervention.

Further complications with a 5 rate (8.8%) comprised arrhythmia, flap dehiscence, pulmonary thromboembolism, and rehospitalization for uncontrolled pain. Two patients required long-term anticoagulation therapy for atrial fibrillation and pulmonary embolism 4 and 15 days after the surgery, respectively. Nevertheless, the surgical procedure cannot be considered the leading cause of these complications because comorbidities such as obesity, hypertension, and dyslipidemia were previously present in both patients, and the anesthetic medication could have triggered these pathologies. The pulmonary embolism was diagnosed because the patient came to the emergency room, but the atrial fibrillation was discovered casually in an undiagnosed patient.

On the other hand, the higher rate of minor complications and the high costs of TORS must also be considered [10]. In the literature, the complications described have usually been rare and transient [2], with the most common being transient hypogeusia, transient pharyngeal oedema, and limited bleeding. In our study, dehydration and pain were the most common minor complications. In most cases, these complications were not severe and resolved with conservative measures.

Finally, regarding dysphagia after TORS, Eesa et al. [20] followed 78 patients operated by the group of Vicini for an average of 20 months (7–32 months). The results showed that dysphagia scales such as Anderson's were not affected beyond the initial period. The mean time to begin with the oral diet was a single day, with a range from 1 to 3 days. None of the patients required a nasogastric tube. In our group, no patients complained of impaired swallowing longer than 2 weeks after the procedure.

We would like to point out that TORS was performed in conjunction with other level surgeries during the intervention, which shows that it is a safe procedure. However, there is a need for close mandatory vigilance in the first 24 h. Recently, Hypoglossal Nerve Stimulation (HNS) was introduced. It represents one of the latest surgical innovations in the OSA field, enhancing the upper airway neuromuscular tone to reduce collapsibility, which is thought to be the primary pathophysiological basis for OSA [21]. It allows an improvement of the airway by providing a stimulus on the genioglossus, geniohyoid, and palatoglossal muscles. On the other hand, TORS improves the airway by resection of the hyperplasic lingual tonsil, modifying the anatomical structures involved in the obstruction. These surgical procedures are not substitutes for each other but might be complementary. TORS is indicated if there is a very large lingual tonsil, but if there is a loss of tone of the tongue muscles, this should be addressed with HNS. Some papers have shown that HNS has many advantages, but significantly fewer complications, faster recovery, and better results [22,23]. In Spain, HNS is not covered by the Health System or insurance companies, and it represents an expensive treatment with a cost of approximately EUR 30.000 per patient. TORS is also costly and has its place, especially in the hospital where the surgeon works. It might be worth using, but most insurance companies do not cover it. Some patients may have to pay out of pocket for TORS, raising the surgery cost by EUR 2.000.

Our results emphasize that it is essential to select the patients adequately and exclude those with AHI > 60 events/h to achieve surgical success. Furthermore, it is also crucial to recommend weight loss in patients with a BMI > 30 kg/m^2. Patients that do not fulfill these criteria should be excluded as surgical candidates. As for limitation of our study, it was a retrospective series, and our sample was not homogenous regarding the surgical procedure performed. Moreover, even though they were multilevel, performing different surgeries could have introduced a bias. It is hard to determine what percentage of reduction was due to TORS and what percentage was due to other surgeries. Finally, we must consider that the higher rate of complications we encountered may have been due to the surgeon's learning curve, which is why most complications appeared in the first operated patients.

5. Conclusions

In patients with OSA due to retrolingual collapse accompanied by a hyperplasic lingual tonsil, confirmed by DISE, TORS is an effective measure in appropriately selected patients. It is a safe technique if performed by an experienced surgeon, with a reduced rate of complications if done correctly. Complications are infrequent and transitory. Postoperative surveillance in an intensive care unit is critical to ensure the control of possible adverse events.

Supplementary Materials: The following supporting information can be downloaded at: https://www.mdpi.com/article/10.3390/jcm11040990/s1, Video S1: Da Vinci Robotic lingual tonsil resection.

Author Contributions: Conceptualization, P.M.B.; methodology, P.M.B. and J.M.A.N.; formal analysis, N.D.Z. and O.G.; data curation, N.D.Z. and O.G.; writing—original draft preparation, A.M. and L.G.; writing—review and editing, M.C., C.O.-R. and G.P. All authors have read and agreed to the published version of the manuscript.

Funding: This research received no external funding.

Institutional Review Board Statement: All procedures performed in studies involving human participants were in accordance with the ethical standards of the institutional and/or national research committee and with the 1964 Helsinki declaration and its later amendments or comparable ethical standards. The study was approved by the Ethics Committee of CLÍNICA UNIVERSIDAD DE NAVARRA on 17/12/2021, code 2021/206.

Informed Consent Statement: Informed consent was obtained from all individual participants included in the study.

Data Availability Statement: The data presented in this study are available on request from the corresponding author. The data are not publicly available due to originality of the work.

Conflicts of Interest: The authors have no other funding, financial relationships, or conflicts of interest to disclose.

References

1. Gottlieb, D.J.; Yenokyan, G.; Newman, A.B.; O'Connor, G.T.; Punjabi, N.M.; Quan, S.F.; Redline, S.; Resnick, H.E.; Tong, E.K.; Diener-West, M.; et al. Prospective study of obstructive sleep apnea and incident coronary heart disease and heart failure: The sleep heart health study. *Circulation* **2010**, *122*, 352–360. [CrossRef] [PubMed]
2. Glazer, T.A.; Hoff, P.T.; Spector, M.E. Transoral robotic surgery for obstructive sleep apnea: Perioperative management and postoperative complications. *JAMA Otolaryngol. Head Neck Surg.* **2014**, *140*, 1207–1212. [CrossRef] [PubMed]
3. Toh, S.T.; Han, H.J.; Tay, H.N.; Kiong, K.L.Q. Transoral robotic surgery for obstructive sleep apnea in Asian patients: A Singapore sleep centre experience. *JAMA Otolaryngol. Head Neck Surg.* **2014**, *140*, 624–629. [CrossRef] [PubMed]
4. Lechien, J.R.; Chiesa-Estomba, C.M.; Fakhry, N.; Saussez, S.; Badr, I.; Ayad, T.; Chekkoury-Idrissi, Y.; Melkane, A.E.; Bahgat, A.; Crevier-Buchman, L.; et al. Surgical, clinical, and functional outcomes of transoral robotic surgery used in sleep surgery for obstructive sleep apnea syndrome: A systematic review and meta-analysis. *Head Neck* **2021**, *43*, 2216–2239. [CrossRef]
5. Chiu, F.H.; Chen, C.Y.; Lee, J.C.; Hsu, Y.S. Effect of Modified Uvulopalatopharyngoplasty without Tonsillectomy on Obstructive Sleep Apnea: Polysomnographic Outcome and Correlation with Drug-Induced Sleep Endoscopy. *Nat. Sci. Sleep* **2021**, *13*, 11–19. [CrossRef] [PubMed]
6. Vicini, C.; Dallan, I.; Canzi, P.; Frassineti, S.; La Pietra, M.G.; Montevecchi, F. Transoral robotic tongue base resection in obstructive sleep apnoea-hypopnoea syndrome: A preliminary report. *ORL J. Otorhinolaryngol. Relat. Spec.* **2010**, *72*, 22–27. [CrossRef] [PubMed]
7. Meccariello, G.; Cammaroto, G.; Montevecchi, F.; Hoff, P.T.; Spector, M.E.; Negm, H.; Shams, M.; Betllini, C.; Zeccalrdo, E.; Vicini, C. Transoral robotic surgery for the management of obstructive sleep apnea: A systematic review and meta-analysis. *Eur. Arch. Otorhinolaryngol.* **2017**, *274*, 647–653. [CrossRef] [PubMed]
8. Vicini, C.; Montevecchi, F.; Gobbi, R.; De Vito, A.; Meccariello, G. Transoral robotic surgery for obstructive sleep apnea syndrome: Principles and technique. *World J. Otorhinolaryngol.—Head Neck Surg.* **2017**, *3*, 97–100. [CrossRef] [PubMed]
9. Moffa, A.; Rinaldi, V.; Mantovani, M.; Pierri, M.; Fiore, V.; Costantino, A.; Pignataro, L.; Baptista, P.; Cassano, M.; Casale, M. Different barbed pharyngoplasty techniques for retropalatal collapse in obstructive sleep apnea patients: A systematic review. In *Sleep and Breathing*; Springer: Cham, Switzerland, 2020; Volume 24, pp. 1115–1127. Available online: https://moh-it.pure.elsevier.com/en/publications/different-barbed-pharyngoplasty-techniques-for-retropalatal-colla (accessed on 2 November 2021).
10. Lara, A.; Plaza, G. Cirugía robótica transoral (TORS) de base de lengua y epiglotis en el síndrome de apnea-hipopnea durante el sueño (SAHS). In *Sleep Disorder Breathing, Diagnosis and Treatment*; Amplifon Ibérica: Hospitalet de Llobregat, Spain, 2017; pp. 405–421.
11. De Vito, A.; Carrasco Llatas, M.; Ravesloot, M.J.; Kotecha, B.; De Vries, N.; Hamans, E.; Maurer, J.; Bosi, M.; Blumen, M.; Heiser, C.; et al. European position paper on drug-induced sleep endoscopy: 2017 Update. *Clin. Otolaryngol.* **2018**, *43*, 1541–1552. [CrossRef] [PubMed]
12. Kezirian, E.J.; Hohenhorst, W.; de Vries, N. Drug-induced sleep endoscopy: The VOTE classification. *Eur. Arch. Otorhinolaryngol.* **2011**, *268*, 1233–1236. [CrossRef] [PubMed]
13. Friedman, M.; Hamilton, C.; Samuelson, C.G.; Kelley, K.; Taylor, D.; Pearson-Chauhan, K.; Maley, A.; Taylor, R.; Venkatesan, T.K. Transoral robotic glossectomy for the treatment of obstructive sleep apnea-hypopnea syndrome. *Otolaryngol. Head Neck Surg.* **2012**, *146*, 854–862. [CrossRef] [PubMed]
14. Miller, S.C.; Nguyen, S.A.; Ong, A.A.; Gillespie, M.B. Transoral robotic base of tongue reduction for obstructive sleep apnea: A systematic review and meta-analysis. *Laryngoscope* **2017**, *127*, 258–265. [CrossRef] [PubMed]
15. Cammaroto, G.; Montevecchi, F.; D'Agostino, G.; Zeccardo, E.; Bellini, C.; Galletti, B.; Shams, M.; Negm, H.; Vicini, C. Tongue reduction for OSAHS: TORSs vs coblations, technologies vs techniques, apples vs oranges. *Eur. Arch. Otorhinolaryngol.* **2017**, *274*, 637–645. [CrossRef] [PubMed]

16. Babademez, M.A.; Gul, F.; Sancak, M.; Kale, H. Prospective randomized comparison of tongue base resection techniques: Robotic vs coblatio. *Clin. Otolaryngol.* **2019**, *44*, 989–996. Available online: https://www.researchgate.net/publication/335477128_Prospective_Randomized_Comparison_of_Tongue_Base_Resection_Techniques_Robotic_vs_Coblation (accessed on 2 November 2021). [CrossRef]
17. Kim, J.; Poole, B.; Cen, S.Y.; Sanossian, N.; Kezirian, E.J. Transoral Robotic Surgery (TORS) Versus Non-TORS Tongue Resection for Obstructive Sleep Apnea. *Laryngoscope* **2021**, *131*, E1735–E1740. [CrossRef] [PubMed]
18. Lee, J.A.; Byun, Y.J.; Nguyen, S.A.; Lentsch, E.J.; Gillespie, M.B. Transoral Robotic Surgery versus Plasma Ablation for Tongue Base Reduction in Obstructive Sleep Apnea: Meta-analysis. *Otolaryngol.—Head Neck Surg.* **2020**, *162*, 839–852. [CrossRef]
19. Tsou, Y.A.; Chang, W.D. Comparison of transoral robotic surgery with other surgeries for obstructive sleep apnea. *Sci. Rep.* **2020**, *10*, 18163. [CrossRef]
20. Eesa, M.; Montevecchi, F.; Hendawy, E.; D'Agostino, G.; Meccariello, G.; Vicini, C. Swallowing outcome after TORS for sleep apnea: Short- and long-term evaluation. *Eur. Arch. Otorhinolaryngol.* **2015**, *272*, 1537–1541. [CrossRef] [PubMed]
21. Baptista, P.M.; Costantino, A.; Moffa, A.; Rinaldi, V.; Casale, M. Hypoglossal Nerve Stimulation in the Treatment of Obstructive Sleep Apnea: Patient Selection and New Perspectives. *Nat. Sci. Sleep* **2020**, *13*, 151–159. [CrossRef]
22. Huntley, C.; Topf, M.C.; Christopher, V.; Doghramji, K.; Curry, J.; Boon, M. Comparing Upper Airway Stimulation to Transoral Robotic Base of Tongue Resection for Treatment of Obstructive Sleep Apnea. *Laryngoscope* **2019**, *129*, 1010–1013. [CrossRef]
23. Neruntarat, C.; Wanichakorntrakul, P.; Khuancharee, K.; Saengthong, P.; Tangngekkee, M. Upper airway stimulation vs other upper airway surgical procedures for OSA: A meta-analysis. *Sleep Breath* **2021**. [CrossRef] [PubMed]

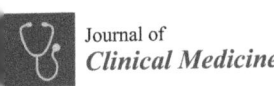

Article

Effect of Continuous Positive Airway Pressure on Lipid Profiles in Obstructive Sleep Apnea: A Meta-Analysis

Baixin Chen [1,2], Miaolan Guo [3], Yüksel Peker [4,5,6,7], Neus Salord [8], Luciano F. Drager [9,10], Geraldo Lorenzi-Filho [11], Xiangdong Tang [12] and Yun Li [1,2,*]

1. Department of Sleep Medicine, Shantou University Mental Health Center, Shantou University Medical College, Shantou 515065, China; 15bxchen@stu.edu.cn
2. Sleep Medicine Center, Shantou University Medical College, Shantou 515041, China
3. Department of Nursing, Shantou University Medical College, Shantou 515041, China; mlguo@stu.edu.cn
4. Department of Pulmonary Medicine, School of Medicine, Koc University, 34010 Istanbul, Turkey; yuksel.peker@lungall.gu.se
5. Sahlgrenska Academy, University of Gothenburg, 40530 Gothenburg, Sweden
6. Department of Clinical Sciences, Respiratory Medicine and Allergology, Faculty of Medicine, Lund University, 22185 Lund, Sweden
7. Division of Pulmonary, Allergy, and Critical Care Medicine, School of Medicine, University of Pittsburgh, Pittsburgh, PA 15213, USA
8. Multidisciplinary Sleep Unit, Department of Respiratory Medicine, Hospital Universitari de Bellvitge, IDIBELL, University of Barcelona, Hospitalet de Llobregat, 08907 Barcelona, Spain; nsalord@bellvitgehospital.cat
9. Unidade de Hipertensao, Instituto do Coraçao (InCor), Hospital das Clinicas HCFMUSP, Faculdade de Medicina, Universidade de São Paulo, São Paulo 05403-904, Brazil; luciano.drager@incor.usp.br
10. Unidade de Hipertensao, Disciplina de Nefrologia, Hospital das Clinicas HCFMUSP, Faculdade de Medicina, Universidade de São Paulo, São Paulo 05403-900, Brazil
11. Laboratorio de Sono, Divisao de Pneumologia, Instituto do Coracao (InCor), Hospital das Clinicas HCFMUSP, Faculdade de Medicina, Universidade de Sao Paulo, Sao Paulo 05508-220, Brazil; geraldo.lorenzi@gmail.com
12. Sleep Medicine Center, Translational Neuroscience Center, West China Hospital, Sichuan University, Chengdu 610041, China; tangxiangdong@scu.edu.cn
* Correspondence: s_liyun@stu.edu.cn; Tel./Fax: +86-(754)-8290-2709

Abstract: Background: Obstructive sleep apnea (OSA) is associated with dyslipidemia. However, the effects of continuous positive airway pressure (CPAP) treatment on lipid profiles are unclear. Methods: PubMed/Medline, Embase and Cochrane were searched up to July 2021. Randomized controlled trials (RCTs) of CPAP versus controls with ≥4 weeks treatment and reported pre- and post-intervention lipid profiles were included. Weighted mean difference (WMD) was used to assess the effect size. Meta-regression was used to explore the potential moderators of post-CPAP treatment changes in lipid profiles. Results: A total of 14 RCTs with 1792 subjects were included. CPAP treatment was associated with a significant decrease in total cholesterol compared to controls (WMD = −0.098 mmol/L, 95% CI = −0.169 to −0.027, $p = 0.007$, $I^2 = 0.0\%$). No significant changes in triglyceride, high-density lipoprotein nor low-density lipoprotein were observed after CPAP treatment (all $p > 0.2$). Furthermore, meta-regression models showed that age, gender, body mass index, daytime sleepiness, OSA severity, follow-up study duration, CPAP compliance nor patients with cardiometabolic disease did not moderate the effects of CPAP treatment on lipid profiles (all $p > 0.05$). Conclusions: CPAP treatment decreases total cholesterol at a small magnitude but has no effect on other markers of dyslipidemia in OSA patients. Future studies of CPAP therapy should target combined treatment strategies with lifestyle modifications and/or anti-hyperlipidemic medications in the primary as well as secondary cardiovascular prevention models.

Keywords: obstructive sleep apnea; continuous positive airway pressure; lipid profile; total cholesterol

1. Introduction

Obstructive sleep apnea (OSA) is one of the most common sleep disorders in adults, affecting nearly 1 billion individuals worldwide [1]. Obesity [2] and dyslipidemia [3] frequently co-exist among patients with OSA. Findings from large cross-sectional studies show increased prevalence of dyslipidemia among OSA patients in a dose-response manner [3]. Several pathological mechanisms including chronic intermittent hypoxia (CIH) [4–7], sympathetic overactivation [8,9] and sleep fragmentation [10,11] may cause lipid profile dysregulation in OSA. For example, consistent evidence from animal models of OSA has shown that CIH induces fasting dyslipidemia due to activation of the transcription factor sterol regulatory element-binding protein 1 (a master transcription factor that controls lipid metabolism) and overexpression of stearoyl-CoA desaturase-1 (an important downstream enzyme of triglyceride and phospholipid biosynthesis) [12]. Moreover, CIH also impaired clearance of triglyceride-rich lipoproteins, inactivating adipose lipoprotein lipase [13,14].

In theory, continuous positive airway pressure (CPAP), the first-line treatment for OSA, eliminates CIH and therefore is expected to improve dyslipidemia. However, findings of previous studies regarding CPAP effects on each lipid profile have been inconsistent. A meta-analysis including 6 randomized controlled trials (RCTs) with 741 participants showed that CPAP treatment decreased total cholesterol (TC) for 0.15 mmol/L, but no changes in levels of low-density lipoprotein (LDL), high-density lipoprotein (HDL) nor triglyceride (TG) [15] were observed. Another meta-analysis including 6 RCTs with 699 participants showed that CPAP treatment decreased the levels of TC for 0.16 mmol/L, HDL for 0.03 mmol/L and TG for 0.32 mmol/L respectively [16]. However, this meta-analysis included an RCT [17], which was retracted later. Furthermore, these two meta-analyses included crossover studies [17–20], and both included data from post crossover periods, which is not recommended by the Cochrane Handbook [21], given that this may induce a carry-over effect. Moreover, most RCTs included in these two meta-analyses have relatively short follow-up durations, i.e., over 80% included RCTs with follow-up durations shorter than 24 weeks. Another meta-analysis including 29 cohort studies with 1958 participants showed that CPAP treatment decreased TC and LDL and increased HDL [22]. In addition, findings from the three aforementioned meta-analyses may be influenced by potential publication bias since their article searches were performed using the specific keywords "lipid profile" and might omit some eligible studies with negative findings of CPAP effects on lipid levels. For example, the study by Nguyen et al. in 2010 [23] analyzed lipid profiles as a secondary outcome, but no significant lipid-lowering effect of CPAP was observed. Taken together, the effect of CPAP treatment on lipid profiles in OSA is yet not well understood.

After publication of the three aforementioned meta-analyses, new RCTs with longer follow-up durations have been published. Because both OSA and dyslipidemia are highly associated with cardiometabolic disease [24–26], here is a need for an update to address the effect of CPAP on lipid profiles in OSA, which was the rationale for the current study.

2. Methods

Search Strategy and Selection Criteria

This meta-analysis was registered in the Prospective Register of Systematic Reviews (CRD 42020201177) and conducted according to Preferred Reporting Items for Systematic Review and Meta-analysis Protocols [27]. We searched PubMed/Medline, Embase and Cochrane Central Register using the following key terms: "obstructive sleep apnea" AND "continuous positive airway pressure" AND "randomized controlled trial". The literature search was up to July 2021 with no language restrictions. Table S1 presents the specific search strategies for each database, Figure 1 shows the study selection process and Table S2 lists the included studies.

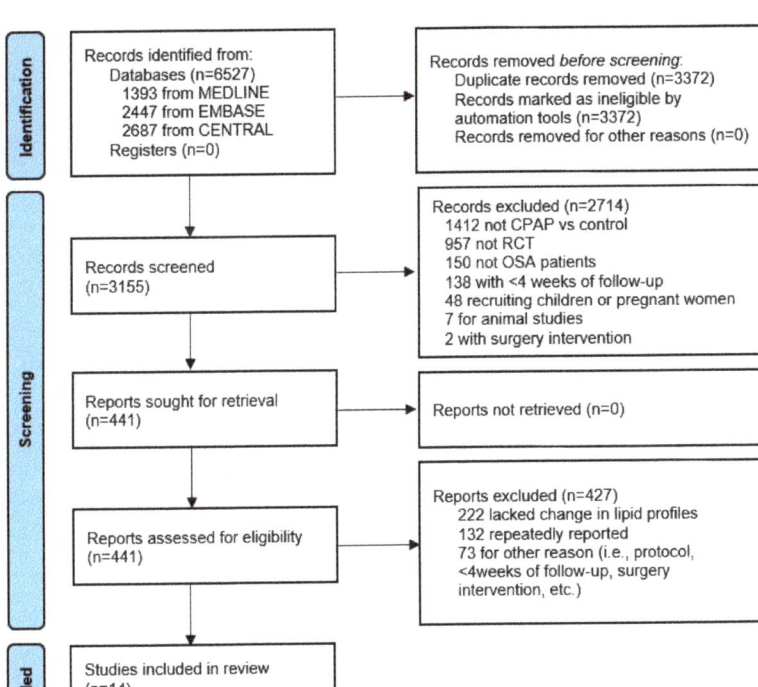

Figure 1. Flow chart of literature search. CPAP = continuous positive airway pressure, OSA = obstructive sleep apnea, RCT = randomized controlled trial.

The review of search results was conducted independently by two researchers (Guo M. and Chen B.). Any inconsistency was adjudicated by the senior author (Li Y.). Studies were eligible if they were: (1) studies recruiting adults with OSA (age ≥ 18 years), (2) RCTs with CPAP and control groups (either sham-CPAP or usual care treatment) with at least 4-week follow-up duration, (3) trials reporting mean and standard deviation (SD)/standard error of any of the 4 plasma lipid profiles (e.g., TC, TG, HDL or LDL) during pre- and post-intervention periods and (4) of any language; there was no restriction. Submitted data from one of the RCTs [28] were provided by the principal investigator of the main study [29]. We excluded studies if they: (1) were designed to examine the effects of anti-hyperlipidemic medications on lipid profiles, (2) involved active weight loss interventions (i.e., vertical banded gastroplasty), (3) included pregnant women, (4) were non-randomized designs or crossover trials or (5) were reviews, editorials, letters or case reports.

3. Data Analysis

Two researchers (Guo M. and Chen B.) independently extracted key characteristics (e.g., first author's name, publication year, sample size, inclusion criteria, percentage of males, percentage of patients on anti-hyperlipidemic medications, et al., Table 1) and target outcomes (e.g., baseline, endpoint and delta values (endpoint minus baseline values) of TC, TG, HDL or LDL) of each trial. Cardiometabolic disease was defined as resistant hypertension, coronary artery disease or diabetes. The Cochrane Collaboration Tool was used to assess quality and risk of bias of included RCTs [30] (Table S3). In this study, we converted all lipid profiles data from mg/dL to mmol/L for meta-analysis (Supplementary Text).

Table 1. Characteristics of the 14 included studies.

Study (First Author, Year)	N, CPAP	N, Control	Inclusion Criteria	Cardiometabolic Disease	Country	Sham-CPAP Controlled	Age (Year)	Male (%)	BMI (kg/m²)	Follow-Up (Week)	Baseline ESS	AHI (Event/Hour)	CPAP Compliance (Hour/Night)	Use of Antihyperlipidemic Medications (%)
Robinson, 2004	108	112	ESS > 9; ODI > 10; Male	No	UK	Yes	45.5	100	29.9	4	16.2	38.7	5	-
Drager, 2007	12	12	AHI > 30; BMI ≤ 35; Age < 60; Non-HT; Non-diabetes; Male	No	Brazil	No	53.4	100	29.8	16	13.5	59	6	-
Nguyen, 2010	10	10	AHI ≥ 15; ESS > 10	No	USA	Yes	57.7	90	32.4	12	-	35.2	5.1	-
Craig, 2012	172	174	ODI > 7.5	No	UK, Canada	No	56	78	32	24	8	13.4	2.65	-
Pedrosa, 2013	19	16	AHI ≥ 15; RHT	Yes	Brazil	No	69.9	77	33.8	24	10	29	6.01	-
McMillan, 2015	114	117	Age ≥ 65; ODI > 7.5; ESS ≥ 9	No	UK	No	53.7	81.7	30.2	48	11.6	28.7	1.9	-
Feres, 2015	22	23	AHI > 5; BMI ≤ 40	No	Brazil	Yes	46.6	-	47.4	24	-	40.2	-	-
Salord, 2016	42	38	AHI > 30; Non-diabetes; BMI ≥ 35 with obesity co-morbidity or BMI ≥ 40	No	Spain	No	62.1	27.5	23.0	12	7.9	60.8	5.4	6.3
Huang, 2016	37	33	AHI ≥ 15; Newly diagnosed coronary artery disease; Non-diabetes; BMI < 25; ESS < 14	Yes	China	No	54.5	83.3	30.8	48	9	28.9	4.2	100
Lam, 2017	32	32	AHI ≥ 15; Diabetes	Yes	Hongkong China	No	57.1	81	33.7	12	7.5	45.3	2.5	-
Rodriguez, 2017	151	156	AHI ≥ 15; Female	No	Spain	No	54.8	0	33	12	9.8	32	4.8	34.5
Pascual, 2018	30	27	AHI > 20; Erectile dysfunction	No	Spain	No	49.4	100	35.8	12	10.2	51.6	5.3	25.3
Silva, 2020	31	23	AHI: 5–5; Age < 65; BMI < 35	No	Brazil	No	47.4	51.9	28.4	48	-	9.7	3.8	-
Celik, 2022	94	102	AHI ≥ 15; ESS < 10; Coronary artery disease	Yes	Sweden	No	66	84.2	28.3	38	5.5	28.8	3.3	95

AHI = apnea–hypopnea index; BMI = body mass index; CPAP = continuous positive airway pressure; DBP = diastolic blood pressure; ESS = Epworth Sleepiness Scale; HT = hypertension; ODI = oxygen desaturation index; SBP = systolic blood pressure; RCT = randomized controlled trial; RHT = resistant hypertension. -indicates that the value was not reported.

4. Statistical Analysis

The mean value and SD of change in TC, TG, HDL or LDL for each group were calculated according to the Cochrane Handbook [30]. The weighted mean difference (WMD) was used to assess the effect size. The heterogeneity was assessed by I^2. Random or fixed effects model was conducted in the presence ($I^2 > 50\%$) or absence ($I^2 \leq 50\%$) of heterogeneity, respectively [30]. To explore the potential moderators of change in lipid profiles after CPAP treatment, meta-regression models were performed by using TC, TG, HDL and LDL as the outcomes and using age, male percentage, body mass index (BMI), obesity (the studies in which mean BMI $\geq$ 30 kg/m^2), Epworth Sleepiness Scale (ESS), apnea–hypopnea index (AHI), follow-up duration, CPAP compliance and studies that recruited only patients with cardiometabolic diseases patients as independent variables, respectively, according to possible clinical relevance. Due to the limited numbers of included studies, only one independent variable was meta-regressed at each time. Publication bias was assessed by the inspection of funnel plot [31]. The trim and fill method was used to assess the influence of potential publication bias in case of absence of heterogeneity ($I^2 \leq 50\%$) [21]. Sensitivity analyses were used to test the stability of results. A level of p-value <0.05 was considered statistically significant. All statistical analyses were conducted by using Stata (STATA 14.0, Stata Corp, College Station, TX, USA) and R Project (R 3.4.2, R Foundation for Statistical Computing, Vienna, Austria).

5. Results

A total of 14 RCTs with 899 patients in the CPAP group and 893 patients in the control group were included. The main characteristics of included studies are presented in Table 1. Among the 1792 subjects included, the mean age was 55.3 $\pm$ 7.1 years, baseline BMI was 32.0 $\pm$ 5.4 kg/m^2 and 78.2% were males. The median follow-up duration of included study was 20 weeks (range: 4 to 48 weeks), and median CPAP compliance was 4.8 hours/night (range: 1.9 to 6.0 hours/night).

A total of 11 studies with 1638 patients provided available data of TC levels at pre- and post-CPAP treatment periods. Fixed-effects meta-analysis showed that CPAP treatment resulted in a significant decrease in TC levels (WMD = -0.098 mmol/L, 95% CI = -0.169 to -0.027, $p = 0.007$, $I^2 = 0.0\%$, Figure 2). No significant publication bias was observed by the inspection of funnel plot (Figure S1). After trim and fill methods, results were similar (Figure S2 and Table S4). Sensitivity analysis confirmed the stability of result that it was not violated after omitting any particular study (Table S5). Moreover, meta-analyses showed no significant differences in changes in TG (14 studies, 1792 patients, WMD = 0.074 mmol/L, 95% CI = -0.056 to 0.205, $p = 0.264$, $I^2 = 75.4\%$), HDL (13 studies, 1572 patients, WMD = -0.032 mmol/L, 95% CI = -0.108 to 0.044, $p = 0.408$, $I^2 = 92.3\%$) and LDL (12 studies, 1492 patients, WMD = -0.064 mmol/L, 95% CI = -0.185 to 0.056, $p = 0.296$, $I^2 = 86.0\%$, Figure 2) between the CPAP group and control group. No significant publication bias of TG, HDL and LDL was observed by the inspection of funnel plot (Figure S1). Sensitivity analyses confirmed the stability of results for TG, HDL and LDL and that they were not violated after omitting any particular study (Table S5).

Meta-regression models were conducted to determine the potential moderators of CPAP treatment effect on the changes in lipid profiles. However, no significant association was found between each lipid profile and age, gender, BMI, obesity, ESS, AHI, follow-up duration, CPAP compliance and studies that recruited only patients with cardiometabolic diseases patients (all p-value > 0.05, Table S6). Furthermore, in the sub-group analyses of follow-up duration with 12, 16 and 20 weeks as cut-off points, respectively, no significant between-group difference of any lipid profile was observed (all p-value > 0.05). Moreover, sub-group analyses by different diagnostic criteria for OSA (using AHI versus using oxygen desaturation index) showed no significant differences between the two groups in each lipid profile (all p-value > 0.1).

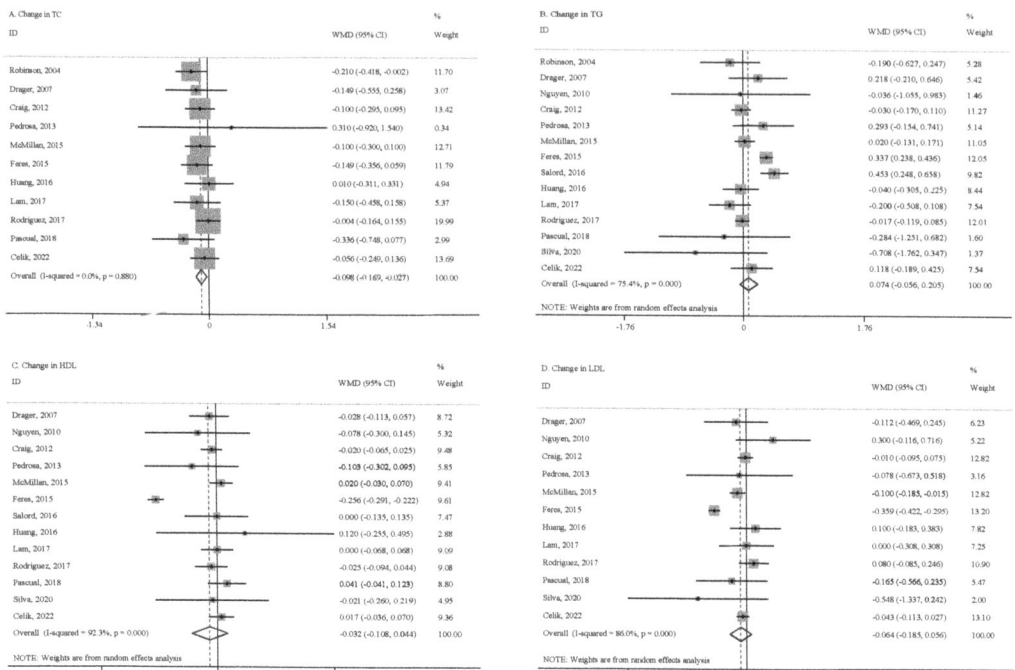

Figure 2. Forest plots for changes in lipid profiles after CPAP treatment. CPAP = continuous positive airway pressure, HDL = high-density lipoprotein, LDL = low-density lipoprotein, TC = total cholesterol, TG = triglyceride, WMD = weighted mean difference. Panel (**A**) Change in TC. Panel (**B**) Change in TG. Panel (**C**) Change in HDL. Panel (**D**) Change in LDL.

6. Discussion

This is an updated meta-analysis including 14 RCTs with a total of 1792 participants (as many as twice the number of RCTs and participants compared to the previous ones). Our findings indicate that CPAP treatment decreases TC in adults with OSA, though only by at a relatively small magnitude. However, there is no effect of CPAP treatment on TG, HDL and LDL levels in adults with OSA.

In 2014, two meta-analyses including RCTs examined the effect of CPAP treatment on lipid profiles in OSA and found that CPAP treatment promoted decreased TC for 0.15 and 0.16 mmol/L, respectively [15,16]. In the current study, we have a similar finding of decreased TC after CPAP treatment, but this effect was of a smaller magnitude. The lower rate of decrease of TC in the current study may be partially interpreted by the fact that we used a less restricted search strategy and included more studies reporting negative findings of CPAP effects on changes in lipid profiles. As for other lipid profiles (i.e., TG, HDL and LDL), no changes after CPAP treatment were observed, which is consistent with the previous meta-analyses [15,16,22], suggesting CPAP therapy promotes limited improvement of dyslipidemia in OSA.

The underlying mechanisms for reduction of TC levels after CPAP treatment in OSA are unclear. First, it could be associated with the improvement of CIH by CPAP. CIH, one of the main pathological conditions in OSA, upregulates the pathways of hepatic liver biosynthesis in a fasting state [4] and delays post-prandial lipid clearance [5,13,14] through inducing activation of the enzyme of triglyceride and phospholipid biosynthesis [12], excessive production of reactive oxygen species [6] and low-grade inflammation [7], which has been proposed as one of the main mechanisms for OSA-inducing hyperlipidemia. Since

TC is one of the first components to respond to the reduction in oxidative stress associated with OSA treatment [32], it is expected that TC levels decrease after CPAP treatment. Second, decreased levels of sympathetic activity [33], cortisol [34] and insulin [35] after CPAP treatment may result in decreased lipid levels. Increased levels of norepinephrine and cortisol, as well as insulin resistance, have been noted to collectively stimulate lipolysis in adipose tissue and induce syntheses of hepatic fatty acid and lipid profiles [8]. Third, it could be associated with the improvement of sleep continuity by CPAP treatment because dyslipidemia may result from sleep fragmentation [11] caused by apneic events. Finally, it could be associated with improvement of fatigue and excessive daytime sleepiness after CPAP treatment [36,37], which may result in increased levels of physical activity. However, a 10-year follow-up cohort study among elderly suggested that worsening of nocturnal oxygen desaturation was independent of changes in circulating lipids and not influenced by lipid-lowering treatments [38]. However, the changes in blood pressure remained associated with waist/hip and LDL/HDL ratios. Taken together, besides sleep apnea, other factors such as age, blood pressure and central obesity may affect lipid levels. However, our findings of meta-regression show that age, cardiometabolic diseases and obesity do not moderate the effect of CPAP on lipid levels. Future studies should be conducted to examine the underlying mechanisms for limited effects of CPAP on lipid levels in patients with OSA.

In the previous two meta-analyses with RCTs examining CPAP effects on lipid profiles, the findings of moderators for CPAP effects on lipid profiles are inconsistent. For example, one reported that a better lipid-lowering effect was observed in studies with longer follow-up duration [16], while the other reported an opposite finding [15]. In the current study, meta-regression models show that post-CPAP treatment changes in TC, as well as other lipid profiles, are not moderated by age, sex, BMI, daytime sleepiness, the severity of OSA, follow-up duration or CPAP compliance, suggesting no single moderator influences the main outcome for lipid profiles.

Our study has several clinical implications. The findings of a decrease in TC suggest that CPAP treatment improves lipid metabolism in OSA. However, such relatively small decrement of TC (-0.098 mmol/L; 3.793 mg/dL) could be the result of slightly decreased LDL and HDL after CPAP treatment. Its clinical significance should be interpreted cautiously. Future longitudinal studies should examine the clinical implications regarding decreasing cardiovascular risk at the relatively small magnitude decrease in TC. Moreover, our findings show no effects of CPAP treatment on HDL and LDL. Thus, it appears that CPAP treatment alone does not improve the lipid profiles in OSA patients with dyslipidemia, and CPAP should be combined with lifestyle modifications and anti-hyperlipidemic medications [39]. Of note, one of the RCTs addressed the effect of CPAP in patients with OSA and coronary artery disease who were already on anti-hyperlipidemic medication without any additional improvement [28,29]. Notwithstanding, the combined effect of CPAP and anti-hyperlipidemic medication might be more effective among patients with OSA free from cardiometabolic disease at baseline compared to the effects in patients who already have developed a cardiometabolic disease. In addition, barbed repositioning pharyngoplasty has been shown to improve chronic inflammation and cardiometabolic disease, which may be regarded as one efficient intervention for obese OSA patients [40,41].

The current study has some strengths to be addressed. Comparing to the previous two meta-analyses with RCTs [15,16], we included as many as twice the number of RCTs, of which seven have relatively long follow-up durations (24-to-48 weeks). Some limitations need to be acknowledged. Lipid levels are associated with diet, medications (i.e., anti-hyperlipidemic medications, insulin and beta-blockers), daily physical activity and lifestyle [42]. Unfortunately, such confounders might not be well-controlled in the current study since most of the included RCTs were not specifically designed to evaluate lipid profiles and did not provide information regarding these confounders. Furthermore, some participants using anti-hyperlipidemic medications were included, and only five studies reported the percentage of using anti-hyperlipidemic medications, which does not allow us to eliminate its confounding effect. Future studies should fully consider the aforementioned confounding effects when examining the effects of CPAP on lipid profile. Moreover, CPAP compliance in this meta-analysis was based on the mean compliance for each study but not for each patient. Therefore, the non-significant relationship between changes in lipid profiles and CPAP compliance in meta-regression models should be interpreted cautiously and be examined in future studies. Finally, since a great part of the included participants were males (78.2%), sex-stratified designed studies are also needed.

7. Conclusions

CPAP treatment decreases TC at a small magnitude in adults with OSA. Since TC is a strong predictor for cardiometabolic diseases, our findings indicate that CPAP combined with lipid-lowering drugs are warranted for OSA patients with dyslipidemia. Future studies should be conducted to explore the potential mechanisms for CPAP treatment effects on lipid profiles.

Supplementary Materials: The following supporting information can be downloaded at: https://www.mdpi.com/article/10.3390/jcm11030596/s1, Supplementary Text. The unit conversion formulas of each lipid profile. Figure S1. Funnel plots of lipid profiles. Figure S2. Funnel plots after trim and fill for total cholesterol. Table S1. Search strategies. Table S2. List of 14 included studies. Table S3. Quality and risk of bias. Table S4 Comparison of total cholesterol before and after trim and fill. Table S5: 1. Sensitivity analyses of total cholesterol, 2. Sensitivity analyses of triglyceride, 3. Sensitivity analyses of high-density lipoprotein, 4. Sensitivity analyses of low-density lipoprotein. Table S6. Meta-regression analyses for lipid profiles.

Author Contributions: B.C. and M.G. conducted the literature search, data extraction, statistical analyses and drafted the first manuscript. Y.P., N.S., L.F.D. and G.L.-F. provided some data sources of the included studies and revised the manuscript. X.T. contributed the idea of this study and revised the manuscript. Y.L. adjudicated any inconsistency in literature search and data extraction, modified statistical analyses and revised the manuscript. All authors have read and agreed to the published version of the manuscript.

Funding: This study was supported by National Natural Science Foundation of China (No. 81970087), Grant for Key Disciplinary Project of Clinical Medicine under the Guangdong High-level University Development Program, Guangdong Province Science and Technology Special Fund project (200115165870512) and 2020 Li Ka Shing Foundation Cross-Disciplinary Research Grant (2020LKSFG05B).

Institutional Review Board Statement: Not applicable.

Informed Consent Statement: Not applicable.

Data Availability Statement: Data that underlie the results reported in this article can be obtained by contacting the corresponding author; s_liyun@stu.edu.cn.

Conflicts of Interest: All authors report no biomedical financial interests or potential conflicts of interest.

References

1. Benjafield, A.V.; Ayas, N.T.; Eastwood, P.R.; Heinzer, R.; Ip, M.S.M.; Morrell, M.J.; Nunez, C.M.; Patel, S.R.; Penzel, T.; Pépin, J.-L.; et al. Estimation of the global prevalence and burden of obstructive sleep apnoea: A literature-based analysis. *Lancet Respir. Med.* **2019**, *7*, 687–698. [CrossRef]
2. Peppard, P.E.; Young, T.; Barnet, J.H.; Palta, M.; Hagen, E.W.; Hla, K.M. Increased Prevalence of Sleep-Disordered Breathing in Adults. *Am. J. Epidemiol.* **2013**, *177*, 1006–1014. [CrossRef] [PubMed]
3. Gunduz, C.; Basoglu, O.K.; Hedner, J.; Zou, D.; Bonsignore, M.R.; Hein, H.; Staats, R.; Pataka, A.; Barbe, F.; Sliwinski, P.; et al. Obstructive sleep apnoea independently predicts lipid levels: Data from the European Sleep Apnea Database. *Respirology* **2018**, *23*, 1180–1189. [CrossRef] [PubMed]
4. Li, J.; Grigoryev, D.N.; Ye, S.Q.; Thorne, L.; Schwartz, A.R.; Smith, P.L.; O'Donnell, C.P.; Polotsky, V.Y. Chronic intermittent hypoxia upregulates genes of lipid biosynthesis in obese mice. *J. Appl. Physiol.* **2005**, *99*, 1643–1648. [CrossRef] [PubMed]
5. Trzepizur, W.; Le Vaillant, M.; Meslier, N.; Pigeanne, T.; Masson, P.; Humeau, M.P.; Goupil, F.; Chollet, S.; Ducluzeau, P.H.; Gagnadoux, F. Independent association between nocturnal intermittent hypoxemia and metabolic dyslipidemia. *Chest* **2013**, *143*, 1584–1589. [CrossRef]

6. Chen, L.; Einbinder, E.; Zhang, Q.; Hasday, J.; Balke, C.W.; Scharf, S.M. Oxidative stress and left ventricular function with chronic intermittent hypoxia in rats. *Am. J. Respir. Crit. Care Med.* **2005**, *172*, 915–920. [CrossRef]
7. Mesarwi, O.A.; Loomba, R.; Malhotra, A. Obstructive Sleep Apnea, Hypoxia, and Nonalcoholic Fatty Liver Disease. *Am. J. Respir. Crit. Care Med.* **2019**, *199*, 830–841. [CrossRef]
8. Brindley, D.N.; McCann, B.; Niaura, R.; Stoney, C.M.; Suarez, E.C. Stress and lipoprotein metabolism: Modulators and mechanisms. *Metabolism* **1993**, *42*, 3–15. [CrossRef]
9. Borovac, J.A.; Dogas, Z.; Supe-Domic, D.; Galic, T.; Bozic, J. Catestatin serum levels are increased in male patients with obstructive sleep apnea. *Sleep Breath.* **2018**, *23*, 473–481. [CrossRef] [PubMed]
10. Toyama, Y.; Chin, K.; Chihara, Y.; Takegami, M.; Takahashi, K.I.; Sumi, K.; Nakamura, T.; Nakayama-Ashida, Y.; Minami, I.; Horita, S.; et al. Association between sleep apnea, sleep duration, and serum lipid profile in an urban, male, working population in Japan. *Chest* **2013**, *143*, 720–728. [CrossRef]
11. Chopra, S.; Rathore, A.; Younas, H.; Pham, L.V.; Gu, C.; Beselman, A.; Kim, I.-Y.; Wolfe, R.R.; Perin, J.; Polotsky, V.Y.; et al. Obstructive Sleep Apnea Dynamically Increases Nocturnal Plasma Free Fatty Acids, Glucose, and Cortisol During Sleep. *J. Clin. Endocrinol. Metab.* **2017**, *102*, 3172–3181. [CrossRef] [PubMed]
12. Savransky, V.; Jun, J.; Li, J.; Nanayakkara, A.; Fonti, S.; Moser, A.B.; Steele, K.E.; Sweitzer, M.E.; Patil, S.P.; Bhanot, S.; et al. Dyslipidemia and atherosclerosis induced by chronic intermittent hypoxia are attenuated by deficiency of stearoyl coenzyme A desaturase. *Circ Res.* **2008**, *103*, 1173–1180. [CrossRef] [PubMed]
13. Drager, L.F.; Li, J.; Shin, M.-K.; Reinke, C.; Aggarwal, N.R.; Jun, J.C.; Bevans-Fonti, S.; Sztalryd, C.; O'Byrne, S.M.; Kroupa, O.; et al. Intermittent hypoxia inhibits clearance of triglyceride-rich lipoproteins and inactivates adipose lipoprotein lipase in a mouse model of sleep apnoea. *Eur. Hear. J.* **2011**, *33*, 783–790. [CrossRef] [PubMed]
14. Drager, L.F.; Yao, Q.; Hernandez, K.L.; Shin, M.-K.; Bevans-Fonti, S.; Gay, J.; Sussan, T.E.; Jun, J.C.; Myers, A.C.; Olivecrona, G.; et al. Chronic Intermittent Hypoxia Induces Atherosclerosis via Activation of Adipose Angiopoietin-like 4. *Am. J. Respir. Crit. Care Med.* **2013**, *188*, 240–248. [CrossRef]
15. Xu, H.; Yi, H.; Guan, J.; Yin, S. Effect of continuous positive airway pressure on lipid profile in patients with obstructive sleep apnea syndrome: A meta-analysis of randomized controlled trials. *Atherosclerosis* **2014**, *234*, 446–453. [CrossRef]
16. Lin, M.T.; Lin, H.H.; Lee, P.L.; Weng, P.H.; Lee, C.C.; Lai, T.C.; Liu, W.; Chen, C.-L. Beneficial effect of continuous positive airway pressure on lipid profiles in obstructive sleep apnea: A meta-analysis. *Sleep Breath* **2015**, *19*, 809–817. [CrossRef]
17. Sharma, S.K.; Agrawal, S.; Damodaran, D.; Sreenivas, V.; Kadhiravan, T.; Lakshmy, R.; Jagia, P.; Kumar, A. Retraction: CPAP for the metabolic syndrome in patients with obstructive sleep apnea. *N. Engl. J. Med.* **2011**, *365*, 2277–2286, Erratum in *N. Engl. J. Med.* **2013**, *369*, 1770. [CrossRef]
18. Coughlin, S.R.; Mawdsley, L.; Mugarza, J.A.; Wilding, J.P.; Calverley, P.M. Cardiovascular and metabolic effects of CPAP in obese males with OSA. *Eur. Respir. J.* **2007**, *29*, 720–727. [CrossRef]
19. Comondore, V.R.; Cheema, R.; Fox, J.; Butt, A.; Mancini, G.B.J.; Fleetham, J.A.; Ryan, C.F.; Chan, S.; Ayas, N.T. The Impact of CPAP on Cardiovascular Biomarkers in Minimally Symptomatic Patients with Obstructive Sleep Apnea: A Pilot Feasibility Randomized Crossover Trial. *Lung* **2008**, *187*, 17–22. [CrossRef]
20. Phillips, C.L.; Yee, B.J.; Marshall, N.S.; Liu, P.Y.; Sullivan, D.R.; Grunstein, R.R. Continuous positive airway pressure reduces postprandial lipidemia in obstructive sleep apnea: A randomized, placebo-controlled crossover trial. *Am. J. Respir. Crit. Care Med.* **2011**, *184*, 355–361. [CrossRef]
21. Cochrane Collaboration. Cochrane Handbook for Systematic Reviews of Interventions. Available online: https://training.cochrane.org/handbook/archive/v5.1/ (accessed on 1 September 2021).
22. Nadeem, R.; Singh, M.; Nida, M.; Kwon, S.; Sajid, H.; Witkowski, J.; Pahomov, E.; Shah, K.; Park, W.; Champeau, D. Effect of CPAP Treatment for Obstructive Sleep Apnea Hypopnea Syndrome on Lipid Profile: A Meta-Regression Analysis. *J. Clin. Sleep Med.* **2014**, *10*, 1295–1302. [CrossRef] [PubMed]
23. Nguyen, P.K.; Katikireddy, C.K.; McConnell, M.V.; Kushida, C.; Yang, P.C. Nasal continuous positive airway pressure improves myocardial perfusion reserve and endothelial-dependent vasodilation in patients with obstructive sleep apnea. *J. Cardiovasc. Magn. Reson.* **2010**, *12*, 10–50. [CrossRef] [PubMed]
24. Ference, B.A.; Graham, I.; Tokgozoglu, L.; Catapano, A.L. Impact of Lipids on Cardiovascular Health: JACC Health Promotion Series. *J. Am. Coll. Cardiol.* **2018**, *72*, 1141–1156. [CrossRef] [PubMed]
25. Marin, J.M.; Carrizo, S.J.; Vicente, E.; Agusti, A.G. Long-term cardiovascular outcomes in men with obstructive sleep apnoea-hypopnoea with or without treatment with continuous positive airway pressure: An observational study. *Lancet* **2005**, *365*, 1046–1053. [CrossRef]
26. Drager, L.F.; Togeiro, S.M.; Polotsky, V.Y.; Lorenzi-Filho, G. Obstructive sleep apnea: A cardiometabolic risk in obesity and the metabolic syndrome. *J. Am. Coll. Cardiol.* **2013**, *62*, 569–576. [CrossRef] [PubMed]
27. Shamseer, L.; Moher, D.; Clarke, M.; Ghersi, D.; Liberati, A.; Petticrew, M.; Shekelle, P.; Stewart, L.A. Preferred reporting items for systematic review and meta-analysis protocols (PRISMA-P) 2015: Elaboration and explanation. *BMJ* **2015**, *350*, g7647. [CrossRef]
28. Peker, Y.; Glantz, H.; Eulenburg, C.; Wegscheider, K.; Herlitz, J.; Thunstrom, E. Effect of Positive Airway Pressure on Cardiovascular Outcomes in Coronary Artery Disease Patients with Nonsleepy Obstructive Sleep Apnea. The RICCADSA Randomized Controlled Trial. *Am. J. Respir. Crit. Care Med.* **2016**, *194*, 613–620. [CrossRef]

29. Celik, Y.; Balcan, B.; Peker, Y. CPAP Intervention as an Add-On Treatment to Lipid-Lowering Medication in Coronary Artery Disease Patients with Obstructive Sleep Apnea in the RICCADSA Trial. *J. Clin. Med.* **2022**, *11*, 273. [CrossRef]
30. Higgins, J.P.; Altman, D.G.; Gøtzsche, P.C.; Jüni, P.; Moher, D.; Oxman, A.D.; Savovic, J.; Schulz, K.F.; Weeks, L.; Sterne, J.A.C. The Cochrane Collaboration's tool for assessing risk of bias in randomised trials. *BMJ* **2011**, *343*, d5928. [CrossRef]
31. Thornton, A.; Lee, P. Publication bias in meta-analysis: Its causes and consequences. *J. Clin. Epidemiol.* **2000**, *53*, 207–216. [CrossRef]
32. Robinson, G.V.; Pepperell, J.C.T.; Segal, H.C.; Davies, R.J.O.; Stradling, J.R. Circulating cardiovascular risk factors in obstructive sleep apnoea: Data from randomised controlled trials. *Thorax* **2004**, *59*, 777–782. [CrossRef] [PubMed]
33. Chen, B.; Somers, V.K.; Tang, X.; Li, Y. Moderating Effect of BMI on the Relationship Between Sympathetic Activation and Blood Pressure in Males with Obstructive Sleep Apnea. *Nat. Sci. Sleep* **2021**, *13*, 339–348. [CrossRef] [PubMed]
34. Schmoller, A.; Eberhardt, F.; Jauch-Chara, K.; Schweiger, U.; Zabel, P.; Peters, A.; Schultes, B.; Oltmanns, K.M. Continuous positive airway pressure therapy decreases evening cortisol concentrations in patients with severe obstructive sleep apnea. *Metabolism* **2009**, *58*, 848–853. [CrossRef] [PubMed]
35. Shang, W.; Zhang, Y.; Wang, G.; Han, D. Benefits of continuous positive airway pressure on glycaemic control and insulin resistance in patients with type 2 diabetes and obstructive sleep apnoea: A meta-analysis. *Diabetes Obes. Metab.* **2021**, *23*, 540–548. [CrossRef]
36. Vasquez, M.M.; Goodwin, J.L.; Drescher, A.A.; Smith, T.W.; Quan, S.F. Associations of dietary intake and physical activity with sleep disordered breathing in the Apnea Positive Pressure Long-Term Efficacy Study (APPLES). *J. Clin. Sleep Med.* **2008**, *4*, 411–418. [CrossRef]
37. Katcher, H.I.; Hill, A.M.; Lanford, J.L.; Yoo, J.S.; Kris-Etherton, P.M. Lifestyle Approaches and Dietary Strategies to Lower LDL-Cholesterol and Triglycerides and Raise HDL-Cholesterol. *Endocrinol. Metab. Clin. N. Am.* **2009**, *38*, 45–78. [CrossRef]
38. Monneret, D.; Barthélémy, J.C.; Hupin, D.; Maudoux, D.; Celle, S.; Sforza, E.; Roche, F. Serum lipid profile, sleep-disordered breathing and blood pressure in the elderly: A 10-year follow-up of the PROOF-SYNAPSE cohort. *Sleep Med.* **2017**, *39*, 14–22. [CrossRef]
39. Chirinos, J.A.; Gurubhagavatula, I.; Teff, K.; Rader, D.J.; Wadden, T.A.; Townsend, R.; Foster, G.D.; Maislin, G.; Saif, H.; Broderick, P.; et al. CPAP, weight loss, or both for obstructive sleep apnea. *N. Engl. J. Med.* **2014**, *370*, 2265–2275. [CrossRef]
40. Binar, M.; Akcam, T.; Karakoc, O.; Sagkan, R.I.; Musabak, U.; Gerek, M. A new surgical technique versus an old marker: Can expansion sphincter pharyngoplasty reduce C-reactive protein levels in patients with obstructive sleep apnea? *Eur. Arch. Otorhinolaryngol.* **2017**, *274*, 829–836. [CrossRef]
41. Iannella, G.; Lechien, J.R.; Perrone, T.; Meccariello, G.; Cammaroto, G.; Cannavicci, A.; Burgio, L.; Maniaci, A.; Cocuzza, S.; Di Luca, M.; et al. Barbed reposition pharyngoplasty (BRP) in obstructive sleep apnea treatment: State of the art. *Am. J. Otolaryngol.* **2022**, *43*, 103197. [CrossRef]
42. Barros, D.; Garcia-Rio, F. Obstructive sleep apnea and dyslipidemia: From animal models to clinical evidence. *Sleep* **2019**, *42*, zsy236. [CrossRef] [PubMed]

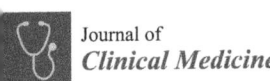

Article

CPAP Intervention as an Add-On Treatment to Lipid-Lowering Medication in Coronary Artery Disease Patients with Obstructive Sleep Apnea in the RICCADSA Trial

Yeliz Celik [1,*], Baran Balcan [2] and Yüksel Peker [1,2,3,4,5]

1. Research Center for Translational Medicine (KUTTAM), Koc University, 34010 Istanbul, Turkey; yuksel.peker@lungall.gu.se
2. Department of Pulmonary Medicine, Koc University Hospital, 34010 Istanbul, Turkey; drbaranbalcan@gmail.com
3. Department of Molecular and Clinical Medicine/Cardiology, Institute of Medicine, Sahlgrenska Academy, University of Gothenburg, 40530 Gothenburg, Sweden
4. Department of Clinical Sciences, Respiratory Medicine and Allergology, School of Medicine, Lund University, 22185 Lund, Sweden
5. Division of Pulmonary, Allergy, and Critical Care Medicine, University of Pittsburgh School of Medicine, Pittsburgh, PA 15213, USA
* Correspondence: ycelik19@ku.edu.tr

Citation: Celik, Y.; Balcan, B.; Peker, Y. CPAP Intervention as an Add-On Treatment to Lipid-Lowering Medication in Coronary Artery Disease Patients with Obstructive Sleep Apnea in the RICCADSA Trial. *J. Clin. Med.* **2022**, *11*, 273. https://doi.org/10.3390/jcm11010273

Academic Editor: David Barnes

Received: 2 December 2021
Accepted: 30 December 2021
Published: 5 January 2022

Publisher's Note: MDPI stays neutral with regard to jurisdictional claims in published maps and institutional affiliations.

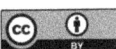

Copyright: © 2022 by the authors. Licensee MDPI, Basel, Switzerland. This article is an open access article distributed under the terms and conditions of the Creative Commons Attribution (CC BY) license (https://creativecommons.org/licenses/by/4.0/).

Abstract: Dyslipidaemia is a well-known risk factor for coronary artery disease (CAD), and reducing lipid levels is essential for secondary prevention in management of these high-risk individuals. Dyslipidaemia is common also in patients with obstructive sleep apnea (OSA). Continuous positive airway pressure (CPAP) is the first line treatment of OSA. However, evidence of a possible lipid-lowering effect of CPAP in CAD patients with OSA is scarce. We addressed the effect of CPAP as an add-on treatment to lipid-lowering medication in a CAD cohort with concomitant OSA. This study was a secondary analysis of the RICCADSA trial (Trial Registry: ClinicalTrials.gov; No: NCT 00519597), that was conducted in Sweden between 2005 and 2013. In total, 244 revascularized CAD patients with nonsleepy OSA (apnea–hypopnea index ≥ 15/h, Epworth Sleepiness Scale score < 10) were randomly assigned to CPAP or no-CPAP. Circulating triglycerides (TG), total cholesterol (TC), high-density lipoprotein (HDL) and low-density lipoprotein (LDL) levels (all in mg/dL) were measured at baseline and 12 months after randomization. The desired TG levels were defined as circulating TG < 150 mg/dL, and LDL levels were targeted as <70 mg/dL according to the recent guidelines of the European Cardiology Society and the European Atherosclerosis Society. A total of 196 patients with available blood samples at baseline and 12-month follow-up were included (94 randomized to CPAP, 102 to no-CPAP). We found no significant between-group differences in circulating levels of TG, TC, HDL and LDL at baseline and after 12 months as well as in the amount of change from baseline. However, there was a significant decline regarding the proportion of patients with the desired TG levels from 87.2% to 77.2% in the CPAP group ($p = 0.022$), whereas there was an increase from 84.3% to 88.2% in the no-CPAP group (n.s.). The desired LDL levels remained low after 12 months in both groups (15.1% vs. 17.2% in CPAP group, and 20.8% vs. 18.8% in no-CPAP group; n.s.). In a multiple linear regression model, the increase in the TG levels was predicted by the increase in body-mass-index ($\beta = 4.1$; 95% confidence interval (1.0–7.1); $p = 0.009$) adjusted for age, sex and CPAP usage (hours/night). CPAP had no lipid-lowering effect in this revascularized cohort with OSA. An increase in body-mass-index predicted the increase in TG levels after 12 months, suggesting that lifestyle modifications should be given priority in adults with CAD and OSA, regardless of CPAP treatment.

Keywords: coronary artery disease; dyslipidaemia; obstructive sleep apnea; CPAP; randomized controlled trial

1. Introduction

Dyslipidaemia, especially low-density lipoprotein (LDL)–cholesterol, is a well-known risk factor for coronary artery disease (CAD), and reducing lipid levels is essential for secondary prevention in management of these high-risk individuals [1]. According to the National Health and Nutrition Examination Survey, 11.7% of people between the ages 20–39, and 41.2% of adults between ages 40–64 have elevated levels of LDL [2].

Obstructive sleep apnea (OSA) is also an important public health problem in developed countries, affecting 9% and 24% of middle-aged women and men, respectively [3]. Based on the longitudinal Wisconsin Sleep Cohort study, published in 2013, the prevalence estimates are even higher (17% of women, and 34% of men) age 30–70 [4]. Moreover, dyslipidemia [5] and obesity [4] co-exist among adult OSA populations. Mechanisms, such as chronic intermittent hypoxia [6–8], sleep fragmentation [9,10] and sympathetic overactivation [11], have been suggested to contribute to dysregulation in lipid profiles among patients with OSA.

OSA along with dyslipidemia has been independently associated with an increase in all-cause mortality, vascular heart disease and stroke, further creating an important demand for efficient treatment [12]. Continuous positive airway pressure (CPAP) is the first line treatment of OSA [13]. An observational study over 30 years has shown that OSA patients treated with CPAP for longer than 5 years were 5.6 times more likely to survive [14]. Notwithstanding, evidence of a possible lipid-lowering effect of CPAP in CAD patients with OSA is scarce. Previous meta-analyzes showed smaller reductions in circulating triglycerides (TG), total cholesterol (TC) and high-density lipoprotein (HDL)–cholesterol levels [15,16], but none of the included studies in those meta-analyzes were conducted in cardiac cohorts. A later study by Huang et al. [17] addressed the impact of CPAP in a small sample of 65 non-obese adults with newly diagnosed CAD, and reported no effect of CPAP on the circulating lipid levels.

In the current study, we addressed the effect of CPAP for 12 months as an add-on treatment to lipid-lowering medication in a CAD cohort with concomitant OSA. We have also examined whether or not the desired TG and LDL levels according to the recent guidelines of the European Cardiology Society (ECS) and the European Atherosclerosis Society (EAS) were reached in this cohort following CPAP treatment [1].

2. Materials and Methods

2.1. Study Population

The present study is a primary analysis of one of the secondary outcomes of the **R**andomized **I**ntervention with **C**PAP in **C**oronary **A**rtery **D**isease and obstructive **S**leep **A**pnea (RICCADSA) trial, which was conducted in Sweden between 2005 and 2013. The RICCADSA cohort has been previously described elsewhere [18]. In brief, adults with a history of percutaneous coronary intervention (PCI) or coronary artery by-pass grafting (CABG) within 6 months prior to study start were consecutively invited to participate. The CAD patients were classified as having OSA (apnea–hypopnea index [AHI] $\geq$ 15/h) and no-OSA (apnea–hypopnea index [AHI] < 5/h) based on the home sleep apnea testing (HSAT). As previously described in detail [18,19], the Embletta® Portable Digital System device (Embla, Broomfield, CO, USA) was used for the HSAT recordings, which included a nasal pressure detector, two respiratory inductance plethysmography belts and pulse-oximetry for recording heart rate and oxyhemoglobin saturation (SpO2). Apnea was defined as at least 90% cessation of airflow, and the hypopnea definition was based on the guidelines from 1999 as at least a 50% reduction in nasal pressure amplitude and/or in thoraco–abdominal movement for at least 10 s [20]. For the current protocol, 196 CAD patients with nonsleepy OSA (AHI $\geq$ 15/h, Epworth Sleepiness Scale (ESS) score < 10) from the randomized controlled trial (RCT) arm were included (Figure 1). As previously described [19], the 1:1 random assignment of the main trial was scheduled with a block size of eight patients (four CPAP, four controls) stratified by gender and revascularization type (PCI/CABG).

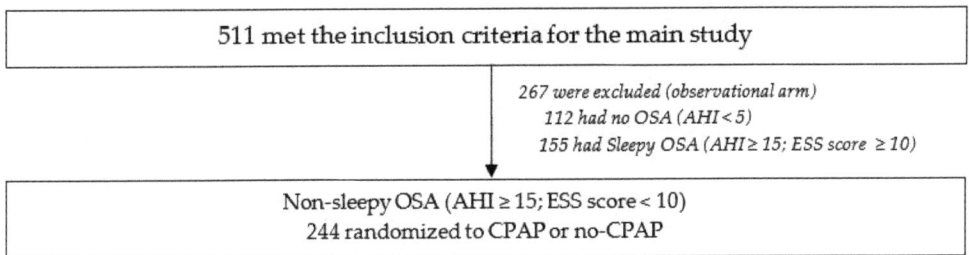

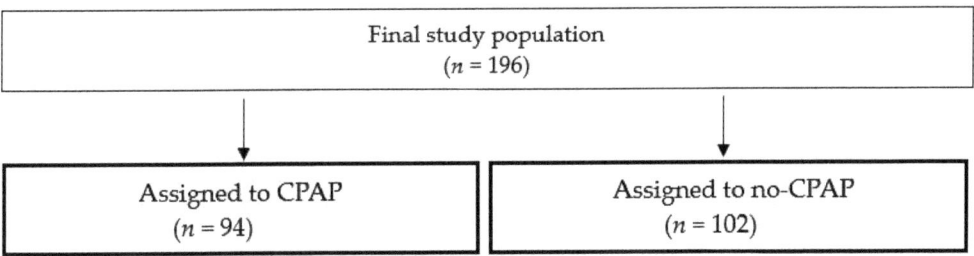

Figure 1. Consort flow chart of the study population.

2.2. Epworth Sleepiness Scale

The ESS is a self-rating questionnaire, which includes eight items estimating the risk of dozing-off under eight different conditions [21]. The subjects who scored less than 10 out of 24 points were categorized as nonsleepy.

2.3. Comorbidities

As previously described [19], anthropometrics, smoking habits, medical history of the study population as well as medications, including the use of lipid-lowering agents were obtained from the medical records. Participants with as a body-mass-index (BMI) ≥ 30 kg/m^2 were categorized as obese [22].

2.4. Circulating Lipid Levels

Blood samples were collected after an overnight fasting using ethylenediaminetetraacetic acid and serum tubes in the morning (07:00–08.00 am). Circulating total cholesterol (TC), high-density lipoprotein (HDL), low-density lipoprotein (LDL) as well as triglycerides (TG) levels (all in mg/dL) were measured at baseline and 12 months after randomization. The desired TG levels were defined as circulating TG < 150 mg/dL, and LDL levels were targeted as <70 mg/dL according to the recent guidelines of the ECS and the EAS [1].

2.5. Statistical Analysis

The study sample distribution of demographics and clinical characteristics at baseline was examined using the descriptive statistics. The Shapiro–Wilk test was used to test normality assumption of the current data for all variables. Continuous variables were reported as median values with boundaries of the interquartile ranges (IQR), and the categorical variables as numbers and percentages. Between-group differences were tested by the Mann–Whitney U test for the continuous variables. The chi-square test was used to compare the subgroups on the categorical variables. The within-group differences were tested by Wilcoxon Signed-Rank test for the continuous variables and McNemar's test for the categorical variables. All statistical tests were two-sided and a p-value < 0.05 was considered significant. Statistical analyses were performed using SPSS® 26.0 for Windows® (SPSS Inc., Chicago, IL, USA).

3. Results

3.1. Baseline Characteristics of the Study Population

A total of 196 patients with available blood samples at baseline and 12-month follow-up, who were on lipid-lowering treatment were included (94 randomized to CPAP, 102 to no-CPAP). As shown in Table 1, demographic and clinical characteristics as well as HSAT and circulating lipid levels at baseline were similar in participants allocated to CPAP vs. no-CPAP. All patients were on statin-treatment at baseline as a part of the secondary cardiovascular prevention guidelines at the time of the study period.

Table 1. Baseline demographic and clinical characteristics of the CAD patients with nonsleepy OSA in the RCT arm.

	CPAP n = 94	No-CPAP n = 102	p
Age, yrs	65.4 (60.4–70.6)	67.3 (61.0–72.7)	0.243
Male,%	84.0	84.3	0.959
BMI, kg/m^2	28.1 (25.7–30.2)	28.7 (26.6–30.6)	0.395
Obesity,%	27.7	29.4	0.786
PCI,%	76.6	76.5	0.984
AHI, events/h	23.5 (17.9–37.0)	24.9 (18.9–32.2)	0.648
ODI, events/h	13.5 (8.5–20.8)	12.6 (6.8–21.1)	0.502
ESS score	6 (4.0–8.0)	5.5 (4.0–7.0)	0.659
Total Cholesterol, mg/dL	158.6 (146.0–181.8)	152.8 (131.5–181.8)	0.107
HDL, mg/dL	47.4 (37.4–55.0)	43.9 (38.7–51.8)	0.290
LDL, mg/dL	90.1 (77.5–107.0)	87.0 (72.1–105.4)	0.309
Triglycerides, mg/dL	112.5 (81.3–151.7)	101.0 (81.4–143.0)	0.422
Glucose, mg/dL	101.0 (90.1–115.3)	97.3 (90.1–104.5)	0.166
Current smoker, %	17.0	14.7	0.657
AMI, %	57.4	48.0	0.188
Hypertension, %	66.0	59.8	0.373
Diabetes, %	26.6	18.6	0.182
Stroke, %	7.4	10.9	0.406
Lung Disease, %	4.3	9.8	0.132
Depression, %	4.3	3.0	0.619

Continuous data are presented as median and 25–75% quartiles. Categorical data are presented as percentage. Abbreviations: AHI, apnea hypopnea index; AMI, acute myocardial infarction; BMI, body mass index; CAD, coronary artery disease; CPAP, continuous positive airway pressure; ESS, Epworth Sleepiness Scale; HDL, high-density lipoprotein; LDL, low-density lipoprotein; OSA, obstructive sleep apnea; PCI, percutaneous coronary intervention; RCT, randomized controlled trial.

3.2. Outcomes

All patients remained on the statin therapy at 1-year follow-up. As illustrated in Figure 2, there were no significant between-group as well as within-group differences regarding the circulating levels of the TG, TC, HDL and LDL levels at 12-month follow-up compared to baseline across the CPAP and no-CPAP groups in the intention-to-treat population.

As shown in Figure 3, the desired TG levels at baseline were similar between the groups. However, there was a significant between-group differences in proportion of patients with the desired TG-levels after 12 months ($p = 0.048$). The significant within-group difference was observed in the CPAP group (87.2% at baseline vs. 77.2% after 12 months; $p = 0.022$). The proportion of participants with the desired LDL levels remained low after 12 months in both groups (15.1% vs. 17.2% in CPAP group, and 20.8% vs. 18.8% in no-CPAP group, respectively) with no significant within- and between-group differences.

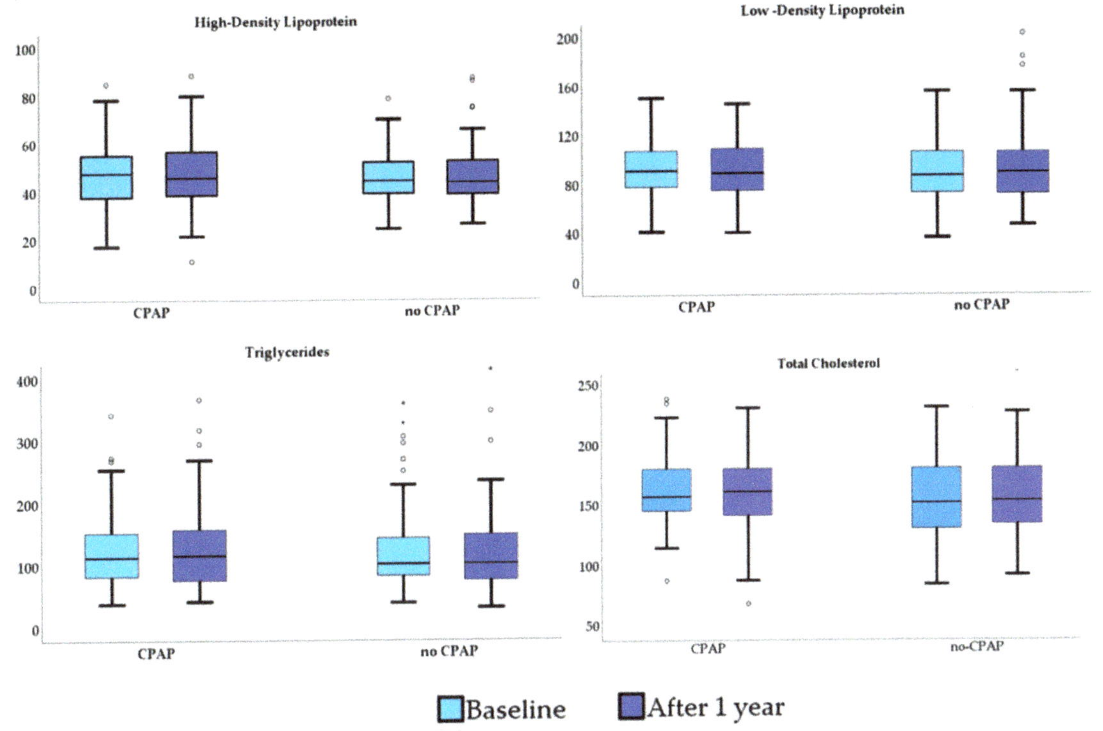

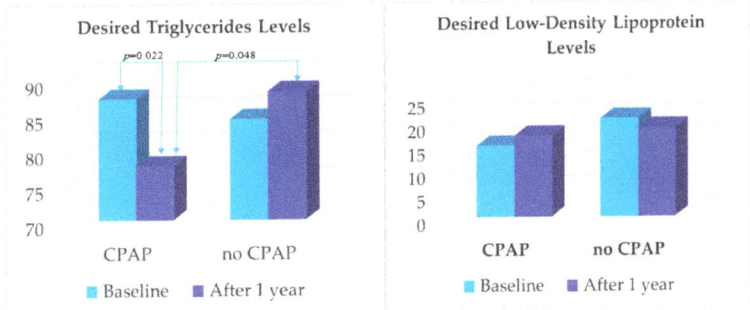

Figure 2. Distribution of the circulating lipid levels at baseline and after 12 months in patients in the CPAP and no-CPAP groups.

Figure 3. Proportion of participants with the desired triglyceride and low-density lipoprotein levels at baseline and after 12 months.

As illustrated in Figure 4, there was a linear association between the changes in TG levels and BMI at 1-year follow-up. In a multiple linear regression model, the increase in the TG levels was predicted by the increase in BMI (β = 4.1; 95% confidence interval (1.0–7.1); p = 0.009) adjusted for age, sex and CPAP usage (hours/night).

In the entire study population randomized to CPAP, the median CPAP usage was 3.8 h/night (IQR 0.0–6.1 h/night), and 47 out 94 (50%) were classified as CPAP adherent. The adherence was defined as at least 4 h/night, corresponding all nights during the 1-yr period. Post-hoc analyzes of the patients stratified by CPAP adherence did not change the main findings of the study (data not shown).

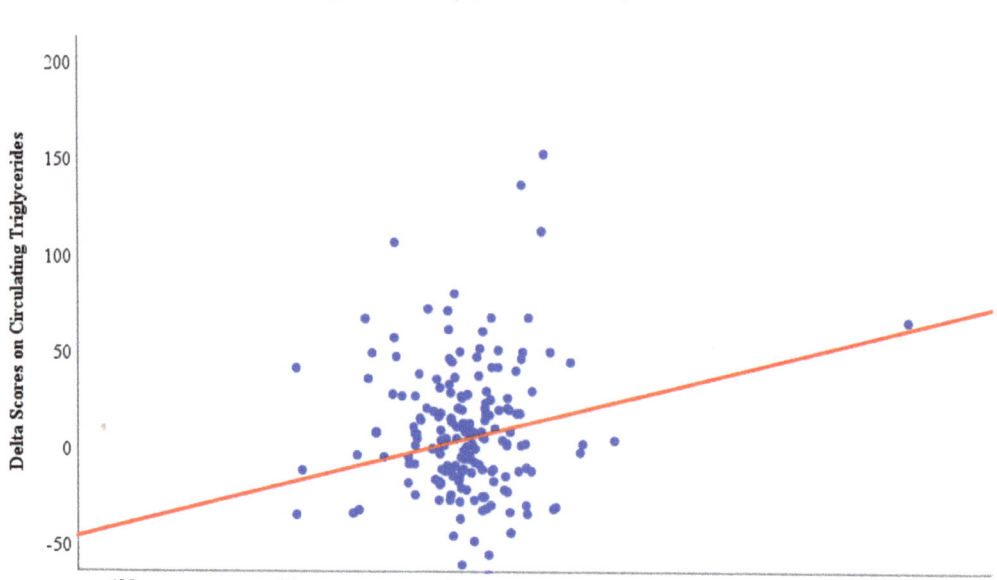

Figure 4. Multiple linear regression line for the association between change in body-mass-index and change in circulating triglyceride levels after 12 months.

4. Discussion

The current study found no additional effect of CPAP therapy on the circulating levels of lipids after 12 months in CAD patients with OSA who were already on lipid-lowering medication. The desired LDL levels remained low in both CPAP and no-CPAP groups, and this was unrelated to OSA severity at baseline and/or CPAP adherence. Moreover, we observed a decrease in the proportion of patients with the desired TG levels, indicating a worsening. However, in a multiple linear regression model, the increase in BMI was the only significant predictor of the increase in TG levels independent of age, sex, AHI at baseline and CPAP adherence.

To the best of our knowledge, this study is the first RCT evaluating the effect of CPAP intervention as an add-on treatment to lipid-lowering medication in revascularized CAD patients with nonsleepy OSA. Previously, Huang et al. [17] addressed the impact of CPAP in a small sample of 65 non-obese adults with newly diagnosed CAD, who were on standardized lipid-lowering medication. The authors reported no effect of CPAP on the circulating lipid levels, which is in line with our results. We additionally showed no improvement regarding the proportion of patients with the desired TG and LDL levels after CPAP treatment. The decrease in the proportion of patients with the desired TG levels after CPAP treatment and its association with the increase in BMI is clinically relevant, and should be taken into consideration in the management of CAD patients with concomitant OSA.

The RCTs in non-cardiac cohorts with concomitant OSA [23–28] have also demonstrated no significant changes in circulating lipid levels except for the study by Phillips et al. [28], in which reductions in the total cholesterol and triglyceride levels have been demonstrated after 2 months of CPAP treatment. Moreover, a previous meta-analysis by Xu et al. [15] included six RCTs with 741 individuals and showed a significant but modest decrease in TC without any changes in the other parameters. Another meta-analysis Lin et al. [16] including 699 participants demonstrated smaller reductions in TG and HDL in addition to the decreased levels of TC following CPAP treatment. Thus, no impact has been shown on the circulating LDL levels, which is the most important target, especially in the secondary cardiovascular prevention models [1].

Chronic intermittent hypoxia is considered to be the main mechanism via systemic inflammation, oxidative distress, endothelial dysfunction and atherosclerosis in the previous literature [29]. It has also been suggested that increased sympathetic system activation may modulate the hormone-sensitive lipoprotein activity in the adipose tissue, which triggers lipolysis [30]. Moreover, Trammell et al. [31] showed in a mice model that sleep fragmentation is related with impaired lipid mechanism. Recently, Martinez-Ceron et al. [32] demonstrated a significant association between dyslipidemia and severe OSA, which might be due to sleep fragmentation and increased sympathetic activity. Although these proposed mechanisms constitute a relevant rationale to expect positive effects of the treatment of OSA by CPAP, our study does not show any significant impact on the circulating lipid levels as an add-on treatment to lipid-lowering medication. A slight decrease in the proportion of patients with the desired TG levels, explained by the increase in BMI at the 1-yr follow-up, as well as the remaining low proportion of patients with the desired LDL levels in spite of medication, strongly emphasizes that lifestyle modifications should be given priority in adults with CAD and OSA, regardless of CPAP treatment.

Lifestyle interventions on the severity of OSA as well as on the metabolic abnormalities in adults with OSA are still being studied, and have been showing promising results [33]. Moreover, although CPAP is recommended as the first therapeutic choice for patients with OSA, there is also data suggesting that pharyngoplasty with barbed sutures may improve the metabolic profile of patients with OSA [34,35].

Of note, our results apply to the CAD patients with the nonsleepy OSA phenotype. The reason for not including the patients with the "sleepy" phenotype in the current analysis was to evaluate the effect of CPAP on circulating levels of lipids in a more scientific manner, since randomization of individuals with the "sleepy phenotype" would not be ethical (risk for traffic and work accidents). Whether or not the response to CPAP treatment regarding the lipid profiles differs between OSA patients with the "sleepy" versus "nonsleepy" phenotype is indeed interesting, and will be further analyzed in the entire RICCADSA population.

The current study has three main limitations. First, the power estimate for the main RICCADSA trial was conducted for the primary outcomes (composite of major cardiovascular and cerebrovascular events) [19] and not for the secondary outcomes, and thus, the sample size may not be sufficient to validate the additional effect of CPAP on the lipid profiles. Second, our results are not generalizable to individuals with OSA in general population or other clinical cohorts. Third, categorization of patients as "nonsleepy" was based on an ESS score less than 10, which may not be precise in a CAD population. However, this questionnaire is a generally accepted tool used in clinical cohorts [21], and objective measurements, such as the Multiple Sleep Latency Test [36], are time consuming, expensive and not realistic to use in large-scale trials in cardiac populations.

5. Conclusions

CPAP had no lipid-lowering effect in this revascularized cohort with OSA. An increase in BMI predicted the increase in TG levels after 12 months, suggesting that lifestyle modifications should be given priority in adults with CAD and OSA, regardless of CPAP treatment.

Author Contributions: Y.P. designed the main RICCADSA trial in 2005. Y.P. performed the patient recruitment and clinical follow-ups. Y.C. and Y.P. performed the statistical analysis. Y.C., B.B. and Y.P. interpreted the data, prepared the manuscript, and drafted the article. All authors have read and agreed to the published version of the manuscript.

Funding: The RICCADSA trial is supported by grants from the Swedish Research Council (521-2011-537 and 521-2013-3439); the Swedish Heart-Lung Foundation (20080592, 20090708 and 20100664); the "Agreement concerning research and education of doctors" of Västra Götalandsregionen (ALFGBG-

11538 and ALFGBG-150801), Research fund at Skaraborg Hospital (VGSKAS-4731, VGSKAS-5908, VGSKAS-9134, VGSKAS-14781, VGSKAS-40271 and VGSKAS-116431); Skaraborg Research and Development Council (VGFOUSKB-46371); the Heart Foundation of Kärnsjukhuset; ResMed Foundation; and ResMed Ltd. ResMed Sweden provided some of the sleep recording devices and technical support. None of the funders had any direct influence on the design of the study, the analysis of the data, the data collection, drafting of the manuscript, or the decision to publish.

Institutional Review Board Statement: The study was conducted according to the guidelines of the Declaration of Helsinki, and approved by the Regional Ethical Review Board in Gothenburg (approval nr 207-05; 13 September 2005; amendment T744-10; 26 November 2010; amendment T512-11; 16 June 2011).

Informed Consent Statement: All patients provided written informed consent.

Data Availability Statement: Individual participant data that underlie the results reported in this article can be obtained by contacting the principal investigator of the RICCADSA trial; yuksel.peker@lungall.gu.se.

Conflicts of Interest: Yüksel Peker received institutional grants from ResMed for the main RICCADSA trial. Yeliz Celik and Baran Balcan report no conflict of interest.

References

1. Mach, F.; Baigent, C.; Catapano, A.L.; Koskinas, K.C.; Casula, M.; Badimon, L.; Chapman, M.J.; De Backer, G.G.; Delgado, V.; Ference, B.A.; et al. 2019 ESC/EAS Guidelines for the management of dyslipidaemias: Lipid modification to reduce cardiovascular risk. *Eur. Heart J.* **2019**, *41*, 111–188. [CrossRef] [PubMed]
2. Navar-Boggan, A.M.; Peterson, E.D.; D'Agostino, S.R.B.; Neely, B.; Sniderman, A.D.; Pencina, M.J. Hyperlipidemia in Early Adulthood Increases Long-Term Risk of Coronary Heart Disease. *Circulation* **2015**, *131*, 451–458. [CrossRef] [PubMed]
3. Young, T.; Palta, M.; Dempsey, J.; Skatrud, J.; Weber, S.; Badr, S. The Occurrence of Sleep-Disordered Breathing among Middle-Aged Adults. *N. Engl. J. Med.* **1993**, *328*, 1230–1235. [CrossRef]
4. Peppard, P.E.; Young, T.; Barnet, J.H.; Palta, M.; Hagen, E.W. Hla, K.M. Increased Prevalence of Sleep-Disordered Breathing in Adults. *Am. J. Epidemiol.* **2013**, *177*, 1006–1014. [CrossRef]
5. Gunduz, C.; Basoglu, O.K.; Kvamme, J.A.; Verbraecken, J.; Anttalainen, U.; Marrone, O.; Steiropoulos, P.; Roisman, G.; Joppa, P.; Hein, H.; et al. Long-term positive airway pressure therapy is associated with reduced total cholesterol levels in patients with obstructive sleep apnea: Data from the European Sleep Apnea Database (ESADA). *Sleep Med.* **2020**, *75*, 201–209. [CrossRef] [PubMed]
6. Trzepizur, W.; Le Vaillant, M.; Meslier, N.; Pigeanne, T.; Masson, P.; Humeau, M.P.; Bizieux-Thaminy, A.; Goupil, F.; Chollet, S.; Ducluzeau, P.H.; et al. Independent Association Between Nocturnal Intermittent Hypoxemia and Metabolic Dyslipidemia. *Chest* **2013**, *143*, 1584–1589. [CrossRef] [PubMed]
7. Chen, L.; Einbinder, E.; Zhang, Q.; Hasday, J.; Balke, C.W.; Scharf, S.M. Oxidative Stress and Left Ventricular Function with Chronic Intermittent Hypoxia in Rats. *Am. J. Respir. Crit. Care Med.* **2005**, *172*, 915–920. [CrossRef]
8. Mesarwi, O.A.; Loomba, R.; Malhotra, A. Obstructive Sleep Apnea, Hypoxia, and Nonalcoholic Fatty Liver Disease. *Am. J. Respir. Crit. Care Med.* **2019**, *199*, 830–841. [CrossRef]
9. Toyama, Y.; Chin, K.; Chihara, Y.; Takegami, M.; Takahashi, K.-I.; Sumi, K.; Nakamura, T.; Nakayama-Ashida, Y.; Minami, I.; Horita, S.; et al. Association Between Sleep Apnea, Sleep Duration, and Serum Lipid Profile in an Urban, Male, Working Population in Japan. *Chest* **2013**, *143*, 720–728. [CrossRef]
10. Chopra, S.; Rathore, A.; Younas, H.; Pham, L.V.; Gu, C.; Beselman, A.; Kim, I.-Y.; Wolfe, R.R.; Perin, J.; Polotsky, V.Y.; et al. Obstructive Sleep Apnea Dynamically Increases Nocturnal Plasma Free Fatty Acids, Glucose, and Cortisol During Sleep. *J. Clin. Endocrinol. Metab.* **2017**, *102*, 3172–3181. [CrossRef]
11. Borovac, J.A.; Dogas, Z.; Supe-Domic, D.; Galic, T.; Bozic, J. Catestatin serum levels are increased in male patients with obstructive sleep apnea. *Sleep Breath.* **2019**, *23*, 473–481. [CrossRef] [PubMed]
12. Marshall, N.S.; Wong, K.K.; Cullen, S.R.; Knuiman, M.W.; Grunstein, R.R. Sleep apnea and 20-year follow-up for all-cause mortality, stroke, and cancer incidence and mortality in the Busselton Health Study cohort. *J. Clin. Sleep Med.* **2014**, *10*, 355–362. [CrossRef] [PubMed]
13. Javaheri, S.; Martinez-García, M.A.; Campos-Rodriguez, F.; Muriel, A.; Peker, Y. Continuous Positive Airway Pressure Adherence for Prevention of Major Adverse Cerebrovascular and Cardiovascular Events in Obstructive Sleep Apnea. *Am. J. Respir. Crit. Care Med.* **2020**, *201*, 607–610. [CrossRef] [PubMed]
14. Dodds, S.; Williams, L.J.; Roguski, A.; Vennelle, M.; Douglas, N.J.; Kotoulas, S.-C.; Riha, R.L. Mortality and morbidity in obstructive sleep apnoea–hypopnoea syndrome: Results from a 30-year prospective cohort study. *ERJ Open Res.* **2020**, *6*, 00057-2020. [CrossRef] [PubMed]
15. Xu, H.; Yi, H.; Guan, J.; Yin, S. Effect of continuous positive airway pressure on lipid profile in patients with obstructive sleep apnea syndrome: A meta-analysis of randomized controlled trials. *Atherosclerosis* **2014**, *234*, 446–453. [CrossRef]

16. Lin, M.-T.; Lin, H.-H.; Lee, P.-L.; Weng, P.-H.; Lee, C.-C.; Lai, T.-C.; Liu, W.; Chen, C.-L. Beneficial effect of continuous positive airway pressure on lipid profiles in obstructive sleep apnea: A meta-analysis. *Sleep Breath.* **2015**, *19*, 809–817. [CrossRef]
17. Huang, Z.; Liu, Z.; Zhao, Z.; Zhao, Q.; Luo, Q.; Tang, Y. Effects of Continuous Positive Airway Pressure on Lipidaemia and High-sensitivity C-reactive Protein Levels in Non-obese Patients with Coronary Artery Disease and Obstructive Sleep Apnoea. *Hear. Lung Circ.* **2016**, *25*, 576–583. [CrossRef]
18. Peker, Y.; Glantz, H.; Thunström, E.; Kallryd, A.; Herlitz, J.; Ejdebäck, J. Rationale and design of the Randomized Intervention with CPAP in Coronary Artery Disease and Sleep Apnoea–RICCADSA trial. *Scand. Cardiovasc. J.* **2009**, *43*, 24–31. [CrossRef]
19. Peker, Y.; Glantz, H.; Eulenburg, C.; Wegscheider, K.; Herlitz, J.; Thunström, E. Effect of Positive Airway Pressure on Cardiovascular Outcomes in Coronary Artery Disease Patients with Nonsleepy Obstructive Sleep Apnea. The RICCADSA Randomized Controlled Trial. *Am. J. Respir. Crit. Care Med.* **2016**, *194*, 613–620. [CrossRef]
20. Quan, S.F.; Gillin, J.C.; Littner, M.R.; Shepard, J.W. Sleep-related breathing disorders in adults: Recommendations for syndrome definition and measurement techniques in clinical research. The Report of an American Academy of Sleep Medicine Task Force. *Sleep* **1999**, *22*, 667–689.
21. Johns, M.W. A New Method for Measuring Daytime Sleepiness: The Epworth Sleepiness Scale. *Sleep* **1991**, *14*, 540–545. [CrossRef] [PubMed]
22. World Health Organization. Obesity: Overview. Available online: https://www.who.int/health-topics/obesity#tab=tab_1 (accessed on 3 January 2022).
23. Coughlin, S.R.; Mawdsley, L.; Mugarza, J.A.; Wilding, J.P.H.; Calverley, P.M.A. Cardiovascular and metabolic effects of CPAP in obese males with OSA. *Eur. Respir. J.* **2007**, *29*, 720–727. [CrossRef] [PubMed]
24. Drager, L.F.; Bortolotto, L.A.; Figueiredo, A.C.; Krieger, E.M.; Lorenzi-Filho, G. Effects of Continuous Positive Airway Pressure on Early Signs of Atherosclerosis in Obstructive Sleep Apnea. *Am. J. Respir. Crit. Care Med.* **2007**, *176*, 706–712. [CrossRef] [PubMed]
25. Robinson, G.V.; Pepperell, J.C.T.; Segal, H.C.; Davies, R.J.O.; Stradling, J.R. Circulating cardiovascular risk factors in obstructive sleep apnoea: Data from randomised controlled trials. *Thorax* **2004**, *59*, 777–782. [CrossRef]
26. Comondore, V.R.; Cheema, R.; Fox, J.; Butt, A.; Mancini, G.B.J.; Fleetham, J.A.; Ryan, C.F.; Chan, S.; Ayas, N.T. The Impact of CPAP on Cardiovascular Biomarkers in Minimally Symptomatic Patients with Obstructive Sleep Apnea: A Pilot Feasibility Randomized Crossover Trial. *Lung* **2009**, *187*, 17–22. [CrossRef] [PubMed]
27. Chirinos, J.A.; Gurubhagavatula, I.; Teff, K.; Rader, D.J.; Wadden, T.A.; Townsend, R.; Foster, G.D.; Maislin, G.; Saif, H.; Broderick, P.; et al. CPAP, Weight Loss, or Both for Obstructive Sleep Apnea. *N. Engl. J. Med.* **2014**, *370*, 2265–2275. [CrossRef]
28. Phillips, C.L.; Yee, B.J.; Marshall, N.S.; Liu, P.Y.; Sullivan, D.R.; Grunstein, R.R. Continuous positive airway pressure reduces postprandial lipidemia in obstructive sleep apnea: A randomized, placebo-controlled crossover trial. *Am. J. Respir. Crit. Care Med.* **2011**, *184*, 355–361. [CrossRef]
29. Adedayo, A.M.; Olafiranye, O.; Smith, D.; Hill, A.; Zizi, F.; Brown, C.; Jean-Louis, G. Obstructive sleep apnea and dyslipidemia: Evidence and underlying mechanism. *Sleep Breath.* **2014**, *18*, 13–18. [CrossRef]
30. Lafontan, M.; Langin, D. Lipolysis and lipid mobilization in human adipose tissue. *Prog. Lipid Res.* **2009**, *48*, 275–297. [CrossRef]
31. Trammell, R.A.; Verhulst, S.; Toth, L.A. Effects of Sleep Fragmentation on Sleep and Markers of Inflammation in Mice. *Comp. Med.* **2014**, *64*, 13–24.
32. Martínez-Cerón, E.; Casitas, R.; Galera, R.; Sánchez-Sánchez, B.; Zamarrón, E.; Garcia-Sanchez, A.; Jaureguizar, A.; Cubillos-Zapata, C.; Garcia-Rio, F. Contribution of sleep characteristics to the association between obstructive sleep apnea and dyslipidemia. *Sleep Med.* **2021**, *84*, 63–72. [CrossRef]
33. Bonsignore, M.R.; Borel, A.-L.; Machan, E.; Grunstein, R. Sleep apnoea and metabolic dysfunction. *Eur. Respir. Rev.* **2013**, *22*, 353–364. [CrossRef] [PubMed]
34. Binar, M.; Akçam, M.T.; Karakoc, O.; Sagkan, R.I.; Musabak, U.H.; Gerek, M. A new surgical technique versus an old marker: Can expansion sphincter pharyngoplasty reduce C-reactive protein levels in patients with obstructive sleep apnea? *Eur. Arch. Oto-Rhino-Laryngol.* **2017**, *274*, 829–836. [CrossRef]
35. Iannella, G.; Lechien, J.R.; Perrone, T.; Meccariello, G.; Cammaroto, G.; Cannavicci, A.; Burgio, L.; Maniaci, A.; Cocuzza, S.; Di Luca, M.; et al. Barbed reposition pharyngoplasty (BRP) in obstructive sleep apnea treatment: State of the art. *Am. J. Otolaryngol.* **2022**, *43*, 103197. [CrossRef] [PubMed]
36. Wise, M.S. Objective measures of sleepiness and wakefulness: Application to the real world? *J. Clin. Neurophysiol.* **2006**, *23*, 39–49. [CrossRef] [PubMed]

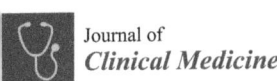

Article

Sleep Apnea Classification Algorithm Development Using a Machine-Learning Framework and Bag-of-Features Derived from Electrocardiogram Spectrograms

Cheng-Yu Lin [1,2,3], Yi-Wen Wang [4], Febryan Setiawan [4], Nguyen Thi Hoang Trang [4] and Che-Wei Lin [4,5,6,*]

1. Department of Otolaryngology, National Cheng Kung University Hospital, College of Medicine, National Cheng Kung University, Tainan 704, Taiwan; yu621109@ms48.hinet.net
2. Department of Environmental and Occupational Medicine, National Cheng Kung University Hospital, College of Medicine, National Cheng Kung University, Tainan 704, Taiwan
3. Sleep Medicine Center, National Cheng Kung University Hospital, College of Medicine, National Cheng Kung University, Tainan 704, Taiwan
4. Department of Biomedical Engineering, College of Engineering, National Cheng Kung University, Tainan 701, Taiwan; yiwen.wtmh@gmail.com (Y.-W.W.); febryans2802@gs.ncku.edu.tw (F.S.); hoangtrangnguyen181@gmail.com (N.T.H.T.)
5. Medical Device Innovation Center, National Cheng Kung University, Tainan 704, Taiwan
6. Institute of Gerontology, College of Medicine, National Cheng Kung University, Tainan 701, Taiwan
* Correspondence: lincw@mail.ncku.edu.tw

Abstract: Background: Heart rate variability (HRV) and electrocardiogram (ECG)-derived respiration (EDR) have been used to detect sleep apnea (SA) for decades. The present study proposes an SA-detection algorithm using a machine-learning framework and bag-of-features (BoF) derived from an ECG spectrogram. Methods: This study was verified using overnight ECG recordings from 83 subjects with an average apnea–hypopnea index (AHI) 29.63 (/h) derived from the Physionet Apnea-ECG and National Cheng Kung University Hospital Sleep Center database. The study used signal preprocessing to filter noise and artifacts, ECG time–frequency transformation using continuous wavelet transform (CWT), BoF feature generation, machine-learning classification using support vector machine (SVM), ensemble learning (EL), k-nearest neighbor (KNN) classification, and cross-validation. The time length of the spectrogram was set as 10 and 60 s to examine the required minimum spectrogram window time length to achieve satisfactory accuracy. Specific frequency bands of 0.1–50, 8–50, 0.8–10, and 0–0.8 Hz were also extracted to generate the BoF to determine the band frequency best suited for SA detection. Results: The five-fold cross-validation accuracy using the BoF derived from the ECG spectrogram with 10 and 60 s time windows were 90.5% and 91.4% for the 0.1–50 Hz and 8–50 Hz frequency bands, respectively. Conclusion: An SA-detection algorithm utilizing BoF and a machine-learning framework was successfully developed in this study with satisfactory classification accuracy and high temporal resolution.

Keywords: sleep apnea; time–frequency transformation; bag-of-features; support vector machine; k-nearest neighbor algorithm; ensemble learning

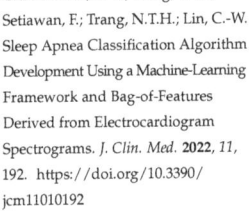

Citation: Lin, C.-Y.; Wang, Y.-W.; Setiawan, F.; Trang, N.T.H.; Lin, C.-W. Sleep Apnea Classification Algorithm Development Using a Machine-Learning Framework and Bag-of-Features Derived from Electrocardiogram Spectrograms. *J. Clin. Med.* **2022**, *11*, 192. https://doi.org/10.3390/jcm11010192

Academic Editors: Yuksel Peker and Gasparri Roberto

Received: 1 November 2021
Accepted: 29 December 2021
Published: 30 December 2021

Publisher's Note: MDPI stays neutral with regard to jurisdictional claims in published maps and institutional affiliations.

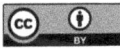

Copyright: © 2021 by the authors. Licensee MDPI, Basel, Switzerland. This article is an open access article distributed under the terms and conditions of the Creative Commons Attribution (CC BY) license (https://creativecommons.org/licenses/by/4.0/).

1. Introduction

Sleep apnea (SA) is a sleep disorder with high prevalence, particularly among middle-aged and elderly subjects. SA prevalence in the overall population ranges from 9% to 38% [1]. Frost and Sullivan (2016) estimated the annual medical cost of undiagnosed SA among U.S. adults to be nearly USD 149.6 billion per year [2]. To reduce the number of undiagnosed SA patients, sleep examinations with fewer channels of physiological signals, such as type III home sleep testing (HST), have received increasing attention in recent years. Facco et al. demonstrated that HST has relatively high intraclass correlation and unconditional agreement with in-lab polysomnography (PSG) testing in SA diagnosis [3].

Dalewski et al. estimated the usefulness of employing modified Mallampati scores (MMP) and the upper airway volume (UAV) to diagnose obstructive SA among patients with breathing-related sleep disorders compared to the more expensive and time-consuming PSG [4]. Philip et al. showed that self-reported sleepiness at the wheel is a better predictor than the apnea hypopnea index (AHI) for sleepiness-related accidents among obstructive SA patients [5]. Furthermore, Kukwa et al. determined that there was no significant difference in the percentage of supine sleep between in-lab PSG and HST. However, women presented more supine sleep with HST than with PSG [6]. Thus, the development of sleep technologies such as type III or type IV monitors may be beneficial for the development of sleep medicines due to the convenience of such medicines compared to PSG.

SA episodes are generally accompanied by abnormal breathing [7] and relative sympathetic nervous system hyperactivity [8]. Several studies attempted to utilize electrocardiogram (ECG) technology to develop automatic SA-detection algorithms since ECG can yield both electrocardiogram-derived respiration (EDR), representing breathing activity [9], and heart rate variability (HRV), representing autonomous nervous function indexes [10]. Most existing automatic SA-detection algorithms using ECG can be categorized into EDR-, HRV-, and cardiopulmonary coupling (CPC)-related approaches.

Many studies have shown that EDR is correlated with respiratory variation [11–14]. EDR is used to estimate respiration based on changes in the morphology of the ECG. Varon et al. proposed a method to detect SA by using an EDR signal derived from a single-lead ECG [12]. In this study, the ECG was transformed into EDR signals in three different ways; moreover, two novel feature sets were proposed (principal components for QRS complexes and orthogonal subspace projections between respiration and heart rate) and compared with the two most popular features in heart rate variability analysis. The accuracy was 85% for the discrimination of both apnea and hypopneas together. An algorithm based on deep learning approaches for automatically extracting features and detecting SA events in an EDR signal was proposed by Steenkiste et al. [14]. The authors employed a balanced bootstrapping scheme to extract efficient respiratory information and trained long short-term memory (LSTM) networks to produce a robust and accurate model.

Several studies have investigated the association between HRV and SA, and many SA-detection algorithms were developed using the HRV parameter [15–20]. HRV assesses the variability in periods between consecutive heartbeats, which change under the control of the autonomous nervous system. Quiceno-Manrique et al. [16] transformed an HRV signal into the time–frequency domain using short-time Fourier transform (STFT) and extracted indices including spectral centroids, spectral centroid energy, and cepstral coefficients to detect SA with 92.67% accuracy. However, these approaches required the collection of at least 3 min of ECG signals to include low-frequency components. Martin-Gonzalez et al. [19] developed a detection algorithm using machine-learning methods to characterize and classify SA based on an HRV feature selection process, focusing on the underlying process from a cardiac-rate point of view. The authors generated linear and nonlinear variables such as Cepstrum coefficients (CCs), Filterbanks (Fbank), and detrended fluctuation analysis (DFA). This algorithm achieved 84.76% accuracy, 81.45% sensitivity, 86.82% specificity, and 0.87 area under the receiver operating characteristic (ROC) curve AUC value. Singh et al. [20] implemented a convolutional neural network (CNN) using a pre-trained AlexNet model in order to improve the detection performance of obstructive SA based on a single-lead ECG scalogram with accuracy of 86.22%, sensitivity of 90%, specificity of 83.8%, and an AUC value of 0.8810.

One of the classic analysis tools for SA disorders is electrocardiogram-derived CPC sleep spectrograms using RR interval and EDR coupling characteristics. Thomas et al. [21] used CPC to evaluate ECG-based cardiopulmonary interactions against standard sleep staging among 35 PSG test subjects (including 15 healthy subjects). Spectrogram features included normal-to-normal sinus inter-beat interval series and corresponding EDR signals. However, using the kappa statistic, agreement with standard sleep staging was poor, with 62.7% for the training set and 43.9% for the testing set. Meanwhile, the cyclic alternating pattern scoring was higher, with 74% for the training set and 77.3% for the testing set. Guo et al. [22] found that CPC high frequency coupling (HFC) proportionally reduced sleep disorder behavior and that HFC durations were negatively correlated with the nasal-flow-derived respiratory disturbance index. Liu et al. [23] developed a CPC method based on the Hilbert–Huang transform (HHT) and found that HHT-CPC spectra provided better temporal and frequency resolution (8 s and 0.001 Hz, respectively) compared to the original CPC (8.5 min and 0.004 Hz, respectively).

Previous studies showed that HRV, EDR, and CPC features can be used to develop automated SA-classification algorithms. However, the RR interval and EDR need a relatively longer time to collect the data; hence, the temporal resolution is poor for algorithms based on HRV or EDR features. Sleep CPC is a good visualization tool for RR interval and EDR coupling since it can indicate sleep quality or sleep-based breathing disorders. However, CPC's temporal resolution for sleep is also poor, as breathing- disorder patterns present large variance, making automated classification difficult. Thus, developing an automated SA algorithm with high temporal resolution was taken as the main research aim of the present study. In this work, we used ECG spectrogram features to develop an algorithm that employs bag-of-features (BoF) techniques and machine-learning classifiers to identify various patterns in SA episodes from ECG spectrograms. Penzel et al. [24] initially exhibited different patterns on the ECG time–frequency spectrogram between normal and SA episodes. However, the authors did not develop automatic classification for SA episodes. Thus, the aim of this study was to develop automatic SA classification based on ECG time–frequency spectrograms.

2. Materials and Methods

2.1. Sleep Apnea ECG Database

Two datasets, the National Cheng Kung University Hospital Sleep Center Apnea Database (NCKUHSCAD) and Physionet Apnea-ECG Database [25] (PAED), were used in this study. NCKUHSCAD was used to observe differences in the apnea and normal periods of the ECG spectrogram. PAED was used to validate the proposed algorithm, as PAED is a public database, which enabled us to compare our results with the existing literature. NCKUHSCAD included information collected from patients who underwent overnight PSG in the Sleep Center of NCKU Hospital (Taiwan) between December 2016 and August 2018. Patients with the following conditions were excluded: PSG recordings for continuous positive airway pressure ventilation titration, the use of hypnotic medicine during the test, and missing data. The study protocol was approved by the Institutional Review Board of NCKUH (protocol number: B-ER-108-426). The database included 50 recordings sampled at 200 Hz, with annotations provided for 10 and 60 s as either normal breathing, hypopnea, or apnea disordered breathing. Hypopnea was defined as a $\geq$30% reduction in baseline airflow for at least 10 seconds combined with either arousal in an electroencephalogram for $\geq$3 seconds or oxygen desaturation $\geq$ 3%. Apnea was defined as a $\geq$90% decrease in airflow over a 10-second period with concomitant respiratory-related chest wall movement for obstructive apnea [26]. In this study, ECG recordings with hypopnea and apnea annotations were merged together as the apnea group.

The 50 recordings from NCKUHSCAD were rearranged into three groups (APEG-A, APEG-B, and APEG-C) (APEG is the abbreviation of APnEa Group) to fulfill different purposes during algorithm performance evaluation.

- NCKUHSCAD-APEG-A included 11 participants who provided severe SA recordings (30 < AHI $\leq$ 45), with an average $\pm$ standard deviation AHI of 39.25 $\pm$ 5.78/h.
- NCKUHSCAD-APEG-B included 35 participants who suffered from SA (AHI $\geq$ 10), with an average $\pm$ standard deviation AHI of 39.83 $\pm$ 23.08/h.
- NCKUHSCAD-APEG-C included the whole database, with an average $\pm$ standard deviation AHI of 29.02 $\pm$ 25.49/h.

PAED [25] was adopted to develop and verify the proposed algorithm's performance. The ECG recordings of PAED were sampled at 100 Hz, and sleep recording durations ranged between 7 and 10 h depending on the participant. The database included 35 recordings, with SA annotations provided on a minute-by-minute basis—i.e., each minute of ECG recording was annotated as either N (normal breathing) or A (disordered breathing including the occurrence of an apnea episode).

PAED included three participant groups: A: apnea, B: borderline, and C: healthy (the control), with 20, 5, and 10 participants, respectively. Those in Group A were known to be related to people definitely suffering from obstructive SA and had total apnea durations > 100 min for each recording. The range of ages among subjects in this group was 38–63, and the AHI of this group's subjects ranged between 21 and 83; those in Group B were borderline and had total apnea episode durations of 10–96 min. The age range within this group was 42–53, and the AHI ranged between 0 and 25; those in Group C had no obstructive SA or very low levels of disease and total apnea durations between 0 and 3 min [27]. Recordings b05 from Group B and c05 from Group C were excluded because recording b05 contained a grinding noise, and c05 was identical to c06. Therefore, only 33 recordings were ultimately included in this study [28].

The remaining 33 recordings from the PAED [28] were also regrouped into three categories:

- PAED-APEG-A included 8 participants with severe SA recordings from group A (30 < AHI ≤ 45, average ± standard deviation AHI: 39.14 ± 3.60/h, age 51.38 ± 6.43 years, and weight 87.88 ± 9.42 kg).
- PAED-APEG-B included participants who suffered from SA—i.e., all of group A (21 < AHI < 83) and group B (0 < AHI < 25, except b05). Thus, APEG-B included 1 female and 23 males, with an average ± standard deviation AHI of 41.55 ± 23.45/h, an age of 51.42 ± 6.50 years, and a weight of 93.04 ± 16.67 kg.
- PAED-APEG-C included the whole database (excluding b05 and c05). Thus, APEG-C included 4 females and 29 males, with an average ± standard deviation AHI of 30.23 ± 27.35/h, an age of 46.85 ± 9.80 years, and a weight of 86.67 ± 18.23 kg. This group featured the same arrangement of participants used in [12,16–18,20,29,30].

Table 1 presents the ECG spectrogram results counted for the different groups after dividing the nocturnal ECG signals into 1 min time windows. The ECG signals were divided into 1 min time window because the sleep expert labelled the ECG signal event (normal vs. apnea) based on a 1 min time window, and some previous studies also employed this database from PhysioNet and used 1 min time window divisions to separate ECG signal events [12,17–19]. Contaminated window ECG spectrograms in PAED (but not in NCKUHSCAD) were removed, which was also done in [12,14,16], since raw ECG signals could contain a wide range of noise caused by the patient's movement, poor patch contact, electrical interference, measurement noise, or other disturbances.

Table 1. General apnea group subject patterns for the proposed frequency bands.

Frequency Band	Normal Breathing Data *			Apnea Data *		
	APEG-A	APEG-B	APEG-C	APEG-A	APEG-B	APEG-C
0.1–50 Hz	4990/1778	11,236/4883	16,941/8383	1638/1799	5173/5886	5538/5895
8–50 Hz	4990/1819	11,236/4985	16,941/8665	1638/1820	5173/5902	5538/5908
0.8–10 Hz	4990/1776	11,236/4803	16,941/8568	1638/1802	5173/5775	5538/5778
0–0.8 Hz	4990/1804	11,236/5060	16,941/8526	1638/1801	5173/5931	5538/5993

* Data are given in order: algorithm performance evaluation databases NCKUHSCAD/PAED. The number before "/" is for the NCKUHSCAD dataset, and the number after "/" is for the PAED dataset.

2.2. Sleep Apnea Detection Algorithm Using a Machine-Learning Framework and Bag-of-Features Derived from ECG Spectrograms

This study proposes an SA-detection algorithm using a machine-learning framework and BoF derived from ECG spectral intensity differences between SA and normal breathing. Figure 1 shows the proposed algorithm flowchart. Single-lead ECG data were input and then divided into consecutive 60 s ECG windows. The time–domain ECG for each window was transformed into the time–frequency spectrogram to obtain ECG spectrograms as the main feature. The BoF technique was then used to obtain features to discriminate ECG spectrograms for SA and normal breathing. Finally, machine-learning classifiers, including support vector machine (SVM), ensemble learning (EL), k-nearest neighbor (KNN), and cross-validation were used to obtain the classification results.

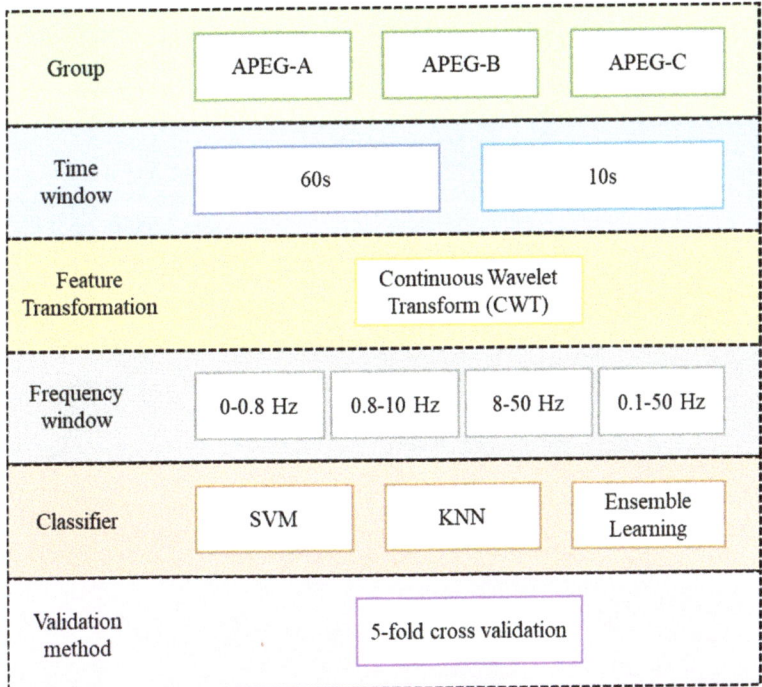

Figure 1. Proposed sleep apnea detection algorithm using machine learning framework and bag-of-features derived from ECG spectrograms (SVM: Support Vector Machine; KNN: k-nearest neighbor).

2.3. Data Preprocessing

In this study, data preprocessing consisted of zero means computation and windowing preprocessing parameters. In this method, the zero-means subtract the mean from the ECG signals to eliminate trend-variation effects, and then nocturnal ECG spectra are segmented into consecutive 60 s windows (to match the database annotation), where windows with large noise are excluded for algorithm development. The PAED [25,28] and NKCUHSCAD utilized in this study labeled every 60 s window as containing an apnea episode or not.

2.4. Time–Frequency Transformation of ECG

The time-domain ECG for each window after data preprocessing was transformed into the time–frequency domain to facilitate better SA-episode classification. Continuous wavelet transform (CWT) [31] was used due to its high-resolution time–frequency components. CWT uses different time lengths to adaptively optimize the resolution in different frequency ranges. A CWT wavelet is a small wave compared to a sinusoidal wave—i.e., a brief oscillation that can be dilated or shifted according to the input signal. Common wavelet types include Meyer, Morlet, and Mexican hat. We selected the Morlet wavelet regime for this study to specify the extraction of several prominent frequency bands. Thus, the CWT regime can be expressed as

$$X_w(s,\tau) = \frac{1}{\sqrt{s}} \int_{-\infty}^{\infty} x(t) \psi^* \left(\frac{t-\tau}{s} \right) dt$$

where $x(t) \in L^2(\mathbb{R})$ is a time series function, $\psi^*(t)$ is the wavelet function, and $s \in \mathbb{R}^+$ ($s > 0$) is a scaling or dilation factor.

To observe the differences between SA episodes and normal breathing (i.e., periods with no SA episode), we used clinical data from the National Cheng Kung University Hospital sleep center for ECG spectrogram observation. Figure 2 shows example benchmark data that include an SA episode, followed by a return to normal breathing and then a subsequent SA episode. ECG spectrogram differences between apnea onset and normal breathing, derived by continuous wavelet transform (CWT), were significant. The power spectrum intensity for normal breathing was much stronger than that for SA episodes in the 5–10 Hz band.

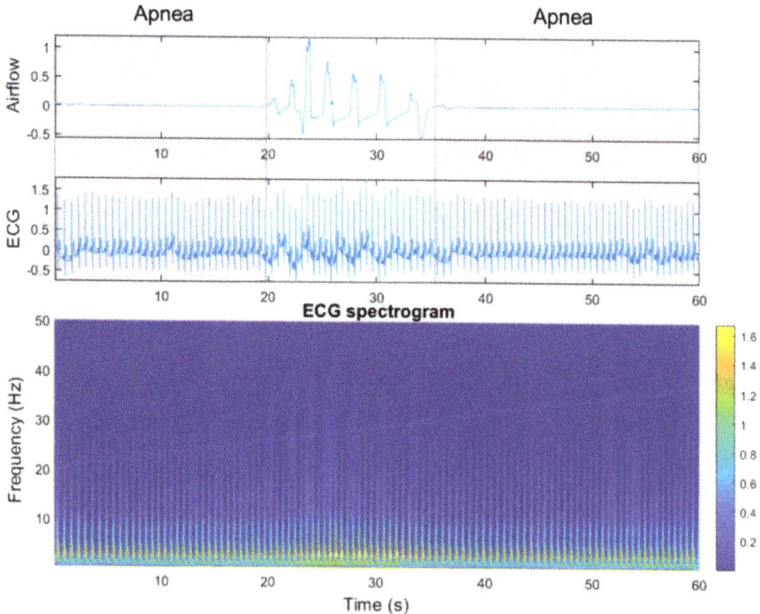

Figure 2. Airflow, electrocardiogram (ECG), and ECG spectrograms from apnea to non-apnea, followed by apnea again.

To achieve high-temporal-resolution pattern visualization, the different spectrogram frequency bands were extracted to classify SA based on other authors' observations and findings [21,22,31]: (1) overall frequency 0.1–50 Hz, (2) high frequency 8–50 Hz, (3) middle frequency 0.8–10 Hz, and (4) low frequency 0–0.8 Hz. Thomas et al. [21,32] and Guo et al. [22] verified that certain frequency bands were associated with periodic respiration during sleep-disorder breathing (0.01–0.1 Hz), as well as physiologic respiratory sinus arrhythmia and deep sleep (0.1–0.4 Hz). As shown in Figure 3, the frequency range definitions of Thomas et al. and Guo et al. do not offer good pattern visualization features between normal ECG and apnea ECG events.

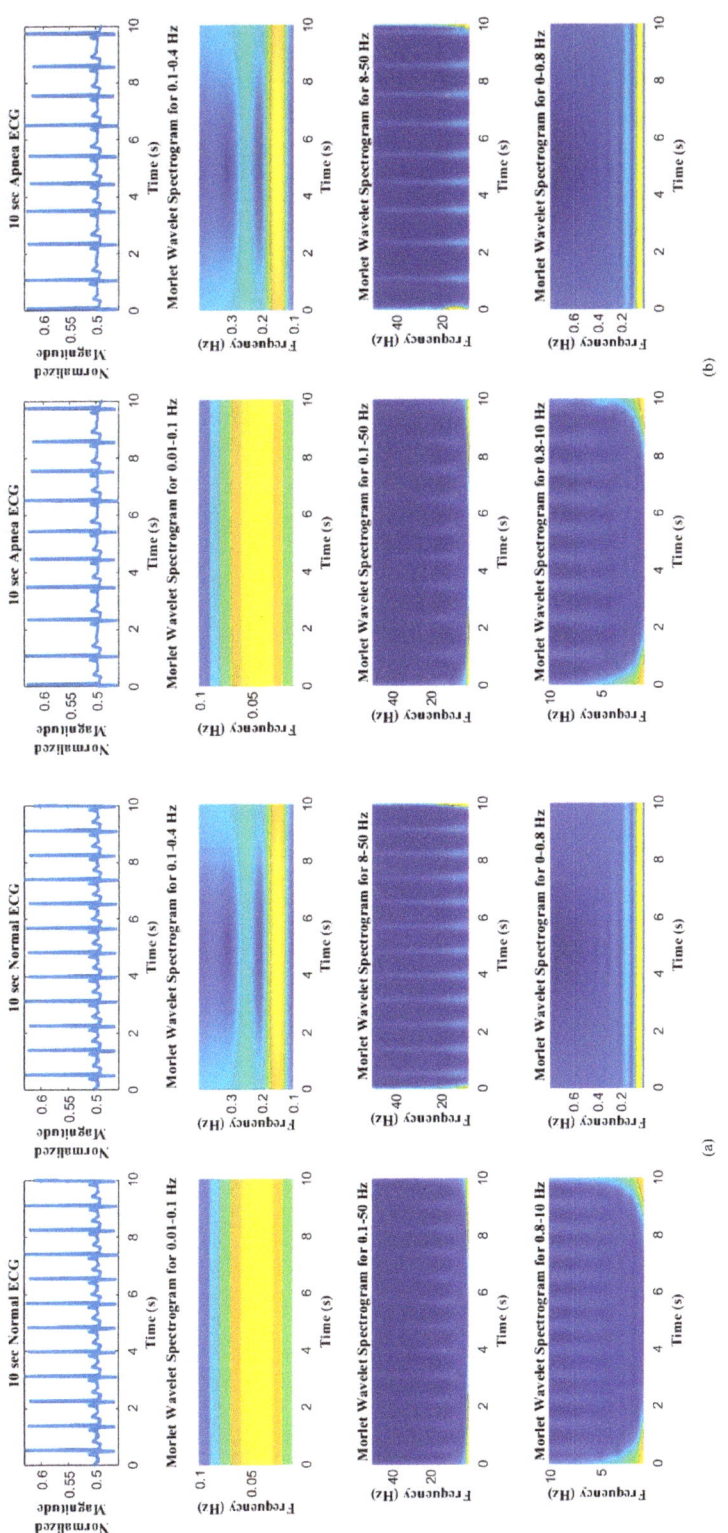

Figure 3. Spectrograms of different frequency bands (0.01–0.1, 0.1–0.4, 0.5–50, 8–50, 0.8–10, and 0–0.8 Hz) [17,18,25] for (**a**) normal ECG and (**b**) apnea ECG events.

2.5. Feature Extraction Using Bag-of-Features

To extract features that best discriminate the spectrogram with apnea onset and normal breathing, we used the bag-of-features (BoF) or bag-of-visual-words [33], a visual classification approach commonly employed for image classification. The BoF corresponds to the frequency histogram of a particular image pattern occurrence in a given image and was also successfully used for text classification. Figure 4 shows the BoF flowchart used in this study.

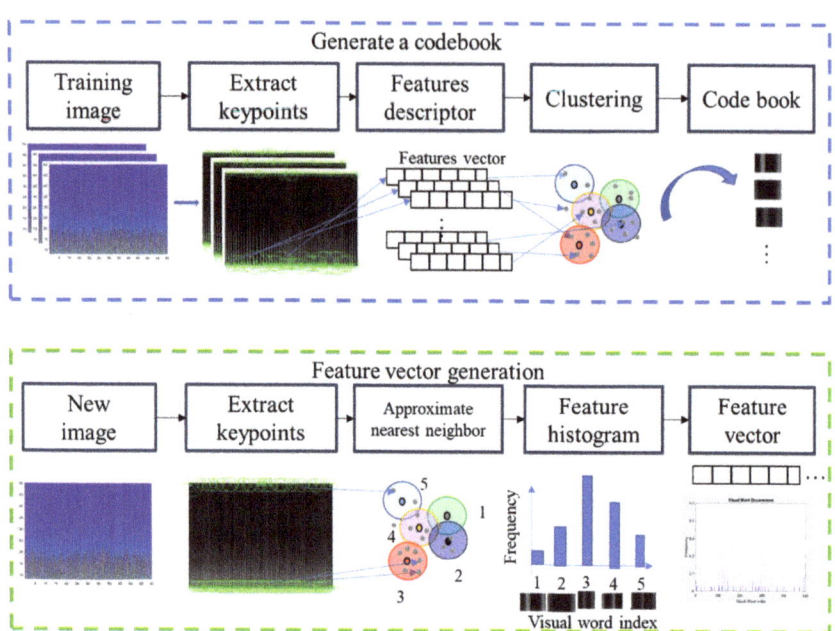

Figure 4. Codebook and feature vector generation for the proposed bag-of-features method.

The two main steps in this process were codebook generation and BoF feature-vector extraction. Codebook generation extracted representative features (visual words) to describe an image. ECG spectrograms were then regarded as images, with visual words being generated as follows. Key points (points of interest) were extracted from training images using a speeded-up robust features (SURF) detector [34], and 64-dimensional descriptors were used to describe the key points. Descriptors were then clustered by k-means clustering, and the resulting clusters were compacted and subsequently separated based on similar characteristics. Each cluster center represented a visual word (analogous to vocabulary), thereby producing a codebook (analogous to a dictionary) [33]. The codebook was then used to obtain the BoF for each ECG spectrogram image. Then, image key points were extracted, and image descriptors were obtained. Here, each descriptor corresponded to the closest visual word, and visual word occurrences in an image were counted to produce a histogram representing the image. Figure 4 shows how these feature vectors were then directly input to machine-learning classifiers for SA classification.

Figures 5 and 6 show the key points automatically extracted by the BoF in the ECG spectrogram algorithm for normal breathing and SA, respectively. Each green circle represents a key point able to best discriminate breathing patterns for each ECG spectrogram. Key points were similar for normal breathing but varied significantly for SA spectrograms.

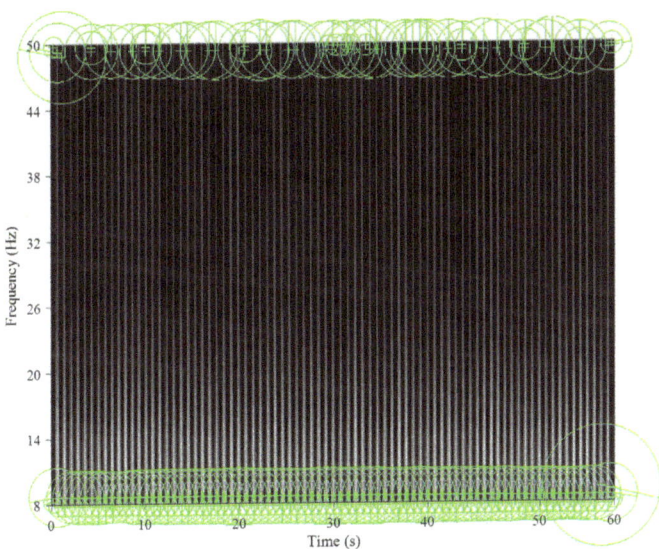

Figure 5. Key points extracted from an ECG spectrogram of normal breathing for a 60 s window and 8–50 Hz band.

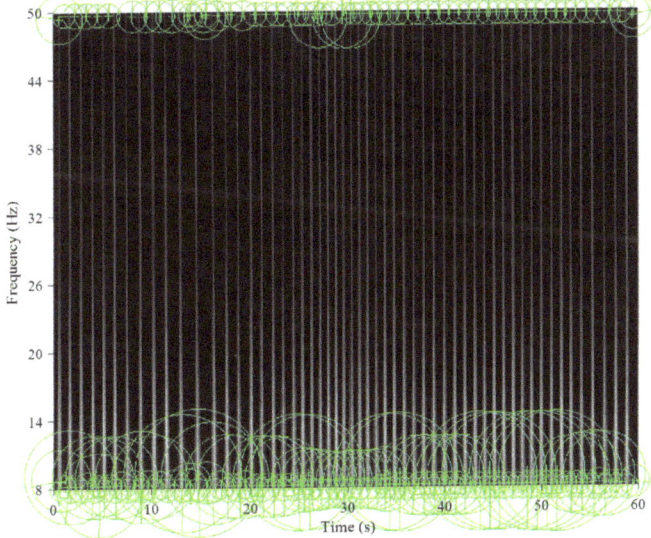

Figure 6. Key points extracted from the sleep apnea ECG spectrogram for a 60 s window and 8–50 Hz band.

2.6. Machine-Learning classifiers

Support vector machine (SVM) is a supervised learning model for classification and regression. The core concept of SVM is to find the hyperplane that best separates data into two classes. In binary classification, generally, p-dimensional data can be separated by a (p-1)-dimensional hyperplane. The best hyperplane is defined as that with the largest margin between the two classes, and the closest point on the hyperplane boundary is considered the support vector [35].

The k-nearest neighbor (KNN) classifier is a simple supervised learning method and uses the nearest distance approach in deciding the group of the new data in the training set. During the training phase, the feature space is split into several regions and the training data are mapped into the similar groups of feature space. The unlabeled testing data are then classified into a certain group of feature space based on the minimum distance. Distance is an important factor for the model and can be determined, e.g., by Euclidean, Mahalanobis, and cosine-distance metrics [36,37].

Ensemble learning (EL) combines multiple learning algorithms and weight sets to construct a better classifier model. Prediction using an ensemble algorithm requires extensive computation compared to using only a single model. Therefore, ensembles can compensate for poor learning algorithms by performing extra computations. EL methods generally use fast algorithms, although slower algorithms can also benefit from ensemble techniques. Many different ensemble models have been proposed, including the Bayes optimal classifier and boosting and bootstrap aggregating (bagging) techniques [38]. EL bagged trees and subspace KNN were employed in this study. The bagged trees method established a set of decision tree models trained on randomly selected portion of data; then, the predictions are merged to achieve final predictions using averaging [38]. Meanwhile, subspace KNN was designed using majority vote rule, where the random subspace ensemble method was used with nearest neighbor learner type of 30 learners [39,40].

2.7. k-Fold Cross-Validation

k-fold cross-validation is a well-developed validation technique [41]. The first step is to divide the data samples into k subgroups. Subsequently, each subgroup can be selected as the testing set with the remaining (k-1) subgroups as the training set. In this way, k-fold cross-validation repeats training and testing k times, and the final accuracy is the average of the k accuracy values for each iteration. In this study, the k-fold cross-validation with k = 5 was performed at the spectrogram-level instead of the participant-level, as some studies have done [16,42–44]. As evaluation criteria, the accuracy, sensitivity, and specificity parameters were computed for classification performance metrics. The definitions of these metrics can be found in Table 2 [45].

Table 2. Confusion matrix and evaluation parameter equations.

Confusion Matrix		Actual Class			
		A	B	Accuracy = $\frac{TP+TN}{P+N}$	Specificity = $\frac{TN}{TN+FP}$
Predicted Class	A	TP	FP		
	B	FN	TN	Sensitivity = $\frac{TP}{TP+FN}$	
Total		P	N		

Note: A = condition positive set; B = condition negative set; TP = true positive; FP = false positive; FN = false negative; TN = true negative; P = TP + FN; N = FP + TN.

3. Experimental Results

The experiments were executed using MATLAB R2020a software on several computers with 24 GB installed RAM, Intel® Core™ i5-8400 CPU @2.80 GHz, and NVIDIA GeForce GTX 1060 6 GB mounted graphic card. The Classification Learner toolbox from MATLAB was utilized to perform the machine-learning classification. Hyperparameter optimization was performed using nested five-fold cross-validation and grid search using a 60 s time window based on the best frequency range, 8~50 Hz, and machine-learning model construction, SVM (see Table 3). Tables 4 and 5 compare the selected APEGs from NCKUHSCAD and PAED for the frequency bands (overall frequency, 0.1–50 Hz; high frequency, 8–50 Hz; middle frequency, 0.8–10 Hz; and low frequency, 0–0.8 Hz) along with SVM, KNN, and EL classifiers using a time-window length of 60 s and five-fold validation. The best classification accuracy for NCKUHSCAD-APEG-A, NCKUSCAD-APEG-B, and NCKUHSCAD-APEG-C was 84.4%, 80.8%, and 83.8% at 8–50 Hz, 8–50 Hz, and 8–50 Hz, respectively, using SVM, EL, and SVM. Conversely, the best classification accuracy for PAED-APEG-A, PAED-APEG-B, and PAED-APEG-C was 88.2%, 88.3%, and 91.4% at 8–50, 8–50, and 8–50 Hz using SVM, EL, and EL, respectively. The PAED-APEG-C classification accuracy for the 0.8–10 Hz band using EL was 89.1%, which was only 2.3% less than the best accuracy (91.4%). Hence, we selected the 8–50 Hz band and EL classifier to classify all SA episodes in the remaining work.

Table 3. Nested five-fold cross-validation training and validation performance using a 60 s time window based on 8~50 Hz frequency range and SVM classifier of PAED and NCKUHSCAD.

Database	Accuracy (%)			Sensitivity (%)			Specificity (%)		
	APEG-A	APEG-B	APEG-C	APEG-A	APEG-B	APEG-C	APEG-A	APEG-B	APEG-C
PAED	87.35	88.06	90.43	89.70	90.40	88.72	85.01	85.32	91.55
NCKUHSCAD	83.40	80.15	83.54	56.78	63.48	57.17	92.14	87.82	92.16

Table 4. Five-fold cross-validation classification performance using a 60 s time window for NCKUHSCAD.

Frequency Band	Accuracy (%)			Sensitivity (%)			Specificity (%)		
	APEG-A	APEG-B	APEG-C	APEG-A	APEG-B	APEG-C	APEG-A	APEG-B	APEG-C
				SVM					
0.1–50 Hz	81.6	77.7	81	50.2	45.4	32.4	91.9	92.5	96.9
8–50 Hz	84.4 #	80.5	83.8 #	57.3	60.6	51.6	93.3	89.6	94.3
0.8–10 Hz	83.3	79.6	82.6	53.8	56.6	42.9	93	90.1	95.5
0–0.8 Hz	79.9	70.9	76.8	18.9	22	6	100	93.4	100
				KNN					
0.1–50 Hz	81	77.8	81.6	49.6	57	47.1	91.3	87.3	92.8
8–50 Hz	83.6	79.3	82.6	56.7	62.5	54.6	92.4	87.1	91.7
0.8–10 Hz	82.7	78	81.3	52.4	53.7	44.6	92.6	89.1	93.4
0–0.8 Hz	78.8	69.9	76.3	29.6	11.4	9	95	96.8	98.2
				EL					
0.1–50 Hz	82.2	78.4	82.5	60.2	61.1	52.2	89.4	86.3	92.4
8–50 Hz	84	80.8 #	83.7	63.7	70.6	65.3	90.6	85.5	89.7
0.8–10 Hz	82.5	78.6	82	60.5	60.8	48.8	89.7	86.8	92.9
0–0.8 Hz	78.8	70.8	76.6	41.1	36.5	20.5	91.2	86.6	95

Note: # denotes the highest accuracy in APEG-A/APEG-B/APEG-C.

SA detection in a short time window was an important consideration for this study. Therefore, we also investigated a shorter window length (10 s). For example, eleven subjects from NCKUHSCAD-APEG-A were selected, and different frequency bands were compared via five-fold cross-validation. The time window length was too short to provide variation in the lower frequency band; hence, that band was not considered in this comparison. Table 6 shows that the 10 s time window provided greater accuracy than the 60 s time window, with the best accuracy reaching 95% for the 8–50 Hz band using SVM.

Table 5. Five-fold cross-validation classification performance using a 60 s time window for PAED.

Frequency Band	Accuracy (%)			Sensitivity (%)			Specificity (%)		
	APEG-A	APEG-B	APEG-C	APEG-A	APEG-B	APEG-C	APEG-A	APEG-B	APEG-C
SVM									
0.1–50 Hz	77.2	82.8	86.5	78.8	81.3	79.1	75.5	84.5	91.3
8–50 Hz	88.2 #	88.3	90.9	90.1	90.7	89.1	86.3	85.6	92.1
0.8–10 Hz	88.2	87.8	90.1	89.8	90.9	87.2	86.7	84.2	92.1
0–0.8 Hz	65.7	68.0	71.4	63.5	73.4	52.4	68.0	61.7	83.8
KNN									
0.1–50 Hz	75.2	81.5	84.9	66.8	77.2	72.2	83.5	86.4	93.3
8–50 Hz	86.1	86.5	89.5	82.3	85.4	82.6	90.0	87.7	94.0
0.8–10 Hz	88.0	86.1	88.5	84.3	83.6	79.7	91.8	89.1	94.3
0–0.8 Hz	59.3	62.5	66.0	52.1	62.1	35.0	66.5	62.9	86.5
EL									
0.1–50 Hz	75.7	81.8	85.6	71.1	81.9	78.0	80.2	81.8	90.7
8–50 Hz	86.9	88.3 #	91.4 #	88.9	90.7	89.8	84.8	85.5	92.4
0.8–10 Hz	87.2	86.5	89.1	87.8	88.6	85.5	86.5	84.0	91.4
0–0.8 Hz	65.2	69.5	69.5	64.7	45.9	45.9	65.8	85.1	85.1

Note: # denotes the highest accuracy in APEG-A/APEG-B/APEG-C.

Table 6. Five-fold cross-validation classification performance using a 10 s time window for NCKUHSCAD.

Frequency Band	Accuracy (%)			Sensitivity (%)			Specificity (%)		
	APEG-A	APEG-B	APEG-C	APEG-A	APEG-B	APEG-C	APEG-A	APEG-B	APEG-C
SVM									
0.1–50 Hz	92.7	93.2	93.9	79.4	80.4	77.4	97	97.4	97.5
8–50 Hz	95 #	93.3 #	94.9 #	84.3	79.2	77.7	98.5	97.8	98.6
0.8–10 Hz	80.1	81.5	85.9	38	40.3	37.3	93.8	94.8	96.5
KNN									
0.1–50 Hz	81.7	84.2	87.3	45.8	53.5	45.5	93.4	94	96.5
8–50 Hz	87.1	85.1	88.2	59.2	52.4	47.3	96.3	95.6	97.1
0.8–10 Hz	76.8	79	84.2	10.8	36	28.8	98.3	92.9	96.2
EL									
0.1–50 Hz	91.3	91.9	92.8	70.5	73.3	64.1	98	97.9	99
8–50 Hz	94	91.8	93.3	79.6	78.4	66.8	98.7	96.1	99.1
0.8–10 Hz	79.3	80.8	85.3	29.6	35.3	29.1	95.5	95.4	97.5

Note: # denotes the highest accuracy in APEG-A/APEG-B/APEG-C.

4. Discussion

To the best of our knowledge, our study is the first to use an ECG spectrogram for SA detection. This proposed algorithm used high-temporal resolution feature visualization of the ECG spectrogram in differentiating normal and SA breathing. Using this high-temporal resolution pattern visualization, the proposed algorithm was able to achieve high accuracy, sensitivity, and specificity in SA detection.

4.1. ECG Variation during Rapid Eye Movement (REM) and Non-REM Sleep Stages

Sleep is a dynamic situation of consciousness characterized by rapid changes in autonomic activity that regulates coronary artery tone, systemic blood pressure, and heart rate. In the analysis of 24-hour heart rate variability (HRV), a nocturnal increase in the standard deviation of mean RR intervals commonly occurrs. In the study by Zemaityte et al. [46] and Raetz et al. [47], they observed that, when compared to the wakefulness stage, non-REM sleep stage was associated with lower overall HRV and during REM sleep stage, the opposite phenomenon was observed, an increase in overall HRV. Otherwise, some studies examined the highest nocturnal activity during REM sleep due to the peripheral sympathetic nerve activity with no difference in heart rates between the sleep stages [48–50].

In this study, by investigating the REM and non-REM partitions on the SA classification using PAED 60 s time window based on the best frequency range (8~50 Hz) and machine-learning model (SVM), it was concluded that the ECG variation (HRV) did not significantly affect the SA classification performance. Both REM and non-REM partitions of imbalanced and balanced datasets generated for PAED-APEG-A, PAED-APEG-B, and PAED-APEG-C groups presented a good classification performance with the average accuracy was up to 81.42% for REM stage and 79.2% for non-REM stage (see Table 7). The balancing data were randomly performed in order to address more imbalanced apnea and normal events as a consequence of partitioning the datasets into REM and non-REM.

Table 7. The REM and Non-REM classification performance using a PAED 60 s time window based on 8~50 Hz frequency range and SVM classifier.

Sleep Stage	Accuracy (%)			Sensitivity (%)			Specificity (%)		
	APEG-A	APEG-B	APEG-C	APEG-A	APEG-B	APEG-C	APEG-A	APEG-B	APEG-C
	Imbalanced Dataset								
REM	83.1	78.7	75	90.5	78.5	84.7	61.3	78.8	59.1
Non-REM	74.8	81.4	77.8	72.3	81.6	78.7	77.1	81.1	77
	Balanced Dataset								
REM	89.6	78.7	83.4	90	78.5	85.3	89.2	78.8	81.5
Non-REM	75.5	86.6	79.1	74.5	86.8	80.8	76.4	86.4	77.5

4.2. Per Subject Classification (Leave-One-Subject-Out Cross-Validation)

A more realistic scenario to the medical application, which is required to classify a new unseen subject into the model, is the so-called per-subject classification. Leave-one-subject-out cross-validation (LOSOCV) was used in this study to perform the per-subject classification. In LOSOCV, one subject is set aside for the evaluation (testing) and the model is trained on remaining subjects. The process is repeated each time with a different subject for evaluation and results are averaged over all folds (subjects).

Results from k-fold cross-validation PAED 60 s time window based on 8~50 Hz frequency range and SVM classifier experimental setting demonstrates that the model almost certainly can detect subjects with disease if training and testing sets are not separated in terms of subjects, leaving data related to a subject in both sets. As the result shows, it can achieve a high level of accuracy (89.13%). With all other experimental settings remaining the same, except PAED-APEG-C group as some subjects in the Group C were excluded since they did not experience anapnea event, when the LOSOCV was applied the accuracy decreased significantly to 70% (Tables 8–10). This probably means that in the case of k-fold cross-validation where subject data are in both training and testing sets, the algorithm is learning the subject rather than the disease condition.

Table 8. Leave-one-subject-out cross-validation classification performance using a PAED-APEG-A 60 s time window based on 8~50 Hz frequency range and SVM classifier.

Evaluation Parameter	APEG-A Subject								Average
	a03	a05	a08	a13	a16	a17	a19	a20	
Accuracy	75.0	54.3	76.5	85.2	73.3	67.2	80.2	52.1	70.48
Sensitivity	98.6	70.1	57.8	77.4	68.4	95.7	66.5	26.4	70.11
Specificity	54.7	32.4	88.4	92.7	83.1	49.5	88.8	93.0	72.83

Table 9. Leave-one-subject-out cross-validation classification performance using a PAED-APEG-B 60 s time window based on 8~50 Hz frequency range and SVM classifier.

Evaluation Parameter	APEG-B Subject												
	a01	a02	a03	a04	a05	a06	a07	a08	a09	a10	a11	a12	a13
Accuracy	92.35	20.83	84.17	58.54	81.90	65.42	72.71	75.83	83.75	77.08	65.95	52.08	81.46
Sensitivity	100	0.26	93.24	56.69	91.80	28.96	85.37	59.36	86.89	87.95	32.97	52.85	65.11
Specificity	21.05	100	76.36	79.49	68.18	87.88	52.69	86.35	73.68	74.81	91.18	43.90	97.14

Evaluation Parameter	APEG-B Subject											Average
	a14	a15	a16	a17	a18	a19	a20	b01	b02	b03	b04	
Accuracy	81.88	75	76.04	78.06	84.38	84.79	73.13	90.63	47.92	63.57	28.81	70.68
Sensitivity	99.74	80.62	72.50	93.48	89.04	68.11	65.08	10.53	88.17	84.62	90.0	70.14
Specificity	11.34	58.87	83.13	68.47	45.10	95.25	85.95	93.93	38.24	59.72	27.32	67.50

Table 10. Leave-one-subject-out cross-validation classification performance using a PAED-APEG-C 60 s time window based on 8~50 Hz frequency range and SVM classifier.

Evaluation Parameter	APEG-C Subject												
	a01	a02	a03	a04	a05	a06	a07	a08	a09	a10	a11	a12	a13
Accuracy	89.80	21.46	83.96	69.17	76.90	64.58	70.83	78.54	79.58	76.25	57.38	44.79	81.25
Sensitivity	94.92	1.0	77.48	67.80	77.05	16.39	85.71	61.50	78.69	79.52	2.75	43.96	65.96
Specificity	42.11	100	89.53	84.62	76.70	94.28	47.31	89.42	82.46	75.57	99.16	53.66	95.92

Evaluation Parameter	APEG-C Subject												
	a14	a15	a16	a17	a18	a19	a20	b01	b02	b03	b04	c02	c06
Accuracy	81.46	73.96	73.33	78.61	88.75	78.96	56.25	93.96	63.54	72.38	41.67	98.54	91.90
Sensitivity	98.43	78.93	70.31	65.94	92.31	57.84	38.98	0	74.19	70.77	50.0	0	0
Specificity	14.43	59.68	79.38	86.49	58.82	92.20	83.78	97.83	60.98	72.68	41.46	98.75	92.12

Evaluation Parameter	APEG-C Subject			Average
	c07	c09	c10	
Accuracy	95.48	90.71	47.86	73.17
Sensitivity	25.0	0	0	50.88
Specificity	96.15	91.15	47.97	76.02

4.3. Performance Comparison with the Existing Literature

Table 11 compares the proposed algorithm with various current best-practice algorithms from the literature using PAED. Quinceno-Manrique et al. [16], Nguyen et al. [17], Sannino et al. [18], and Hassan [29] used HRV-extracted features in the time domain and frequency domain along with non-linear methods, such as features from spectral centroids, spectral centroid energy, recurrence statistics, and wavelet transform, while Varon et al. [12] used EDR as the feature (84.74% accuracy, 84.71% sensitivity, and 84.69% specificity). Singh et al. [20] proposed a CNN-based deep learning approach using the time–frequency scalogram transformation of an ECG signal (86.22% accuracy, 90% sensitivity, and 83.8% specificity). Surrel et al. [30] used RR intervals and RS amplitude series (85.70% accuracy, 81.40% sensitivity, and 88.40% specificity). The proposed method achieved significantly better performance in accuracy, sensitivity, and specificity compared to all other considered methods for 1 min time windows and also achieved comparable accuracy to the compared methods (90.5%) for the 10 s time windows, indicating that the proposed method offers higher temporal resolution.

Quinceno-Manrique et al. (89.02% accuracy) [16], Nguyen et al. (85.26% accuracy, 86.37% sensitivity, and 83.47% specificity) [17], Sannino et al. (85.76% accuracy, 65.82% sensitivity, and 66.03% specificity) [18], Hassan (87.33% accuracy, 81.99% sensitivity, and 90.72% specificity) [29], and Surrel et al. [30] used HRV features to analyze ECG signals, which had two major disadvantages. First, the HRV frequency band was low, meaning that the time windows had to be extended to ensure that signal variation was properly expressed (e.g., Quinceno-Manrique et al. used 3 min time windows, and HRV features required 5 min windows [16]). OSA onsets and offsets could occur several times within windows of these lengths, significantly limiting the practical applications of these approaches. Second, HRV features use simplified information from the original ECG (QRS complexes), so considerable physiological information, such as ECG signal morphology, could be lost. The same situation occurs for EDR [12], as EDR was derived from the R-wave amplitude, which also used simplified ECG information. Conversely, the proposed algorithm directly used ECG spectrograms to classify SA and normal breathing. Hence, the main advantage of the proposed method is the identification of significant variations in the occurrence of apnea episodes.

Similar to the proposed method, Singh et al. [20] also employed time–frequency transformation using CWT to obtain the scalogram of an ECG signal. The deep learning layers of CNN-pre-trained AlexNet were used for feature extraction. At the final layer, the decision fusion of some machine-learning approaches (SVM, KNN, EL, and Linear Discriminant Analysis (LDA)) was utilized for classification. However, the main difference and advantage of this study algorithm is the application of a more sophisticated time–frequency transformation using the Morlet wavelet in order to observe significant variations between several frequency ranges and obtain high temporal resolution. Moreover, the use of bag-of-features in the proposed method enables robust features called SURFs to be generated and outperformed the Singh et al. study performance with 91.4% accuracy and 92.4% specificity.

Table 11. Proposed algorithm comparison with current best-practice algorithms.

Author (Year)	Database (Population)	Time-Window Length	Method	Accuracy (%)	Sensitivity (%)	Specificity (%)
Lin et al. (this paper)	Physionet Apnea-ECG (APEG-A: 3660 min, APEG-B: 11,160 min, APEG-C *: 15,180 min)	1 min	CWT + SVM/KNN/EL	91.4	89.8	92.4
Quinceno-Manrique et al. [16] (2009)	Physionet Apnea-ECG (all observations: 8928 intervals, best observations: 4000 intervals)	3 min	SPWVD + PCA + KNN	89.02	Not mentioned	Not mentioned
Nguyen et al. [17] (2014)	Physionet Apnea-ECG (whole database: Group A, B, and C)	1 min	RQA + greedy forward feature selection + SVM and neural network	85.26	86.37	83.47
Sannino et al. [18] (2014)	Physionet Apnea-ECG (whole database: Group A, B, and C)	1 min	Frequency domain, time domain, and non-linear parameters + DEREx	85.76	65.82	66.03
Varon et al. [12] (2015)	Physionet Apnea-ECG (34,324 annotated min)	1 min	EDR (Ramp/PCA/kPCA) + LS-SVM	84.74	84.71	84.69
Hassan [29] (2016)	Physionet Apnea-ECG (whole database: Group A, B, and C)	1 min	TQWT + NIG + AdaBoost	87.33	81.99	90.72
Surrel et al. [30] (2018)	Physionet Apnea-ECG (34,313 recorded min)	1 min	Apnea scoring (energy) + SVM	85.70	81.40	88.40
Singh et al. [20] (2019)	Physionet Apnea-ECG (whole database: Group A, B, and C)	1 min	CWT + AlexNet CNN + Decision Fusion (SVM, KNN, Ensemble, LDA)	86.22	90	83.8

Note: CWT: continuous wavelet transform; SVM: support vector machine; KNN: k-nearest neighbor; EL: ensemble learning; TQWT: tunable-Q factor wavelet transform; NIG: normal inverse gaussian; AdaBoost: adaptive boosting; SPWVD: smoothed pseudo Wigner-Ville distribution; PCA: principal component analysis; RQA: Recurrence Quantification Analysis; DEREx: Differential Evolution-based Rule Extractor; EDR: ECG derived respiration; Ramp: R-peak amplitude; kPCA: kernel principal component analysis; LS-SVM: least-squares support vector machine. * The APEG-C classification result was chosen because this dataset was comparable with the existing literature, consisting of the whole PhysioNet database (Groups A, B, and C).

4.4. Limitations and Future Developments

Although the proposed algorithm exhibited excellent performance, there were several limitations in this study. First, a limited sample size from PAED was used to validate the proposed algorithm. Second, in PAED, insufficient physiological data and subject disease history was available for further analysis since such information was not provided. Mass data collection from the Sleep Center NCKUH could be a solution for these drawbacks. Third, the proposed algorithm could not be applied to patients with cardiovascular disease complications since their ECG spectrograms tended to be somewhat irregular and not affected only by SA.

Future works could identify physiological meanings for the OSA features automatically extracted from the AI algorithm, test a large-scale group of participants from the sleep center database, and develop an algorithm to discriminate SA and cardiovascular disease using ECG data.

5. Conclusions

This paper proposed a new algorithm to classify SA patterns from ECG spectrograms. Four different frequency bands were considered along with three classifiers. High accuracy was obtained when applying time–frequency spectrograms to SA, and the features extracted by visual classification revealed previously unknown physiological significance, such that SA detection was feasible.

The algorithm provided superior accuracy compared to current common-practice approaches over generally shorter time windows (60 s) compared to those used in earlier models. Acceptable accuracy was also derived for very short time windows (10 s), highlighting the considerable flexibility in potential applications for this algorithm.

Author Contributions: Conceptualization, C.-Y.L. and C.-W.L.; methodology, C.-Y.L., C.-W.L., Y.-W.W. and F.S.; software, Y.-W.W., F.S. and N.T.H.T.; validation, Y.-W.W., F.S. and N.T.H.T.; investigation, C.-Y.L., C.-W.L., Y.-W.W. and F.S.; resources, C.-W.L.; writing—original draft preparation, Y.-W.W. and F.S.; writing—review and editing, C.-Y.L. and C.-W.L.; supervision, C.-Y.L. and C.-W.L. All authors have read and agreed to the published version of the manuscript.

Funding: This research was funded by grants from National Cheng Kung University Hospital (grant number NCKUH-10802018, NCKUH-10904006).

Institutional Review Board Statement: The study protocol was approved by the Institutional Review Board of NCKUH (protocol number: B-ER-108-426).

Informed Consent Statement: Not applicable.

Data Availability Statement: The Physionet Apnea-ECG Database (PAED) is openly available at Physionet at https://doi.org/10.13026/C23W2R (accessed on 15 October 2021). However, the National Cheng Kung University Hospital Sleep Center Apnea Database (NCKUHSCAD) is not publicly available due to privacy and ethical issues.

Acknowledgments: The authors thank Wen-Kuei Lin, Li-Zhen Lin, Yen-Su Lin, Fu-Hsin Liao, Shin-Ru Hou, and Yi-Chun Lin (the staff of the sleep medicine center at National Cheng Kung University Hospital).

Conflicts of Interest: The authors declare no conflict of interest.

References

1. Senaratna, C.V.; Perret, J.L.; Lodge, C.J.; Lowe, A.J.; Campbell, B.E.; Matheson, M.C.; Hamilton, G.S.; Dharmage, S.C. Prevalence of obstructive sleep apnea in the general population: A systematic review. *Sleep Med. Rev.* **2017**, *34*, 70–81. [CrossRef]
2. American Academy of Sleep Medicine. Hidden health crisis costing America billions. In *Underdiagnosing and Undertreating Obstructive Sleep Apnea Draining Healthcare System*; Frost & Sullivan: Mountain View, CA, USA, 2016.
3. Facco, F.L.; Lopata, V.; Wolsk, J.M.; Patel, S.; Wisniewski, S.R. Can We Use Home Sleep Testing for the Evaluation of Sleep Apnea in Obese Pregnant Women? *Sleep Disord.* **2019**, *2019*, 3827579. [CrossRef] [PubMed]

4. Dalewski, B.; Kamińska, A.; Syrico, A.; Kałdunska, A.; Pałka, Ł.; Sobolewska, E. The Usefulness of Modified Mallampati Score and CT Upper Airway Volume Measurements in Diagnosing OSA among Patients with Breathing-Related Sleep Disorders. *Appl. Sci.* **2021**, *11*, 3764. [CrossRef]
5. Philip, P.; Bailly, S.; Benmerad, M.; Micoulaud-Franchi, J.; Grillet, Y.; Sapène, M.; Jullian-Desayes, I.; Joyeux-Faure, M.; Tamisier, R.; Pépin, J. Self-reported sleepiness and not the apnoea hypopnoea index is the best predictor of sleepiness-related accidents in obstructive sleep apnoea. *Sci. Rep.* **2020**, *10*, 16267. [CrossRef]
6. Kukwa, W.; Migacz, E.; Lis, T.; Ishman, S.L. The effect of in-lab polysomnography and home sleep polygraphy on sleep position. *Sleep Breath. Schlaf Atm.* **2021**, *25*, 251. [CrossRef]
7. Young, T.; Palta, M.; Dempsey, J.; Skatrud, J.; Weber, S.; Badr, S. The occurrence of sleep-disordered breathing among middle-aged adults. *N. Eng. J. Med.* **1993**, *328*, 1230–1235. [CrossRef]
8. Guilleminault, C.; Poyares, D.; Rosa, A.; Huang, Y.-S. Heart rate variability, sympathetic and vagal balance and EEG arousals in upper airway resistance and mild obstructive sleep apnea syndromes. *Sleep Med.* **2005**, *6*, 451–457. [CrossRef]
9. Babaeizadeh, S.; Zhou, S.H.; Pittman, S.D.; White, D.P. Electrocardiogram-derived respiration in screening of sleep-disordered breathing. *J. Electrocardiol.* **2011**, *44*, 700–706. [CrossRef]
10. Berntson, G.G.; Thomas Bigger, J., Jr.; Eckberg, D.L.; Grossman, P.; Kaufmann, P.G.; Malik, M.; Nagaraja, H.N.; Porges, S.W.; Saul, J.P.; Stone, P.H. Heart rate variability: Origins, methods, and interpretive caveats. *Psychophysiology* **1997**, *34*, 623–648. [CrossRef]
11. Langley, P.; Bowers, E.J.; Murray, A. Principal component analysis as a tool for analyzing beat-to-beat changes in ECG features: Application to ECG-derived respiration. *IEEE Trans. Biomed. Eng.* **2009**, *57*, 821–829. [CrossRef]
12. Varon, C.; Caicedo, A.; Testelmans, D.; Buyse, B.; Van Huffel, S. A novel algorithm for the automatic detection of sleep apnea from single-lead ECG. *IEEE Trans. Biomed. Eng.* **2015**, *62*, 2269–2278. [CrossRef]
13. Hwang, S.H.; Lee, Y.J.; Jeong, D.-U.; Park, K.S. Apnea–hypopnea index prediction using electrocardiogram acquired during the sleep-onset period. *IEEE Trans. Biomed. Eng.* **2016**, *64*, 295–301.
14. Van Steenkiste, T.; Groenendaal, W.; Deschrijver, D.; Dhaene, T. Automated sleep apnea detection in raw respiratory signals using long short-term memory neural networks. *IEEE J. Biomed. Health Inform.* **2018**, *23*, 2354–2364. [CrossRef]
15. Penzel, T.; Kantelhardt, J.W.; Grote, L.; Peter, J.-H.; Bunde, A. Comparison of detrended fluctuation analysis and spectral analysis for heart rate variability in sleep and sleep apnea. *IEEE Trans. Biomed. Eng.* **2003**, *50*, 1143–1151. [CrossRef]
16. Quiceno-Manrique, A.; Alonso-Hernandez, J.; Travieso-Gonzalez, C.; Ferrer-Ballester, M.; Castellanos-Dominguez, G. Detection of obstructive sleep apnea in ECG recordings using time-frequency distributions and dynamic features. In Proceedings of the 2009 Annual International Conference of the IEEE Engineering in Medicine and Biology Society, Minneapolis, MN, USA, 3–6 September 2009; IEEE: Manhattan, NY, USA, 2009; pp. 5559–5562.
17. Nguyen, H.D.; Wilkins, B.A.; Cheng, Q.; Benjamin, B.A. An online sleep apnea detection method based on recurrence quantification analysis. *IEEE J. Biomed. Health Inform.* **2013**, *18*, 1285–1293. [CrossRef]
18. Sannino, G.; De Falco, I.; De Pietro, G. Monitoring obstructive sleep apnea by means of a real-time mobile system based on the automatic extraction of sets of rules through differential evolution. *J. Biomed. Inform.* **2014**, *49*, 84–100. [CrossRef]
19. Martín-González, S.; Navarro-Mesa, J.L.; Juliá-Serdá, G.; Kraemer, J.F.; Wessel, N.; Ravelo-García, A.G. Heart rate variability feature selection in the presence of sleep apnea: An expert system for the characterization and detection of the disorder. *Comput. Biol. Med.* **2017**, *91*, 47–58. [CrossRef]
20. Singh, S.A.; Majumder, S. A novel approach osa detection using single-lead ECG scalogram based on deep neural network. *J. Mech. Med. Biol.* **2019**, *19*, 1950026. [CrossRef]
21. Thomas, R.J.; Mietus, J.E.; Peng, C.-K.; Goldberger, A.L. An electrocardiogram-based technique to assess cardiopulmonary coupling during sleep. *Sleep* **2005**, *28*, 1151–1161. [CrossRef] [PubMed]
22. Guo, D.; Peng, C.-K.; Wu, H.-L.; Mietus, J.E.; Liu, Y.; Sun, R.-S.; Thomas, R.J. ECG-derived cardiopulmonary analysis of pediatric sleep-disordered breathing. *Sleep Med.* **2011**, *12*, 384–389. [CrossRef]
23. Liu, D.; Yang, X.; Wang, G.; Ma, J.; Liu, Y.; Peng, C.-K.; Zhang, J.; Fang, J. HHT based cardiopulmonary coupling analysis for sleep apnea detection. *Sleep Med.* **2012**, *13*, 503–509. [CrossRef]
24. Penzel, T.; McNames, J.; De Chazal, P.; Raymond, B.; Murray, A.; Moody, G. Systematic comparison of different algorithms for apnoea detection based on electrocardiogram recordings. *Med. Biol. Eng. Comput.* **2002**, *40*, 402–407. [CrossRef] [PubMed]
25. Goldberger, A.L.; Amaral, L.A.N.; Glass, L.; Hausdorff, J.M.; Ivanov, P.C.; Mark, R.G.; Mietus, J.E.; Moody, G.B.; Peng, C.-K.; Stanley, H.E. PhysioBank, PhysioToolkit, and PhysioNet: Components of a New Research Resource for Complex Physiologic Signals. *Circulation* **2003**, *101*, e215–e220. [CrossRef]
26. American Academy of Sleep Medicine (AASM). AASM Clarifies Hypopnea Scoring Criteria. 2013. Available online: https://aasm.org/aasm-clarifies-hypopnea-scoring-criteria/ (accessed on 2 December 2021).
27. Ruehland, W.R.; Rochford, P.D.; O'Donoghue, F.J.; Pierce, R.J.; Singh, P.; Thornton, A.T. The new AASM criteria for scoring hypopneas: Impact on the apnea hypopnea index. *Sleep* **2009**, *32*, 150–157. [CrossRef]
28. Penzel, T.; Moody, G.B.; Mark, R.G.; Goldberger, A.L.; Peter, J.H. The apnea-ECG database. In Proceedings of the Computers in Cardiology 2000. Vol. 27 (Cat. 00CH37163), Cambridge, MA, USA, 24–27 September 2000; IEEE: Manhattan, NY, USA, 2000; pp. 255–258.
29. Hassan, A.R. Computer-aided obstructive sleep apnea detection using normal inverse Gaussian parameters and adaptive boosting. *Biomed. Signal Process. Control* **2016**, *29*, 22–30. [CrossRef]

30. Surrel, G.; Aminifar, A.; Rincón, F.; Murali, S.; Atienza, D. Online obstructive sleep apnea detection on medical wearable sensors. *IEEE Trans. Biomed. Circuits Syst.* **2018**, *12*, 762–773. [CrossRef] [PubMed]
31. Rioul, O.; Duhamel, P. Fast algorithms for discrete and continuous wavelet transforms. *IEEE Trans. Inf. Theory* **1992**, *38*, 569–586. [CrossRef]
32. Thomas, R.J.; Mietus, J.E.; Peng, C.-K.; Gilmartin, G.; Daly, R.W.; Goldberger, A.L.; Gottlieb, D.J. Differentiating obstructive from central and complex sleep apnea using an automated electrocardiogram-based method. *Sleep* **2007**, *30*, 1756–1769. [CrossRef]
33. Csurka, G.; Dance, C.; Fan, L.; Willamowski, J.; Bray, C. Visual categorization with bags of keypoints. In Proceedings of the Workshop on Statistical Learning in Computer Vision, ECCV, Prague, Czech Republic, 11–14 May 2004; pp. 1–2.
34. Bay, H.; Ess, A.; Tuytelaars, T.; Van Gool, L. Speeded-up robust features (SURF). *Comput. Vis. Image Underst.* **2008**, *110*, 346–359. [CrossRef]
35. Hearst, M.A.; Dumais, S.T.; Osuna, E.; Platt, J.; Scholkopf, B. Support vector machines. *IEEE Intell. Syst. Appl.* **1998**, *13*, 18–28. [CrossRef]
36. Peterson, L.E. K-nearest neighbor. *Scholarpedia* **2009**, *4*, 1883. [CrossRef]
37. Dasarathy, B.V. *Nearest Neighbor (NN) Norms: NN Pattern Classification Technique*; IEEE Computer Society Tutorial: Ann Arbor, MI, USA, 1991.
38. Dietterich, T.G. Ensemble methods in machine learning. In *Proceedings of the International Workshop on Multiple Classifier Systems*; Springer: Berlin/Heidelberg, Germany, 2000; pp. 1–15.
39. Gul, A.; Perperoglou, A.; Khan, Z.; Mahmoud, O.; Miftahuddin, M.; Adler, W.; Lausen, B. Ensemble of a subset of k NN classifiers. *Adv. Data Anal. Classif.* **2018**, *12*, 827–840. [CrossRef]
40. Ho, T.K. The random subspace method for constructing decision forests. *IEEE Trans. Pattern Anal. Mach. Intell.* **1998**, *20*, 832–844.
41. Bengio, Y.; Grandvalet, Y. No unbiased estimator of the variance of k-fold cross-validation. *J. Mach. Learn. Res.* **2004**, *5*, 1089–1105.
42. Sadek, I.; Heng, T.T.S.; Seet, E.; Abdulrazak, B. A new approach for detecting sleep apnea using a contactless bed sensor: Comparison study. *J. Med. Internet Res.* **2020**, *22*, e18297. [CrossRef] [PubMed]
43. Singh, H.; Tripathy, R.K.; Pachori, R.B. Detection of sleep apnea from heart beat interval and ECG derived respiration signals using sliding mode singular spectrum analysis. *Digit. Signal Process.* **2020**, *104*, 102796. [CrossRef]
44. Niroshana, S.I.; Zhu, X.; Nakamura, K.; Chen, W. A fused-image-based approach to detect obstructive sleep apnea using a single-lead ECG and a 2D convolutional neural network. *PLoS ONE* **2021**, *16*, e0250618. [CrossRef] [PubMed]
45. Fawcett, T. An introduction to ROC analysis. *Pattern Recognit. Lett.* **2006**, *27*, 861–874. [CrossRef]
46. Žemaitytė, D.; Varoneckas, G.; Sokolov, E. Heart rhythm control during sleep. *Psychophysiology* **1984**, *21*, 279–289. [CrossRef]
47. Raetz, S.L.; Richard, C.A.; Garfinkel, A.; Harper, R.M. Dynamic characteristics of cardiac RR intervals during sleep and waking states. *Sleep* **1991**, *14*, 526–533. [CrossRef]
48. Hornyak, M.; Cejnar, M.; Elam, M.; Matousek, M.; Wallin, B.G. Sympathetic muscle nerve activity during sleep in man. *Brain* **1991**, *114*, 1281–1295. [CrossRef] [PubMed]
49. Somers, V.K.; Dyken, M.E.; Mark, A.L.; Abboud, F.M. Sympathetic-nerve activity during sleep in normal subjects. *N. Eng. J. Med.* **1993**, *328*, 303–307. [CrossRef] [PubMed]
50. Valoni, E.; Adamson, P.; Piann, G. A comparison of healthy subjects with patients after myocardial infarction. *Circulation* **1995**, *91*, 1918–1922.

Article

A Pilot Randomized Controlled Trial of Effect of Genioglossus Muscle Strengthening on Obstructive Sleep Apnea Outcomes

Maryam Maghsoudipour [1], Brandon Nokes [1], Naa-Oye Bosompra [1], Rachel Jen [2], Yanru Li [3], Stacie Moore [1], Pamela N. DeYoung [1], Janelle Fine [1], Bradley A. Edwards [4,5], Dillon Gilbertson [1], Robert Owens [1], Todd Morgan [6] and Atul Malhotra [1,*]

1. Department of Medicine, University of California, La Jolla, San Diego, CA 92161, USA; mamaghsoudipour@health.ucsd.edu (M.M.); bnokes@health.ucsd.edu (B.N.); nabosompra@health.ucsd.edu (N.-O.B.); s3moore@health.ucsd.edu (S.M.); pdeyoung@health.ucsd.edu (P.N.D.); jfine@health.ucsd.edu (J.F.); dcgilbertson@health.ucsd.edu (D.G.); rowens@health.ucsd.edu (R.O.)
2. Department of Medicine, University of British Columbia, Vancouver, BC V6T 1Z4, Canada; rachjen@gmail.com
3. Department of Otorhinolaryngology Head and Neck Surgery, Beijing Tongren Hospital, Capital Medical University, Beijing 100730, China; liyanruru@mail.ccmu.edu.cn
4. Department of Physiology, School of Biomedical Sciences and Biomedical Discovery Institute, Monash University, Melbourne, VIC 3800, Australia; bradley.edwards@monash.edu
5. Turner Institute for Brain and Mental Health, Monash University, Melbourne, VIC 3800, Australia
6. Department of Dentistry, Scripps Encinitas Hospital, Encinitas, CA 92024, USA; todd@toddmorgan.com
* Correspondence: amalhotra@health.ucsd.edu

Abstract: The genioglossus is a major upper airway dilator muscle. Our goal was to assess the efficacy of upper airway muscle training on Obstructive Sleep Apnea (OSA) as an adjunct treatment. Sixty-eight participants with OSA (AHI > 10/h) were recruited from our clinic. They fall into the following categories: (a) Treated with Automatic Positive Airway Pressure (APAP), (n = 21), (b) Previously failed APAP therapy (Untreated), (n = 25), (c) Treated with Mandibular Advancement Splint (MAS), (n = 22). All subjects were given a custom-made tongue strengthening device. We conducted a prospective, randomized, controlled study examining the effect of upper airway muscle training. In each subgroup, subjects were randomized to muscle training (volitional protrusion against resistance) or sham group (negligible resistance), with a 1:1 ratio over 3 months of treatment. In the baseline and the final visit, subjects completed home sleep apnea testing, Epworth Sleepiness Scale (ESS), Pittsburgh Sleep Quality Index (PSQI), SF-36 (36-Item Short Form Survey), and Psychomotor Vigilance Test (PVT). Intervention (muscle training) did not affect the AHI (Apnea-Hypopnea Index), (p-values > 0.05). Based on PSQI, ESS, SF-36 scores, and PVT parameters, the changes between the intervention and sham groups were not significant, and the changes were not associated with the type of treatment (p-value > 0.05). The effectiveness of upper airway muscle training exercise as an adjunct treatment requires further study.

Keywords: obstructive sleep apnea; adjunctive treatment; genioglossus muscle; continuous positive airway pressure; mandibular advancement splint

1. Introduction

Obstructive sleep apnea (OSA) is defined by repetitive episodes of pharyngeal collapse during sleep [1,2]. OSA leads to excessive daytime sleepiness because of sleep fragmentation and other factors. Continuous positive airway pressure (CPAP) therapy reduces daytime sleepiness and the risk of cardiovascular morbidity and mortality, and it is known as the most effective intervention for sleep disordered breathing in severely affected patients [3,4]. Of note, incomplete adherence to CPAP treatment in some patients results in sub-optimal treatment outcomes. Oral appliances (mandibular advancement splints) are also considered to be a modality of treatment, but efficacy is variable and unpredictable [5,6].

The genioglossus muscle has a crucial role in the pathogenesis of OSA and is a major upper airway dilator. Studies evaluating genioglossus (GG) muscle activity at sleep onset suggest that patients with OSA have a marked reduction in activity in comparison with healthy individuals [7,8]. Mandibular advancement splints (MAS) pull the patient's mandible in a forward and downward position to increase the airway patency in OSA patients [6,9].

The biomechanical behavior of the upper airway muscles is complicated [10,11]. Although using various modalities of increasing upper airway muscle tone has been controversial in the treatment of OSA [12], oropharyngeal exercises have shown promising results in some previous studies [13].

To our knowledge, there have been no controlled studies assessing the adjunct effect of tongue-muscle training on CPAP or MAS treatment, as a combination therapy. Therefore, we performed a randomized, double-blind, sham-controlled study to evaluate the efficacy of tongue-muscle training on Automatic Positive Airway Pressure (APAP) treatment, MAS treatment, or Untreated groups in OSA patients. We assessed the effectiveness of the intervention on the objective sleep measurements (e.g., polysomnography), as well as subjective sleep symptoms, including daytime sleepiness, sleep quality, and quality of life.

2. Materials and Methods

2.1. Participants

In this randomized clinical trial, patients previously diagnosed with obstructive sleep apnea (Apnea Hypopnea Index (AHI) > 10/h) were recruited from our sleep laboratory. The University of California San Diego Institutional Review Board approved all protocols and methods described adhered to the tenets of the Declaration of Helsinki and the Health Insurance Portability and Accountability Act. Written informed consents were obtained from all participants after the procedure had been explained. Our trial was registered on Clinical Trials (service of NIH): http://www.clinicaltrials.gov/NCT02502942 (accessed on 25 August 2021).

The inclusion criteria were the diagnosis of OSA with AHI > 10 events/h in patients 18–79 years of age. The exclusion criteria were patients with medically unstable status, pregnant women, current smokers, use of alcohol >3 oz/day or illicit drugs, consuming >10 cups of beverages with caffeine per day, and untreated sleep apnea with Epworth Sleepiness Scale (ESS) >18.

Participants were recruited from three subgroups of patients who were (a) Treated with APAP ($n = 21$), (b) Previously failed or refused CPAP therapy (Untreated), ($n = 25$), (c) Currently being treated with an oral appliance (MAS) who still have residual OSA ($n = 22$).

In the APAP group, participants were on APAP treatment for at least 3 months with good compliance (at least 4 h a day on average). In the "Untreated" group, untreated participants with OSA who have previously tried but were not currently using PAP therapy or an oral appliance. In "MAS" group, OSA patients had residual AHI > 10 events/h during oral appliance therapy. Participants in each group were randomized to upper airway muscle training group or sham group with ratio of 1:1 (35 patients received muscle training and 33 patients received a sham).

2.2. Procedure and Measurements

OSA patients who were interested in participating in our study were asked to review the informed consent at the sleep clinic for screening home sleep apnea testing (HSAT) to determine their eligibility. Our home sleep apnea test was Apnea Link (ResMed, Inc, San Diego, CA, USA). If they agreed to proceed and sign the informed consent for pre-screening HSAT, the patient was given a standard HSAT device with instructions to conduct one-night home sleep apnea testing. Apneas and hypopneas were defined according to the American Academy of Sleep Medicine (AASM) criteria [14]. Participant eligibility was determined based on their pre-screening HSAT results or a prior sleep study. If the patients were eligible, we then explained the study activities and obtained informed consent for the main study. The eligible patients had a known diagnosis of sleep apnea and were either untreated or on Automatic Positive Airway Pressure for at least 3 months or using Mandibular Advancement Splint (MSA) for at least 3 months.

At the baseline visit, the informed consent was obtained prior to the experimental visits. The anthropomorphic characteristics (height; weight; body mass index (BMI); neck, waist, and hip circumferences), sleep questionnaires (Epworth Sleepiness Scale (ESS) [15], Pittsburgh Sleep Quality Index (PSQI) [16], Short form 36 health survey questionnaire (SF-36) [17], and Psychomotor Vigilance Test (PVT) [18] were assessed at baseline and after 110 ($\pm$34) days of intervention.

The following OSA parameters were evaluated in first HSAT and the follow up HSAT for all patients: Apnea Hypopnea Index (AHI), Apnea Index (AI), Hypopnea Index (HI), and Oxygen Desaturation Index (ODI). Our primary outcomes defined in our clinical trial were changes in OSA, measured by AHI following intervention, and for the APAP group, changes in OSA pharyngeal mechanics as measured by change in the 95th percentile pressure level.

2.3. Upper Airway Muscle Training

2.3.1. Pharyngeal Exercise Device

Following dental screening by a dentist, standard impressions were made for laboratory fabrication of a novel dental device that was designed to guide strength exercise to the lingual and pharyngeal muscles. The device is comprised of an acrylic-based plate worn on the palate, similar to a simple retainer, and secured to the upper arch using traditional orthodontic clasps, (Figure 1). The active device differs from the inactive device by having a hinge-related anterior palatal "flap" with orthodontic elastics, which provide resistance to pushing upwardly to contact the anterior portion of the palate. The control group was provided a sham device palatal plate without a hinge; they were told simply to clench on the occlusal acrylic periodically.

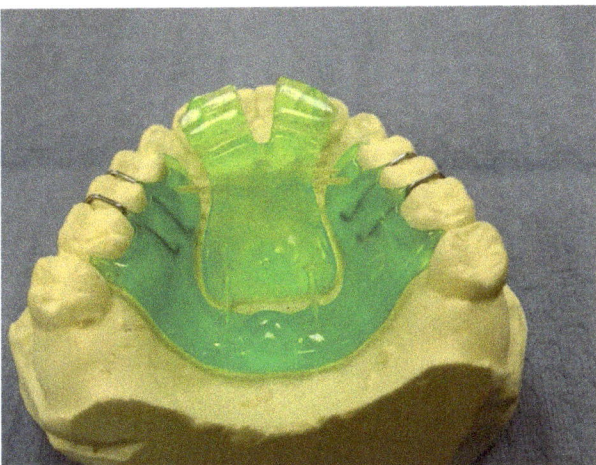

Figure 1. Oral muscle training device.

2.3.2. Mode of Action (Intervention)

Depressing the hinge flap upward against the anterior palate for 10 min, twice a day, and meanwhile using 1–2 s compression bursts was one of the two active exercises. The second exercise required the participant to hold the flap up and then raise to posterior part of the tongue to reach a Target "bump" (shown) for a count of 2 s. In combination, these exercises engage the genioglossus muscle and then the lateral pharyngeal muscles, respectively [19].

2.4. Statistics

All statistical analysis was conducted at a confidence level of 95% using the software Stata version 15.0 (Stata Corp., College Station, TX, USA). We based power calculation on detecting a significant difference between AHI after intervention or sham. Assuming a final sample size of 34 patients in each group. We had an 80% power at the 0.05 significance level to detect a difference with an effect size as subtle as 0.7.

The distribution of numeric variables was assessed by inspecting histograms and using Shapiro–Wilk W tests of normality. Categorical variables were compared using the χ^2 test. Test of significance was performed using Student's t-test to compare the mean values of normally distributed variables: independent t-test for differences between the two study groups and paired t-test for changes of baseline to final IOP. Non-parametric tests such as Mann–Whitney U test and Wilcoxon signed-rank test were used whenever the variables were not normally distributed. The effect of the intervention on AHI, ODI, ESS subjective sleepiness ratings, PVT performance, and PSQI score were assessed with linear mixed model using time, intervention, and their interaction as factors. Subject ID was included as a random effect to account for individual differences. The models were also adjusted for age, gender, and treatment group and the effect of intervention in each treatment group was explored.

The models were refitted with possible confounders (that were borderline significant predictors (p-value < 0.1) of measurement magnitude in univariate models) to adjust for the effect of these variables.

3. Results

From the 121 patients who were recruited initially, 68 patients were included in the final analysis (Figure 2). The demographic characteristics of the patients are presented in Table 1. In the sham group, the participants were significantly younger (63.2 ± 9.1 versus 56.0 ± 13.1 years, p-value, 0.038). The changes of snoring were not different between the intervention and sham groups (p-value, 0.505) (Table 1).

Table 1. Characteristics of participants according to allocation to intervention and Sham groups.

Intervention/Sham (No.)	Intervention (n = 35) (Mean ± SD)	Sham (n = 33) (Mean ± SD)	p-Value
Age (mean ±SD)	63.2 ± 9.1	56.0 ± 13.1	**0.038** *
Gender (M: F)	26:9	17:16	0.052 †
Group of Treatment			
APAP	11	10	0.986 †
MAS	11	11	
Untreated	13	12	
Initial BMI	30.0 ± 4.5	30.9 ± 7.1	0.930 *
Final BMI	30.1 ± 4.5	30.8 ± 6.8	0.979 *
p value of Change	0.681 ‡	0.750 ‡	0.615 §
Initial neck circumference	40.1 ± 3.5	39.3 ± 4.5	0.411 *
Final neck circumference	40.3 ± 4.1	39.3 ± 4.5	0.823 *
p value of Change	0.431 ‡	0.975 ‡	0.674 §
Initial Heart Rate	71.2 ± 14.5	72.1 ± 9	0.411 *
Final Heart Rate	68.3 ± 14.6	69.9 ± 12.5	0.823 *
p value of Change	0.591 ‡	**0.046** ‡	0.935 §
Initial Snoring (total number)	1056.4 ± 1093.7	1021.2 ± 1266.6	0.619 *
Final Snoring (total number)	1014 ± 1070.2	784.4 ± 1554.1	0.103 *
p value of Change	0.869 ‡	**0.028** ‡	0.505 §

* Student's t-test or Mann–Whitney U test for normally or non-normally distributed variables, respectively. † Chi-squared test is used for categorized variable. ‡ Paired t-test or Wilcoxon signed-rank test for normally or non-normally distributed variables, respectively. § Linear mixed model. Bold fonts indicate significant differences.

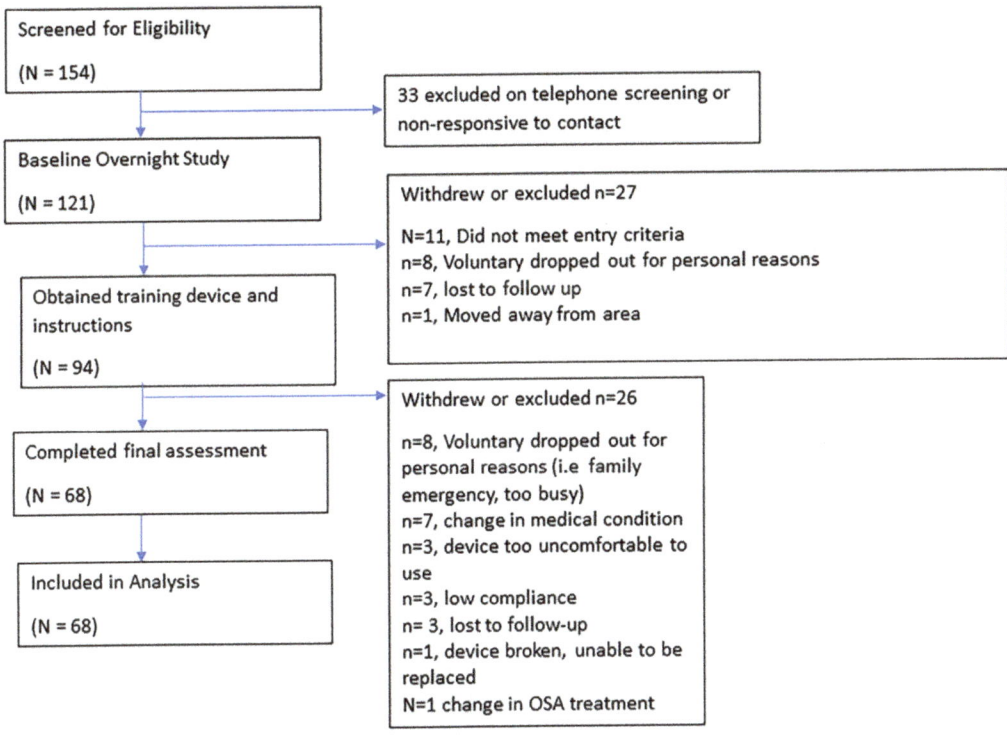

Figure 2. Enrollment flowchart.

Intervention (muscle training) did not affect the change in AHI, AI, and HI (Table 2), but the changes in AHI were different between the treatment groups (p-value, 0.006). A greater decrease in AHI was found in the APAP group compared to the MAS and Untreated groups (p-value, 0.023) (Figure 3A). Intervention (muscle training) did not affect the changes in the 95% APAP level (Table 2). Moreover, intervention (muscle training) was not associated with the changes in ODI (Table 2). The changes in ODI and OD-total were different among the treatment groups (p-value, 0.001 and 0.041, respectively), with a greater decrease in ODI and OD-total in the APAP group (Figure 3B). The results for the factors contributing to the change of AHI over time and tested in the multivariable mixed model are presented in Table 3.

Table 2. Polysomnography results in intervention and Sham groups.

Intervention/Sham	Intervention (n = 35) (Mean ±SD)	Sham (n = 33) (Mean ±SD)	p-Value
Initial AHI	23.8 ± 21.3	17.9 ± 17.6	0.250 *
Final AHI	19.9 ± 18.3	17.7 ± 16.2	0.611 *
Change	0.475 †	0.728 †	0.682 ‡
Initial AI	9.8 ± 13	5.5 ± 11.4	0.070 *
Final AI	8 ± 13.4	6.2 ± 9.3	0.865 *
Change	0.106 †	0.585 †	0.555 ‡
Initial HI	14 ± 13.1	12.4 ± 9.6	0.787 *
Final HI	11.9 ± 9.9	11.9 ± 11.7	0.621 *
Change	0.982 †	0.522 †	0.863 ‡
Initial AHI$_4$	20 ± 14.8	19.6 ± 17.4	0.741 *
Final AHI$_4$	17.9 ± 13.9	18 ± 12.8	0.844 *

Table 2. Cont.

Intervention/Sham	Intervention (n = 35) (Mean ±SD)	Sham (n = 33) (Mean ±SD)	p-Value
Change	0.637 [†]	0.820 [†]	0.749 [‡]
Initial ODI	20.7 ± 17.2	16 ± 13.1	0.401 [*]
Final ODI	18.1 ± 15.3	15.9 ± 12.3	0.788 [*]
Change	0.788 [†]	0.788 [†]	0.764 [‡]
Initial OD total	150.7 ± 135.6	118.4 ± 109.1	0.455 [*]
Final OD total	129.5 ± 116.5	99.8 ± 78.6	0.674 [*]
Change	0.674 [†]	0.506 [†]	0.488 [‡]
Initial APAP 95p	10.7 ± 2.6	11.9 ± 2.6	0.506 [*]
Final APAP 95p	10.5 ± 2.5	10.8 ± 2	0.772 [*]
change	0.593 [†]	0.177 [†]	0.649 [§]

[*] Student's t-test or Mann–Whitney U test for normally or non-normally distributed variables, respectively. [†] Paired t-test or Wilcoxon signed-rank test for normally or non-normally distributed variables, respectively. [‡] Linear mixed model adjusted for treatment, age, and gender. [§] Linear mixed model adjusted for age and gender.

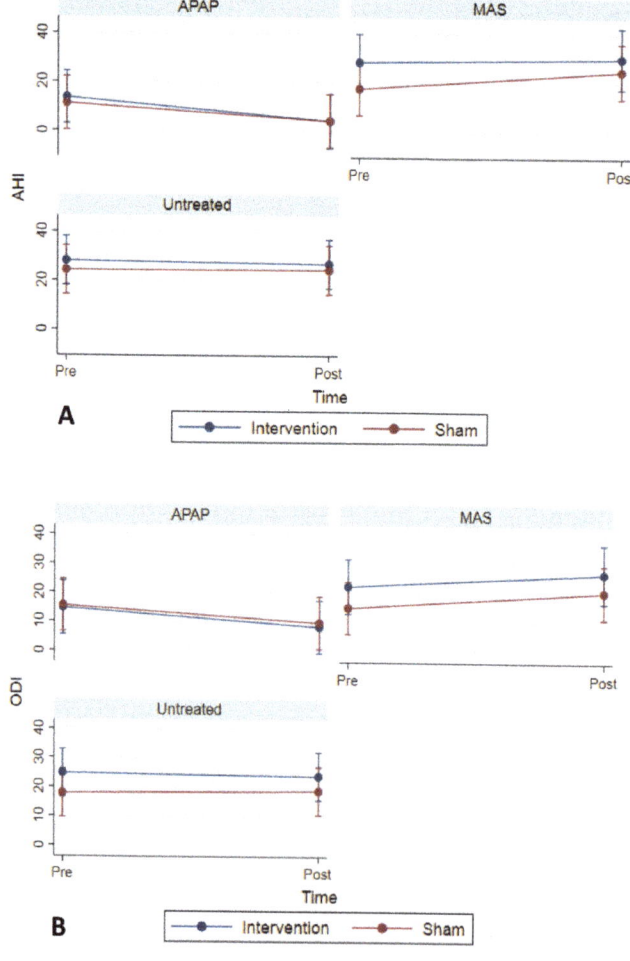

Figure 3. (**A**) Change in Apnea Hypopnea Index (AHI) across treatment groups. (**B**) Change in Oxygen Desaturation Index (ODI) across treatment groups.

Table 3. Factors Contributing to the Change of AHI over time by Mixed Model Analysis.

Variables	Univariable Model	
	β, 95% CI	p-Value
Age	−0.19 (−0.57, 0.19)	0.243
Gender: Female	−3.33 (−12.28, 5.63)	0.466
Group (baseline: Untreated)		
APAP	−5.11 (−14.65, 4.43)	0.294
MAS	7.97 (−1.72, 17.67)	0.107
Intervention (Muscle training)	−1.75 (−10.13, 6.63)	0.682

ESS tended to decrease in both the intervention and sham groups (p-values, 0.072 and 0.084, respectively). However, the change was not significantly different between the intervention and sham groups (p-value, 0.397) (Table 4). The change in ESS was not different across the treatment groups (p-value, 0.850), (Figure 4A). The PSQI score in the sham group was significantly decreased (p-value, 0.004), but the changes between the intervention and sham groups were not significantly different (p-value, 0.056) (Table 4). While the change in the PSQI score was not different across the treatment groups (p-value, 0.590), in the APAP group, the decrease in the PSQI score was greater in the sham group compared to the intervention group (p-value, 0.022), (Figure 4B).

Table 4. Subjective sleep measurements and PVT (Psycho-motor Vigilance Test) results in intervention and Sham groups.

Intervention/Sham	Intervention (n = 35) (Mean ± SD)	Sham (n = 33) (Mean ± SD)	p-Value
Initial ESS Score	7.9 ± 5	8.8 ± 5.2	0.506 *
Final ESS Score	6.8 ± 4.4	7.5 ± 5.4	0.926 *
Change	0.072 †	0.084 †	0.397 ‡
Initial PSQI score	6.9 ± 3.5	8.1 ± 4	0.405 *
Final PSQI score	6.9 ± 3.5	6.4 ± 3.8	0.538 *
Change	0.476 †	**0.004** †	0.056 ‡
Initial PVT_RT	334.4 ± 48.8	329.7 ± 43.1	0.689 *
Final PVT_RT	317.1 ± 36.2	310.5 ± 31.6	0.450 *
Change	0.111 †	**0.003** †	0.653 ‡
Initial PVT_slow10	431.4 ± 44.6	426.6 ± 39.2	0.655 *
Final PVT_slow10	423.2 ± 32	402.2 ± 41.6	**0.030** *
Change	0.413 †	**0.003** †	0.058 ‡
Initial PVT lapses	3.8 ± 5.8	3.2 ± 5.7	0.640 *
Final PVT lapses	1.8 ± 2.9	1.3 ± 1.2	0.3051 *
Change	**0.013** †	0.060 †	0.272 ‡
Initial PVT false starts	0.5 ± 0.7	0.3 ± 0.4	0.220 *
Final PVT false starts	1 ± 1.1	0.4 ± 0.9	**0.043** *
Change	**0.003** †	0.404 †	0.213 ‡

* Student's t-test or Mann–Whitney U test for normally or non-normally distributed variables, respectively. † Paired t-test or Wilcoxon signed-rank test for normally or non-normally distributed variables, respectively. ‡ Linear mixed model adjusted for treatment, age, and gender. Bold fonts indicate significant differences.

Generally, the PVT parameters improved at the final visit compared to the initial visit in both the intervention and sham groups. However, the changes between the intervention and sham groups were not significant (PVT_RT mean, PVT_slow10 mean, PVT lapses mean, and PVT false start); (p-values, 0.653, 0.058, 0.272, and 0.213, respectively) (Table 4). PVT lapses decreased significantly in the intervention group (p-value, 0.013). Improvements in PVT_RT mean, PVT_slow10 mean, PVT lapses mean, and PVT false start were not different among the treatment groups (p-values, 0.864, 0.894, 0.836, and 0.529, respectively). Changes in the PVT lapses were not different between the treatment groups.

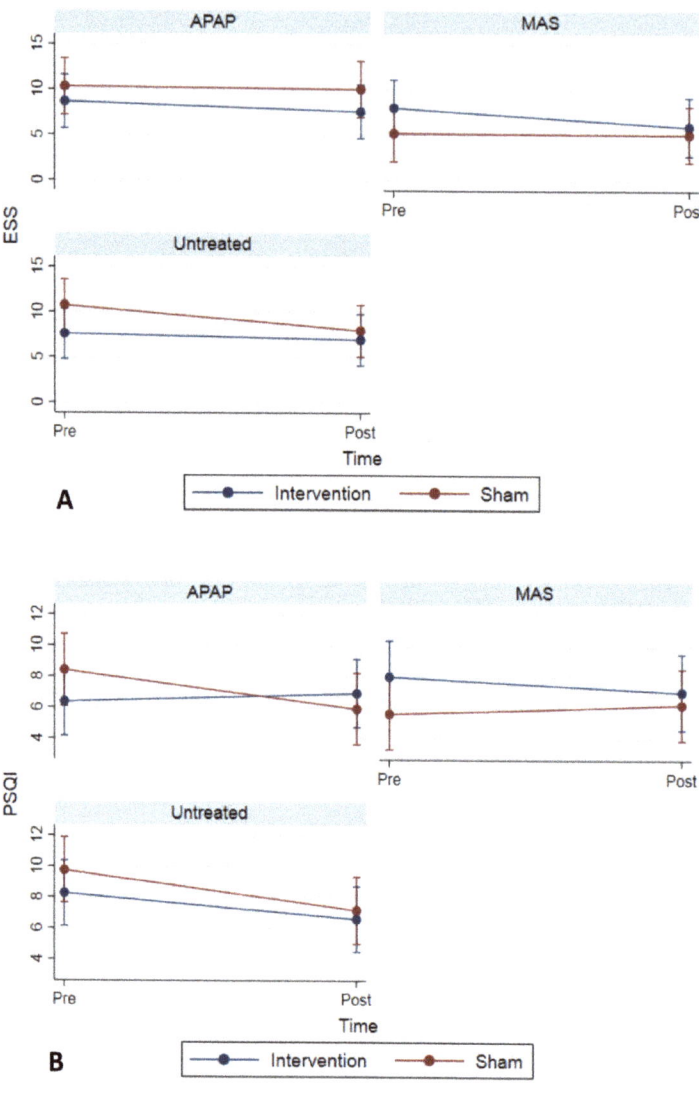

Figure 4. (**A**) Change in Epworth Sleepiness Scale (ESS) across treatment groups. (**B**) Change in Pittsburgh Sleep Quality Index (PSQI) across treatment groups.

In Table 5, the changes of subscales scores of the SF-36 questionnaires between initial and final visits are shown. "Energy/fatigue" increased significantly in the sham group (p-value, 0.037). Although "emotional well-being" increased significantly in the intervention group (p-value, 0.040), it was also increased in the sham group (p-value, 0.040). In addition, "Role limitations due to physical health" increased significantly in the sham group (p-value, 0.020) and the change between the intervention and sham groups was not significant (p-value, 0.078). However, none of the nine subscales show significant changes between the intervention and sham groups (Table 5).

Table 5. Short form survey (SF-36) scoring results in intervention and Sham groups.

Intervention/Sham	Intervention (n = 35) (Mean ± SD)	Sham (n = 33) (Mean ± SD)	p-Value
Initial "Physical functioning"	76.6 ± 27.8	76.5 ± 24.2	0.673 *
Final "Physical functioning"	78.7 ± 23.7	79.2 ± 22.9	0.994 *
Change	0.370 †	0.426 †	0.457 ‡
Initial "Role limitations due to physical health"	75.7 ± 38.6	60.6 ± 42.9	0.130 *
Final "Role limitations due to physical health"	74.2 ± 41.7	79.7 ± 35	0.571 *
Change	>0.99 †	**0.020 †**	0.078 ‡
Initial "Role limitations due to emotional problems"	81 ± 35.5	71.7 ± 39.2	0.311 *
Final "Role limitations due to emotional problems"	85.9 ± 31.2	80.2 ± 33.7	0.486 *
Change	0.280 †	0.324 †	0.834 ‡
Initial "Energy/fatigue"	55.5 ± 20.9	48.7 ± 25.3	0.228 *
Final "Energy/fatigue"	57 ± 24.4	56.9 ± 24.3	0.987 *
Change	0.671 †	**0.037 †**	0.635 ‡
Initial "Emotional well-being"	73.1 ± 19.8	73.2 ± 18.3	0.993 *
Final "Emotional well-being"	80.2 ± 17.2	79.1 ± 16.5	0.790 *
Change	**0.040 †**	**0.040 †**	0.561 ‡
Initial "Social functioning"	80.7 ± 25.4	73.9 ± 27.5	0.294 *
Final "Social functioning"	83.3 ± 25.5	79.3 ± 25.9	0.527 *
Change	0.287 †	0.120 †	0.793 ‡
Initial "Pain"	72.9 ± 24.3	73.3 ± 24.5	0.990 *
Final "Pain"	74.3 ± 22.2	73.3 ± 26.4	0.884 *
Change	0.330 †	0.620 †	0.505 ‡
Initial "General health"	63.3 ± 21.5	64.2 ± 22.4	0.857 *
Final "General health"	63.6 ± 21.7	66.9 ± 21.3	0.538 *
Change	0.733 †	0.388 †	0.901 ‡
Initial "Health change"	57.1 ± 19.7	51.5 ± 22.5	0.275 *
Final "Health change"	57.6 ± 23	53.9 ± 22.1	0.514 *
Change	0.275 †	0.441 †	0.908 ‡

* Student's t-test or Mann–Whitney U test for normally or non-normally distributed variables, respectively. † Paired t-test or Wilcoxon signed-rank test for normally or non-normally distributed variables, respectively. ‡ Linear mixed model adjusted for treatment, age, and gender. Bold fonts indicate significant differences.

4. Discussion

In the present study, pharyngeal muscle training was not associated with improvements in the objective and subjective sleep measurements in OSA patients. In the sham group, compared to the intervention group, the quality of life was decreased to a greater extent during the time of the follow-up period, demonstrated by increased role limitations and increased fatigue. Our results indicate that this particular training device was not effective for OSA treatment, and these results may inform future device designs as well as future studies regarding pharyngeal muscle training.

A systematic review evaluating new strategies targeted to increase upper airway patency in OSA patients assessed the studies that explored the effects of oropharyngeal exercises, as a complementary technique for treating OSA, and identified them to be effective, especially when the severity of the disease is moderate [2]. Although the effectiveness of hypoglossal nerve stimulation (HNS) is promising and has been accepted as a modality of treatment [20], the process is more invasive compared to oropharyngeal exercises. In turn, the attainment of more successful protocols of oropharyngeal exercises could be more beneficial.

The most extensive oropharyngeal exercises were described by Guimarães et al. In their study, patients had a significant decrease in neck circumference, snoring, daytime sleepiness, sleep quality, and OSA severity. The patients performed 30 min of daily exercise for 3 months [13]. Another study reported apnea-hypopnea index, snoring index, and minimum oxygen saturation improvements after oropharyngeal exercises in post-stroke apnea patients. Additionally, their exercise protocol improved subjective measurements of sleep quality, daily sleepiness, and performance [21]. The results of our study are in contrast with them, as we could not see any improvement in the apnea-hypopnea index and oxygen saturations. The different timing of therapy between the protocols and the specific muscles activated could be an explanation for the discrepancies.

In another study, the researchers instructed patients to perform oropharyngeal exercises three times a day, including six mastication patterns for approximately 8 min. Oropharyngeal exercises were effective in reducing objective measures such as snoring [19]. This was in contrast with our results, as we did not find any effects on snoring. Although their exercise protocol was similar to ours, their patients performed it three times a day in contrast with our twice a day protocol.

In a study assessing the effect of didgeridoo playing, daytime sleepiness and apnea-hypopnea index improved significantly. There was no effect on the quality of sleep and the health-related quality of life (SF-36) was not different between groups [22]. However, woodwind instrument methods may not be a fair comparison for isolated oropharyngeal training, given their concurrent role as a means of breathing exercise. One of the challenges in the treatment of OSA is poor compliance. In the present study, the exercises were selected based on previous studies, with a goal to improve the compliance [19]. During the experimental period, the subjects were assessed weekly to evaluate compliance. Convenience of use for the patient is a key factor for compliance. The other reason to choose this protocol with shorter time is that, in our study, the myofunctional therapy of oropharyngeal muscles was adopted as an adjunct therapy, and we tried to evaluate the combination of treatments. The device was built to mimic existing techniques deployed by Myo-functional therapy (MT), supported by previous studies [13,19,22].

In a recent meta-analysis evaluating the benefits of myofunctional therapy for the treatment of OSA, the authors concluded that myofunctional therapy may reduce daytime sleepiness and may increase sleep quality in the short term, and the certainty of the evidence ranges from moderate to very low, due to a lack of blinding, incomplete data and imprecision [23].

Although continuous positive airway pressure (CPAP) is considered the most efficient treatment for OSA [3], studies aiming to document the neurobehavioral outcomes of patients treated by CPAP have shown diverse results, and, of the SF-36 subscales, only the vitality subscale has shown significant improvement in more-adherent patients [24]. Patel and colleagues performed a meta-analysis showing that CPAP reduced the Epworth Sleepiness Scale (ESS) score in patients with OSA. The patients with moderate to severe OSA had a greater fall in ESS compared to those with mild OSA [25]. OSA severity might be a reason we did not see a significant effect of intervention in our patients, as most of our participants had mild or moderate OSA. Moreover, some studies suggest that OSA might lead to permanent structural brain abnormalities that contribute to neurobehavioral deficits in patients. Thus, cognitive symptoms and function may not be reversible with treatment, even if adherence is optimal [26]. This notion of irreversibility of some OSA consequences might be an explanation we could not see significant improvements of PVT parameters in the intervention group compared to the sham group.

Moreover, there is a study that has shown that the physiological traits that cause OSA also influence long-term CPAP adherence among those with OSA and coronary artery disease. A lower arousal threshold was associated with a marked reduction in CPAP use. Additionally, both high and low pharyngeal muscle compensation are linked to poor CPAP adherence. Therefore, identifying patients who are likely to benefit from genioglossus muscle strengthening, and future studies on more efficient genioglossus muscle strengthening protocols, might help the CPAP adherence in OSA patients [27].

Our study had certain limitations. First, the sample size was modest. Although we had a sufficient sample size for detecting the differences between the intervention and sham groups, we are not powered for the subgroups (APAP/MAS/Untreated). Second, our intervention was not universally tolerated, and our conclusions are limited to the population studied. Third, we did not examine dose–response relationships for the duration and frequency of pharyngeal muscle-training time in OSA patients as the intervention group only followed one protocol. Fourth, we acknowledge that most of our participants had mild or moderate OSA and patients with severe OSA may differ regarding the effect of genioglossus muscle strengthening on ESS or other parameters.

5. Conclusions

In the present study, we failed to prove the efficiency of upper airway muscle training exercise as an adjunct treatment in OSA. The exercise device might not adequately target the muscles important to airway patency. It is also possible that the dose (frequency, duration) of the exercise was not sufficient to strengthen the oropharyngeal muscles to reduce airway obstruction. Further research is recommended to determine the efficacy and the best modality for oropharyngeal muscle strengthening in OSA.

Author Contributions: Conceptualization: A.M. and T.M.; data curation: A.M., M.M., P.N.D., N.-O.B., D.G. and J.F.; formal analysis: M.M. and A.M.; funding acquisition: A.M.; investigation: P.N.D., N.-O.B. and D.G.; methodology: A.M. and M.M.; project administration: A.M. and P.N.D.; writing—original draft: A.M. and M.M.; writing—review and editing: A.M., M.M., B.N., R.J., Y.L., S.M., P.N.D., B.A.E., R.O. and T.M. All authors have read and agreed to the published version of the manuscript.

Funding: Malhotra is PI or CoI on NIH RO1 HL085188, K24 HL132105, T32 HL134632 RO1 HL154026; R01 AG063925; R01 HL148436, R21 HL121794, R21 HL138075, RO1 HL 119201, RO1 HL081823, RO1 HL 142114, UG1 HL139117-01, CPLGO (Center for Physiological Genomics of Low Oxygen), RO1 CA215405, RO1 HL133847. He reports medical education income from Livanova, Equillium and Corvus. The project described was partially supported by the NIH Grant UL1TR001442. The content is solely the responsibility of the authors and does not necessarily represent the official view of the NIH. Edwards is supported by a Heart Foundation of Australia Future Leader Fellowship (101167). Edwards has received research support from Apnimed (Australia) and personal fees from Signifier Medical. Nokes is supported by the NIH (T32 grant HL134632), Sleep Research Society Career Development Award, as well as the American Thoracic Society ASPIRE grant. This project utilized REDCap, which was supported by grant UL1TR001442.

Institutional Review Board Statement: The study was conducted according to the guidelines of the Declaration of Helsinki and approved by the Ethics Committee of University of California San Diego. The ID number is 130780.

Informed Consent Statement: Informed consent was obtained from all the subjects involved in the study.

Data Availability Statement: The data that support the findings of this study are available on request from the corresponding author. The data are not publicly available due to privacy or ethical restrictions.

Conflicts of Interest: All authors declare no conflict of interest.

References

1. Dempsey, J.A.; Veasey, S.C.; Morgan, B.J.; O'Donnell, C.P. Pathophysiology of sleep apnea. *Physiol. Rev.* **2010**, *90*, 47–112. [CrossRef]
2. Mediano, O.; Romero-Peralta, S.; Resano, P.; Cano-Pumarega, I.; Sanchez-de-la-Torre, M.; Castillo-Garcia, M.; Martinez-Sanchez, A.B.; Ortigado, A.; Garcia-Rio, F. Obstructive Sleep Apnea: Emerging Treatments Targeting the Genioglossus Muscle. *J. Clin. Med.* **2019**, *8*, 1754. [CrossRef]
3. Giles, T.L.; Lasserson, T.J.; Smith, B.J.; White, J.; Wright, J.; Cates, C.J. Continuous positive airways pressure for obstructive sleep apnoea in adults. *Cochrane Database Syst. Rev.* **2006**, *1*, Cd001106. [CrossRef]
4. Marin, J.M.; Carrizo, S.J.; Vicente, E.; Agusti, A.G. Long-term cardiovascular outcomes in men with obstructive sleep apnoea-hypopnoea with or without treatment with continuous positive airway pressure: An observational study. *Lancet* **2005**, *365*, 1046–1053. [CrossRef]
5. Cao, M.T.; Sternbach, J.M.; Guilleminault, C. Continuous positive airway pressure therapy in obstructive sleep apnea: Benefits and alternatives. *Expert Rev. Respir. Med.* **2017**, *11*, 259–272. [CrossRef]

6. Doff, M.H.; Hoekema, A.; Wijkstra, P.J.; van der Hoeven, J.H.; Huddleston Slater, J.J.; de Bont, L.G.; Stegenga, B. Oral appliance versus continuous positive airway pressure in obstructive sleep apnea syndrome: A 2-year follow-up. *Sleep* **2013**, *36*, 1289–1296. [CrossRef] [PubMed]
7. Mezzanotte, W.S.; Tangel, D.J.; White, D.P. Influence of sleep onset on upper-airway muscle activity in apnea patients versus normal controls. *Am. J. Respir. Crit. Care Med.* **1996**, *153 Pt 1*, 1880–1887. [CrossRef] [PubMed]
8. Fogel, R.B.; Trinder, J.; White, D.P.; Malhotra, A.; Raneri, J.; Schory, K.; Kleverlaan, D.; Pierce, R.J. The effect of sleep onset on upper airway muscle activity in patients with sleep apnoea versus controls. *J. Physiol.* **2005**, *564 Pt 2*, 549–562. [CrossRef] [PubMed]
9. Matsuda, M.; Ogawa, T.; Sitalaksmi, R.M.; Miyashita, M.; Ito, T.; Sasaki, K. Effect of mandibular position achieved using an oral appliance on genioglossus activity in healthy adults during sleep. *Head Face Med.* **2019**, *15*, 26. [CrossRef]
10. Bilston, L.E.; Gandevia, S.C. Biomechanical properties of the human upper airway and their effect on its behavior during breathing and in obstructive sleep apnea. *J. Appl. Physiol.* **2014**, *116*, 314–324. [CrossRef]
11. Bailey, E.F.; Rice, A.D.; Fuglevand, A.J. Firing patterns of human genioglossus motor units during voluntary tongue movement. *J. Neurophysiol.* **2007**, *97*, 933–936. [CrossRef]
12. Valbuza, J.S.; de Oliveira, M.M.; Conti, C.F.; Prado, L.B.; de Carvalho, L.B.; do Prado, G.F. Methods for increasing upper airway muscle tonus in treating obstructive sleep apnea: Systematic review. *Sleep Breath.* **2010**, *14*, 299–305. [CrossRef]
13. Guimaraes, K.C.; Drager, L.F.; Genta, P.R.; Marcondes, B.F.; Lorenzi-Filho, G. Effects of oropharyngeal exercises on patients with moderate obstructive sleep apnea syndrome. *Am. J. Respir. Crit. Care Med.* **2009**, *179*, 962–966. [CrossRef] [PubMed]
14. Berry, R.; Brooks, R.; Gamaldo, C.E.; Harding, S.M.; Lloyd, R.M.; Marcus, C.L.; Vaughn, B.V.; for the American Academy of Sleep Medicine. *The AASM Manual for the Scoring of Sleep and Associated Events: Rules, Terminology and Technical Specifications*, Version 2.2 ed.; American Academy of Sleep Medicine: Darien, IL, USA, 2015.
15. Johns, M.W. A new method for measuring daytime sleepiness: The Epworth sleepiness scale. *Sleep* **1991**, *14*, 540–545. [CrossRef] [PubMed]
16. Buysse, D.J.; Reynolds, C.F., 3rd; Monk, T.H.; Hoch, C.C.; Yeager, A.L.; Kupfer, D.J. Quantification of subjective sleep quality in healthy elderly men and women using the Pittsburgh Sleep Quality Index (PSQI). *Sleep* **1991**, *14*, 331–338. [PubMed]
17. Brazier, J.E.; Harper, R.; Jones, N.M.; O'Cathain, A.; Thomas, K.J.; Usherwood, T.; Westlake, L. Validating the SF-36 health survey questionnaire: New outcome measure for primary care. *BMJ* **1992**, *305*, 160–164. [CrossRef]
18. Basner, M.; Dinges, D.F. Maximizing sensitivity of the psychomotor vigilance test (PVT) to sleep loss. *Sleep* **2011**, *34*, 581–591. [CrossRef]
19. Ieto, V.; Kayamori, F.; Montes, M.I.; Hirata, R.P.; Gregorio, M.G.; Alencar, A.M.; Drager, L.F.; Genta, P.R.; Lorenzi-Filho, G. Effects of Oropharyngeal Exercises on Snoring: A Randomized Trial. *Chest* **2015**, *148*, 683–691. [CrossRef]
20. Remmers, J.E.; deGroot, W.J.; Sauerland, E.K.; Anch, A.M. Pathogenesis of upper airway occlusion during sleep. *J. Appl. Physiol. Respir. Environ. Exerc. Physiol.* **1978**, *44*, 931–938. [CrossRef] [PubMed]
21. Ye, D.; Chen, C.; Song, D.; Shen, M.; Liu, H.; Zhang, S.; Zhang, H.; Li, J.; Yu, W.; Wang, Q. Oropharyngeal Muscle Exercise Therapy Improves Signs and Symptoms of Post-stroke Moderate Obstructive Sleep Apnea Syndrome. *Front. Neurol.* **2018**, *9*, 912. [CrossRef] [PubMed]
22. Puhan, M.A.; Suarez, A.; Lo Cascio, C.; Zahn, A.; Heitz, M.; Braendli, O. Didgeridoo playing as alternative treatment for obstructive sleep apnoea syndrome: Randomised controlled trial. *BMJ* **2006**, *332*, 266–270. [CrossRef] [PubMed]
23. Rueda, J.R.; Mugueta-Aguinaga, I.; Vilaró, J.; Rueda-Etxebarria, M. Myofunctional therapy (oropharyngeal exercises) for obstructive sleep apnoea. *Cochrane Database Syst. Rev.* **2020**, *11*, Cd013449. [CrossRef] [PubMed]
24. Antic, N.A.; Catcheside, P.; Buchan, C.; Hensley, M.; Naughton, M.T.; Rowland, S.; Williamson, B.; Windler, S.; McEvoy, R.D. The effect of CPAP in normalizing daytime sleepiness, quality of life, and neurocognitive function in patients with moderate to severe OSA. *Sleep* **2011**, *34*, 111–119. [CrossRef] [PubMed]
25. Patel, S.R.; White, D.P.; Malhotra, A.; Stanchina, M.L.; Ayas, N.T. Continuous positive airway pressure therapy for treating sleepiness in a diverse population with obstructive sleep apnea: Results of a meta-analysis. *Arch. Intern. Med.* **2003**, *163*, 565–571. [CrossRef] [PubMed]
26. Morrell, M.J.; McRobbie, D.W.; Quest, R.A.; Cummin, A.R.; Ghiassi, R.; Corfield, D.R. Changes in brain morphology associated with obstructive sleep apnea. *Sleep Med.* **2003**, *4*, 451–454. [CrossRef]
27. Zinchuk, A.V.; Chu, J.H.; Liang, J.; Celik, Y.; Op de Beeck, S.; Redeker, N.S.; Wellman, A.; Yaggi, H.K.; Peker, Y.; Sands, S.A. Physiological Traits and Adherence to Sleep Apnea Therapy in Individuals with Coronary Artery Disease. *Am. J. Respir. Crit. Care Med.* **2021**, *204*, 703–712. [CrossRef]

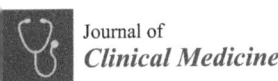

Article

Telemedicine Strategy to Rescue CPAP Therapy in Sleep Apnea Patients with Low Treatment Adherence: A Pilot Study

Onintza Garmendia [1], Ramon Farré [2,3,4], Concepción Ruiz [1], Monique Suarez-Girón [1], Marta Torres [3,5,6], Raisa Cebrian [7], Laura Saura [7], Carmen Monasterio [8], Miguel A. Negrín [9] and Josep M. Montserrat [1,3,4,*]

1. Sleep Unit, Hospital Clínic-Universitat de Barcelona, 08036 Barcelona, Spain; onintzag@gmail.com (O.G.); csanchez@clinic.cat (C.R.); mcsuarezgiron@gmail.com (M.S.-G.)
2. Unitat de Biofisica i Bioenginyeria, Facultat de Medicina i Ciencies de la Salut, Universitat de Barcelona, 08036 Barcelona, Spain; rfarre@ub.edu
3. CIBER de Enfermedades Respiratorias, 28029 Madrid, Spain; torreslopezmarta@gmail.com
4. Institut Investigacions Biomediques August Pi Sunyer, 08036 Barcelona, Spain
5. Agency for Health Quality and Assessment of Catalonia (AQuAS), 08005 Barcelona, Spain
6. CIBER de Epidemiología y Salud Pública, 28029 Madrid, Spain
7. Esteve Teijin, 08029 Barcelona, Spain; rcebrian@esteveteijin.com (R.C.); lsaura@esteveteijin.com (L.S.)
8. Multidisciplinary Sleep Unit, Department of Respiratory Medicine, Hospital Universitari de Bellvitge, 08907 L'Hospitalet de Llobregat, Spain; cmonasterio@bellvitgehospital.cat
9. Quantitative Methods Department, TiDES Institute, Las Palmas de Gran Canaria University, 35001 Las Palmas de Gran Canaria, Spain; miguel.negrin@ulpgc.es
* Correspondence: jmmontserrat@ub.edu

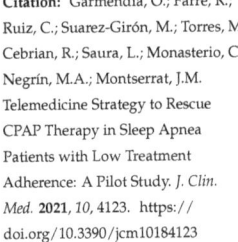

Abstract: Patients with sleep apnea are usually treated with continuous positive airway pressure (CPAP). This therapy is very effective if the patient's adherence is satisfactory. However, although CPAP adherence is usually acceptable during the first months of therapy, it progressively decreases, with a considerable number of patients accepting average treatment duration below the effectiveness threshold (4 h/night). Herein, our aim was to describe and evaluate a novel telemedicine strategy for rescuing CPAP treatment in patients with low adherence after several months/years of treatment. This two-week intervention includes (1) patient support using a smartphone application, phone and voice recorder messages to be answered by a nurse, and (2) daily transmission and analysis of signals from the CPAP device and potential variation of nasal pressure if required. On average, at the end of the intervention, median CPAP adherence considerably increased by 2.17 h/night (from 3.07 to 5.24 h/night). Interestingly, the procedure was able to markedly rescue CPAP adherence: the number of patients with poor adherence (<4 h/night) was considerably reduced from 38 to 7. After one month, adherence improvement was maintained (median 5.09 h/night), and only 13 patients had poor adherence (<4 h/night). This telemedicine intervention (103€ per included patient) is a cost-effective tool for substantially increasing the number of patients with CPAP adherence above the minimum threshold for achieving positive therapeutic effects.

Keywords: obstructive sleep apnea; sleep breathing disorders; nasal pressure; patient adherence; compliance; telemedicine interventions

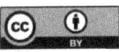

1. Introduction

The obstructive sleep apnea (OSA) syndrome is a highly prevalent chronic disorder associated with substantial morbidity, resulting in considerable healthcare costs [1–3]. Continuous positive airway pressure (CPAP) is by far the most widespread and effective therapy for OSA and is thus the gold standard treatment for this sleep breathing disorder [4]. However, suboptimal patient adherence to CPAP is common [5,6] despite using conventional interventions to increase it [7]. Regarding the clinical effectiveness of CPAP, it is important to mention that treatment adherence of 4 h per night is currently considered the minimum required. However, data in the literature describing the dose-response relationship between CPAP usage and improved clinical outcomes (including sleepiness, functional status, and hypertension) strongly suggest setting an adherence threshold of >5 h/night [8–10]. Therefore, it is of crucial importance to increase CPAP adherence as much as possible to achieve optimal treatment effectiveness.

Telemedicine is a strategic approach to address public health challenges in chronic diseases, offering potential cost-effective management options [11]. In the case of sleep medicine, and particularly in OSA, multiple telemedicine modalities can be used, including telediagnosis, teleconsultation, and telemonitoring of patients being treated with CPAP. However, it is crucial to carefully select clinical outcomes and adequately target those patients who may benefit from telemedicine interventions [12–14]. Currently, and especially after experiencing a global pandemic with COVID-19, the use of telemedicine has been markedly increased. Telemetric monitoring of OSA patients allows remote CPAP titration [14,15]. Moreover, telemedicine allows that most patients can be remotely contacted (by phone or video-visits) for satisfactorily managing OSA [14,16]. Recently described telemedicine interventions focused on improving CPAP adherence are applied during the first weeks/months after CPAP is prescribed, when adherence is relatively acceptable [15,16]. However, it is well known that the patient's adherence with this treatment decreases [16–22] over time. Therefore, novel interventions addressed to improve CPAP adherence in patients already in long-term treatment are required.

Hence, the aim of this research was to set a specific telemedicine procedure for rescuing CPAP adherence in patients already on treatment who, regardless of being conventionally followed up by hospital or CPAP provider staff, are poorly compliant as indicated by a low number of hours per night on CPAP. The primary end-point was to increase the percentage of rescued patients presenting at baseline treatment adherence lower than 4 h/night (considered poor). The secondary end-point was to also improve the percentage of patients who achieve optimal adherence among those with acceptable adherence (4–5.5 h/night).

2. Materials and Methods

2.1. Patients

This was a prospective, pre-post intervention, single-arm study that evaluated patients (18–75 years old) that had a CPAP prescription from September 2016 to June 2020. The research and analysis of the telemedicine application was performed from November 2020 to April 2021 on patients who did not comply with either a minimum (<4 h) or suboptimal (4–5.5 h/night) CPAP treatment despite careful follow-up by the hospital and the service provider. To this end, the value of CPAP adherence registered in the home CPAP device used by the patient was considered.

Before entering the study, the patients were followed up according to our usual protocol. Briefly, before starting CPAP treatment, patients participated in a 1.5-h educational and training session (theoretical and practical use of CPAP and selection of an adequate mask). After starting with CPAP treatment, the first visit was at 15–30 days, the second one after 3 months, the third visit was after 6 months, and finally a fourth visit 1 year after prescription. If treatment was satisfactory, the patient was visited alternately by the specialized nurse and the provider each year. Patients attended their regular medical visits depending on medical needs and problems about CPAP. According to nurse or physician criteria, patients with inadequate adherence were visited (individually or in a group), usually every 3 months. If required, the CPAP provider company increased the number of patient visits.

Patients who met the inclusion criteria and signed the informed consent were included. The exclusion criteria were severe associated comorbidities or coexisting severe psychiatric disease, central apneas, pregnancy, regular use of sedatives or narcotics, uvulopalatopharyngoplasty, incapacity to carry out questionnaires, and any contraindication for CPAP therapy. Importantly, low experience in the use of smartphones or internet applications was not an exclusion criterion. Thus, only patients with no previous experience in using these communication tools were excluded.

2.2. Intervention

The intervention was based on the following three components: (1) Each patient received an automatic-CPAP device (Dreamstation, Respironics) which was able to remotely transmit data on CPAP pressure, breathing flow, air leaks, treatment adherence, and residual respiratory events to a commercially available web server providing remote monitoring to the health care provider. The setting also allowed remotely changing the value of CPAP pressure applied, thus performing home accurate titration/retitration if required [15]. The patient was asked to use a specially designed smartphone application (APPnea) [12] to promote patient self-monitoring of CPAP treatment. APPnea asked the patient simple questions on adherence, sleep improvement, CPAP side effects, and general lifestyle perception each other day. This questionnaire is provided as a Supplementary File Table S1. All answers were sent to a web server and evaluated by a specialized nurse who contacted the patient if required [12]. The patient was invited to use a voicemail available 24 h to collect the patient's questions or problems. Patients were encouraged to leave voicemail messages to be checked and eventually answered by a specialized nurse.

The nurse communicated with the patient if data transmitted by the CPAP device showed problems (air leaks, high residual events, or poor adherence). The telemedicine intervention using the described procedure lasted 15 days. CPAP adherence was measured immediately after the intervention and after a 30-day subsequent period. Moreover, the costs of the intervention as well as the patient's satisfaction were assessed.

2.3. Data Analysis

A per-protocol analysis of improvement in CPAP adherence after the intervention (pre-post analysis) was carried out. Data were characterized by mean (SD) for continuous variables with normal distribution, median (Q1; Q3) for those with nonnormal distribution, and number and percentage of patients for categorical variables. Ninety-five percent confidence intervals for overall incidence in adherence rate and mean change from baseline in adherence measured in hours were computed. Paired adherence data before the intervention (PRE), after the intervention (POST), and 1 month after the end of intervention (1-MONTH) was analyzed with nonparametric ANOVA using the Friedman test followed by Dunn's multiple comparisons test (Prism, GraphPad, CA, USA). If the Friedman test was significant, post hoc paired comparison was made using the Wilcoxon signed-rank test. The McNemar–Bowker test was used to determine differences on a categorical variable between two related groups. All tests were two-tailed, and significance was set at 0.05. All analyses were performed with IBM SPSS Statistics version 26.0 (Armonk, New York, NY, USA).

2.4. Cost Analysis

The cost of the different steps followed in the intervention were considered: before the start of the intervention, a total cost of 3000 € corresponding to the APPnea application was distributed among the 56 patients. Change to an automatic-CPAP was also necessary for 17 patients. Both items resulted in a baseline cost of 4330.25 € (3000 + 78.25 × 17), 77 € per-protocol patient. The other costs include the remote monitoring time (in minutes) by a specialized nurse; the cost of the first phone visit (in minutes), and the other contacts with a specialized nurse through voice mail messages, emails (assumed 5 min per message) and phone calls (in minutes); and time (in minutes) of the two visits of the service company providing CPAP equipment plus additional visits for mask replacements. Unit costs were the same used in similar recent studies [11,15]: 16.2 €/hour for a specialized nurse, 19 €/hour for a technician of the provider company, and 24 € for mask replacement.

3. Results

Table 1 shows the patient's characteristics and their mild comorbidities (patients with severe comorbidities were excluded). Sixty-one patients participated in the study, of which five dropped out from the protocol because they voluntarily abandoned the telemedicine procedure, thus 56 patients completed the study as indicated by the flow chart in Figure 1. Only 7% of patients required CPAP retitration and, in that case, nasal pressure was remotely adjusted, 23% of patients used the nurse call line and only one patient needed a new mask.

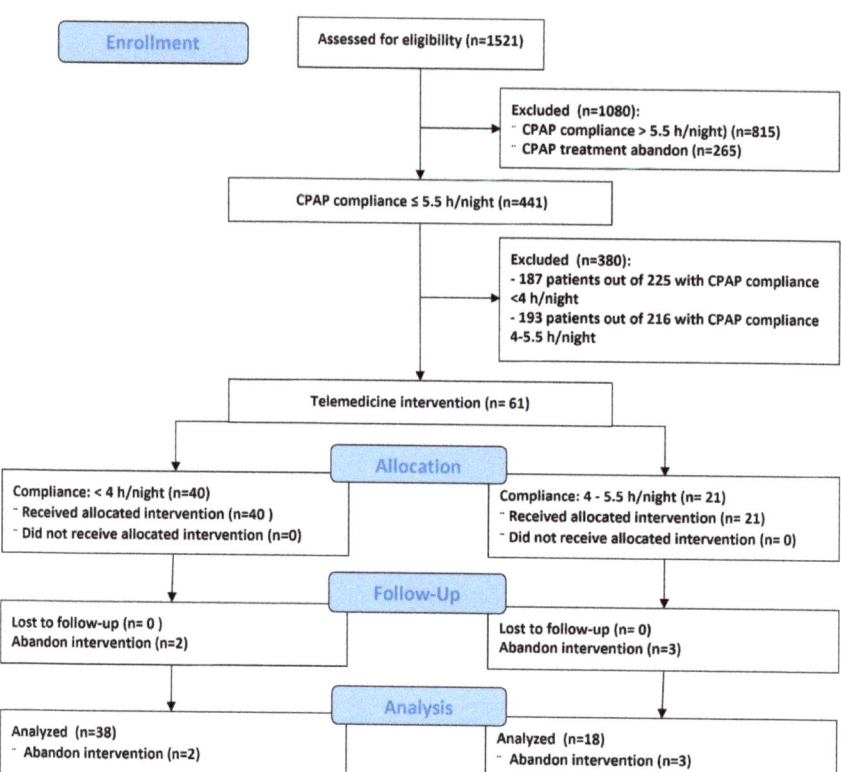

Figure 1. Flow chart of the study.

Table 1. Patient characteristics.

Number	56
Gender (male; %)	78.6
Age (yr; m ± SD)	57.9 ± 8.9
Apnea-hypopnea index (events/h; m ± SD)	45.8 ± 20.1
Time on CPAP therapy (yr; m ± SD)	2.46 ± 0.90
Main Comorbidity:	
Cardiovascular (%)	41.1
Metabolic (%)	39.3
Neurological (%)	1.8
Respiratory (%)	19.6
Depression (%)	12.5
Neurological (%)	1.8

Figure 2 shows the CPAP therapy adherence quantified as the number of hours per night. By considering all patients, on average, the telemedicine intervention considerably increased median treatment adherence by 2.17 h/night (from 3.07 to 5.24 h/night). Among the group of patients with baseline adherence < 4 h/night, the median increase was even higher: 3.79 h/night (from 1.44 to 5.23 h/night). Even patients with already acceptable adherence (4–5.5 h/nigh) experienced an increase of 0.72 h/night (from 4.55 to 5.27 h/night). All these changes were statistically significant. Most interestingly, the general pattern of increase in adherence observed just at the end of the intervention did not significantly change after 1 month: median adherences were 4.55, 5.27, and 5.21 h/night in the three groups respectively (Figure 2). Full raw data on CPAP adherence are provided in a Supplementary File Table S2.

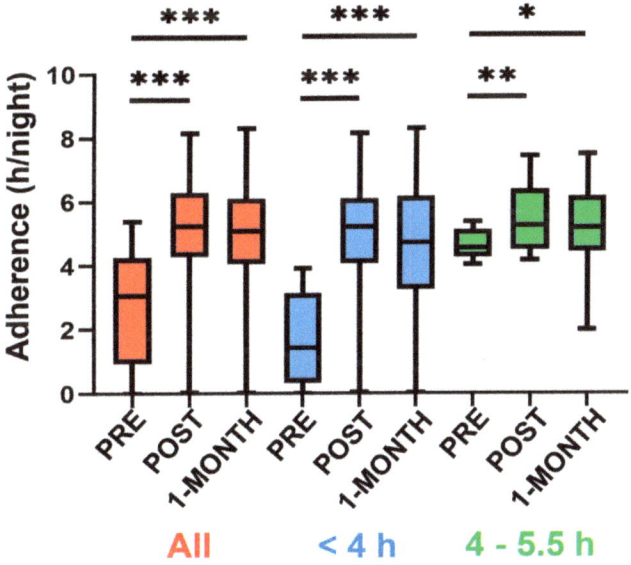

Figure 2. Adherence of CPAP is expressed as the number of hours per night on treatment (median, 25–75% percentiles and smallest and largest values). Data are shown for the whole group of patients (red), for those patients with preintervention (PRE) adherence of <4 h/night (blue), and for those with preintervention adherence between 4 and 5.5 h/night (green). Labels "POST" and "1-MONTH" indicate values measured immediately at the end of the intervention and 1 month later, respectively. All changes from PRE to POST and from PRE to 1-MONTH were statistically significant, and none of the minor changes from POST to 1-MONTH were statistically significant. ***, **, and * indicate $p < 0.001$, $p < 0.01$ and $p < 0.05$, respectively.

The marked increase in adherence (Figure 2) resulted in a considerable number of patients with rescued CPAP treatment.

Figure 3 shows, for each time (preintervention, postintervention and 1 month later) what was the number of patients exhibiting three different levels of adherence: poor adherence (<4 h/night), good adherence (4–5.5 h/night) and excellent adherence (>5.5 h/night). Remarkably, the most important result is that the number of patients with poor adherence (<4 h/night) was considerably reduced from 38 to 7 and 13 after the intervention and after a subsequent month, respectively. In addition to markedly reducing the number of patients with poor adherence, the intervention increased the number of patients with good adherence (4–5.5 h/night) from 18 to 27 and 26, respectively. Finally, whereas before the intervention no patient had optimal adherence (>5.5 h/night), after the intervention and 1 month later the number increased to 22 and 17, respectively. The number of patients within three different levels of adherence when comparing PRE vs. POST and PRE vs. 1-MONTH was significantly different ($p < 0.001$ in both cases; Figure 3).

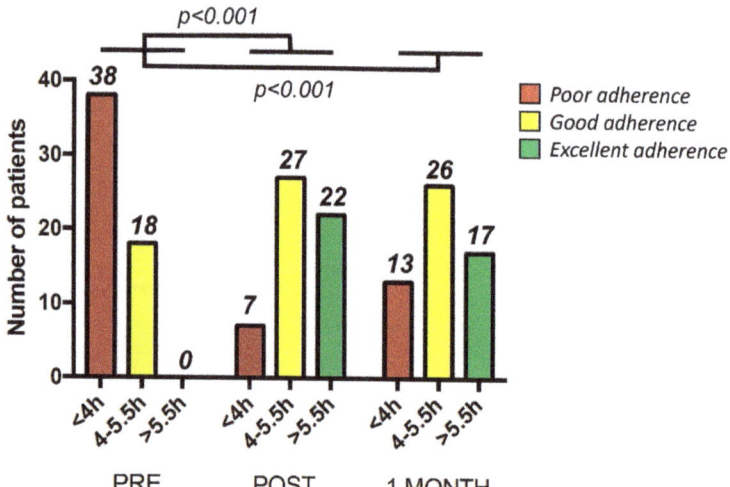

Figure 3. Number of patients within three different levels of adherence: poor and thus poor adherence (<4 h/night) (red), good adherence (4–5.5 h/night) (yellow) and excellent adherence (>5.5 h/night) (green) at three different time points: prior to the telemedicine intervention (Pre), after the intervention (Post) and one month later (1 month). The *p* values refer to differences in the number of patients within three different levels of adherence when comparing PRE vs. POST and PRE vs. 1-MONTH.

Patients showed considerable satisfaction with the intervention: they answered that the questions periodically posed to them by the smartphone App were partially (39%) or totally (60%) useful, with only one patient answering negatively (Figure 4). Interestingly, 82% of patients would recommend the application to other patients and, 85% would like to regularly use the application to control their CPAP therapy (Figure 4).

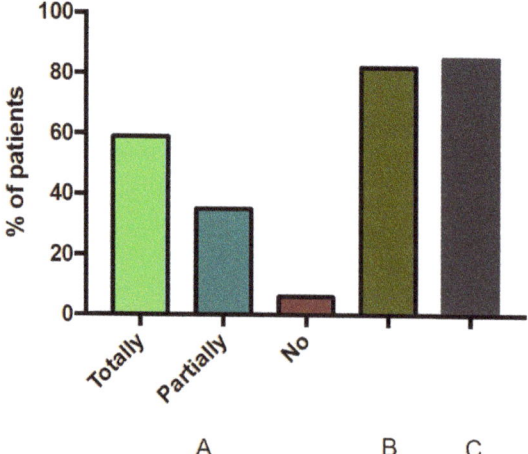

Figure 4. Patient satisfaction with the telemedicine intervention. Left section (**A**) shows the percentage of patient's responses when asked whether the App was totally, partially or not useful. (**B**) and (**C**), on the right, show the percentage of patients who would recommend using the App to other patients and who would like to use the App regularly along their CPAP treatment, respectively.

The total cost of the intervention was on, average 103 €, per included patient. Figure 5 shows the cost distribution among the different intervention actions. No differences in individual costs were observed between patients with and without rescued CPAP adherence.

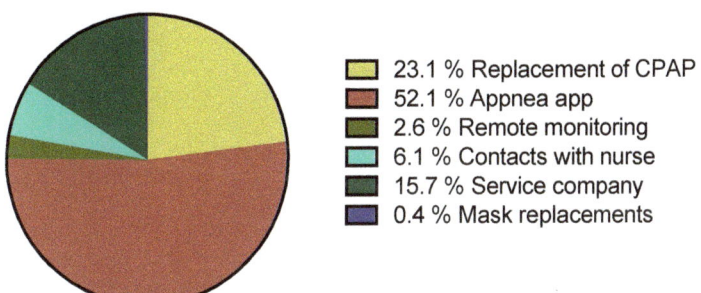

Figure 5. Cost distribution of the proposed telemedicine intervention.

4. Discussion

In this study, we report that noncompliant CPAP treatment in patients with OSA who are under long-term therapy (average 2.5 yr) can be markedly rescued by means of a two-week telemedicine intervention which is based on two different points. First, personal support by using a smartphone application [12], phone and voice recorder where the patients could leave messages that were answered by a nurse. Second, CPAP device signal transmission from the patient's home (e.g., pressure, residual events, adherence, air leaks) which allows remotely adjusting the nasal pressure applied if required. As shown in Figures 2 and 3, the intervention was able to considerably increase the time that patients were on CPAP and thereby improving the level of adherence, in many cases above the threshold for therapeutic effectiveness (4 h/night).

Several previous publications have raised the clinical problem of poor adherence of CPAP in OSA. Pepin et al. [22] analyzed the CPAP therapy of OSA patients from a French nationwide database analysis (n: 480,000 subjects) and found that overall CPAP termination rates after 1, 2 and 3 years were 23.1, 37.1 and 47.7% respectively and raised the importance of phenotyping and personalized care approaches that determine the most appropriate. In the SAVE study, McEvoy et al. [6] found that CPAP adherence at the beginning of the study was 5.3 h/night, and after 24 months of follow-up, it was reduced to 3.4 h/night (n:1121, 5 different countries). In a similar study, Peker et al. [23] described that cardiovascular improvement was found only in subjects with good adherence. Bakker et al. [24] raised two important points: how many hours of CPAP use per night are necessary to improve symptoms and to reduce cardiovascular risk, and what strategies could be implemented to optimize adherence in clinical settings. The main conclusions were that combining theory-driven behavioral approaches with telemedicine technology could hold the answer to increasing real-world CPAP adherence rates, although randomized studies are still required, and socioeconomic barriers to telemedicine will need to be addressed to promote health equity. Accordingly, there is ample consensus on the need to improve the adherence of CPAP treatment to levels higher than the commonly observed in clinical practice.

Given the importance of the problem of poor CPAP adherence, different telemedicine interventions have been proposed to diminish or solve it. Aardoom et al. performed a meta-analysis [21] designed to investigate the effectiveness of a broad range of eHealth interventions in improving CPAP treatment adherence. The main conclusions were that eHealth interventions for adults with OSA could improve adherence to CPAP at the initial weeks/months after the start of treatment, increasing the mean nightly duration of usage by about half an hour. Uncertainty still exists regarding the timing, duration, intensity, and specific types of health interventions that could be most effectively implemented by health care providers [18]. In a recent randomized study, the effect of telemedicine applied after 3 months of regular treatment was analyzed. After 6 months of follow-up, the telemedicine group improved adherence [25]. However, to the best of our knowledge, data in the literature do not describe any procedure that, similar to the one presented herein, successfully rescues CPAP therapy adherence in patients with no recent prescription of CPAP but on therapy for a long period.

In the performed cost analysis, we estimated 103 € per-protocol patient, resulting in a cost per recovered patient of 152 €. It is noteworthy that these costs are overestimated since we divided the total cost of the smartphone application used in the intervention (APPnea) (3000 €) among the only 56 patients of the study. If this intervention was implemented for much more patients, the distributed cost of the App (which in this study was the most expensive contribution in total cost, as shown in Figure 5), would become negligible and then would virtually disappear. Therefore, the effective cost of the intervention per patient would be considerably reduced. To more precisely evaluate whether this intervention is cost-effective, it would be required to also consider that the associated increase in patient's health represents fewer costs to the society, which seems to be proven in the literature. Indeed, Rossi et al. [26] showed that untreated OSA used more medical services and more medicines. Specifically, Guest et al. [27] and Kapur et al. [28] estimated that untreated OSA leads to a twofold increase in medical expenses in Europe and the USA, and Knauert et al. [29] obtained a similar conclusion by reviewing the topic.

The current study has limitations. One of them is that, although being multicentric, the number of patients is relatively reduced. The reason is that patients who were acceptable according to the inclusion criteria were very difficult to recruit since the protocol was carried out during the COVID-19 pandemic. This fact explains why 380 patients were excluded (Figure 1). However, under these conditions the telemedicine approach was tested in a realistic scenario characterized by severely reduced possibility of in person interaction between patients and health care staff. Another limitation is that the time of the follow-up after the intervention (one month) was reduced. However, in this pilot study we have demonstrated that the intervention is feasible and useful, and as such it can be easily reproduced to rescue CPAP treatment in patients poorly complying with the treatment. Regardless of the specific limitations of this study, it should be considered that telemedicine per se has limitations and cannot be applied without previously considering its potential drawbacks and requirements, specifically in the field of CPAP for OSA patients [30]. For instance, the requirement of training the health care professionals involved, the need of phenotyping which patients should be included in a telemedicine program, or better defining not only the cost for the health system but the social and labor costs saved by correctly treated patients.

5. Conclusions

To our knowledge, this is the first study that deals with the CPAP adherence rescue concept in patients under long-term treatment. The results obtained demonstrate that it is possible that a significant proportion of patients with poor, and thus inefficient, adherence achieve the minimum threshold of 4 h/night on CPAP. Moreover, patients already on an adherence range which was satisfactory but not optimal (4–5.5 h/night) increased adherence to optimal values (>5.5 h/night). The fact that the procedure is cost-effective and the very positive patient satisfaction strongly suggests that the proposed telemedicine intervention will be a powerful tool for improving CPAP usage in the clinical arena of OSA treatment.

Supplementary Materials: The following are available online at https://www.mdpi.com/article/10.3390/jcm10184123/s1, Table S1: Follow up patient questionnaire with 9 single-choice questions (Yes/No) concerning: (a) CPAP use and effectiveness (1–3), (b) common side effects (4–6), c) exercise, diet (7–9) and a final question to write down current weight (10). Table S2: CPAP compliance (h/night).

Author Contributions: Conceptualization, O.G., R.F. and J.M.M.; patient study and data acquisition, O.G., C.R., M.T., M.S.-G., R.C. and L.S.; data analysis, O.G., R.F. and J.M.M.; data discussion, M.T., M.S.-G., L.S. and C.M.; cost analysis, M.A.N.; writing—original draft preparation, O.G.; writing—review and editing, R.F., J.M.M.; funding acquisition, J.M.M. All authors have read and agreed to the published version of the manuscript.

Funding: This research was partially funded by Instituto de Salud Carlos III (Spain), grant number PI17/01068.

Institutional Review Board Statement: The study was conducted according to the guidelines of the Declaration of Helsinki, and approved by the Ethics Committee of Hospital Clínic de Barcelona (protocol code HCB/2017/1055, updated version approval date: 14 July 2020).

Informed Consent Statement: Informed consent was obtained from all subjects involved in the study.

Data Availability Statement: The details of data presented in this study are available on request from the corresponding author.

Acknowledgments: The authors wish to thank Albert Gabarrús for his help in statistical analysis, Andreu Vilalta and Hermes Carretero for their technical contribution to the development of APPnea, and Cristina Embid for her insightful comments on the work. The authors also thank the companies Esteve Teijin and Philips for giving unconditional partial support to the clinical research of the lab.

Conflicts of Interest: The authors declare no conflict of interest. The funders had no role in the design of the study, in the collection, analyses, or interpretation of data, in the writing of the manuscript, or in the decision to publish the results.

References

1. Bruyneel, M. Telemedicine in the diagnosis and treatment of sleep apnoea. *Eur. Respir. Rev.* **2019**, *28*, 180093. [CrossRef] [PubMed]
2. Benjafield, A.V.; Ayas, N.T.; Eastwood, P.R.; Heinzer, R.; Ip, M.S.M.; Morrell, M.J.; Nunez, C.M.; Patel, S.R.; Penzel, T.; Pépin, J.L.; et al. Estimation of the global prevalence and burden of obstructive sleep apnoea: A literature-based analysis. *Lancet Respir. Med.* **2019**, *7*, 687–698. [CrossRef]
3. Jordan, A.S.; McSharry, D.G.; Malhotra, A. Adult obstructive sleep apnoea. *Lancet* **2014**, *383*, 736–747. [CrossRef]
4. Sullivan, C.E.; Issa, F.G.; Berthon-Jones, M.; Eves, L. Reversal of obstructive sleep apnoea by continuous positive airway pressure applied through the nares. *Lancet* **1981**, *1*, 862–865. [CrossRef]
5. Van Ryswyk, E.; Anderson, C.S.; Antic, N.A.; Barbe, F.; Bittencourt, L.; Freed, R.; Heeley, E.; Liu, Z.; Loffler, K.A.; Lorenzi-Filho, G.; et al. Predictors of long-term adherence to continuous positive airway pressure in patients with obstructive sleep apnea and cardiovascular disease. *Sleep* **2019**, *42*, zsz152. [CrossRef]
6. McEvoy, R.D.; Antic, N.A.; Heeley, E.; Luo, Y.; Ou, Q.; Zhang, X.; Mediano, O.; Chen, R.; Drager, L.F.; Liu, Z.; et al. CPAP for Prevention of Cardiovascular Events in Obstructive Sleep Apnea. *N. Engl. J. Med.* **2016**, *375*, 919–931. [CrossRef]
7. Askland, K.; Wright, L.; Wozniak, D.R.; Emmanuel, T.; Caston, J.; Smith, I. Educational, supportive and behavioural interventions to improve usage of continuous positive airway pressure machines in adults with obstructive sleep apnoea. *Cochrane Database Syst. Rev.* **2020**, *4*, CD007736. [CrossRef]
8. Martínez-García, M.A.; Capote, F.; Campos-Rodríguez, F.; Lloberes, P.; Díaz de Atauri, M.J.; Somoza, M.; Masa, J.F.; González, M.; Sacristán, L.; Barbé, F.; et al. Effect of CPAP on blood pressure in patients with OSA and resistant hypertension: The HIPARCO trial. *JAMA* **2013**, *310*, 2407–2415. [CrossRef]
9. Barbé, F.; Durán-Cantolla, J.; Capote, F.; de la Peña, M.; Chiner, E.; Masa, J.F.; Gonzalez, M.; Marín, J.M.; Garcia-Rio, F.; de Atauri, J.D.; et al. Long-term effect of continuous positive airway pressure in hypertensive patients with sleep apnea. *Am. J. Respir. Crit. Care Med.* **2010**, *181*, 718–726. [CrossRef]
10. Weaver, T.E.; Maislin, G.; Dinges, D.F.; Bloxham, T.; George, C.F.; Greenberg, H.; Kader, G.; Mahowald, M.; Younger, J.; Pack, A.I. Relationship between hours of CPAP use and achieving normal levels of sleepiness and daily functioning. *Sleep* **2007**, *30*, 711–719. [CrossRef]
11. Isetta, V.; Negrín, M.A.; Monasterio, C.; Masa, J.F.; Feu, N.; Álvarez, A.; Campos-Rodriguez, F.; Ruiz, C.; Abad, J.; Vazquez-Polo, F.J.; et al. A Bayesian cost-effectiveness analysis of a telemedicine-based strategy for the management of sleep apnoea: A multicentre randomised controlled trial. *Thorax* **2015**, *70*, 1054–1061. [CrossRef]
12. Suarez-Giron, M.; Garmendia, O.; Lugo, V.; Ruiz, C.; Salord, N.; Alsina, X.; Farré, R.; Montserrat, J.M.; Torres, M. Mobile health application to support CPAP therapy in obstructive sleep apnoea: Design, feasibility and perspectives. *ERJ Open Res.* **2020**, *6*, 00220-2019. [CrossRef]
13. Pépin, J.L.; Tamisier, R.; Hwang, D.; Mereddy, S.; Parthasarathy, S. Does remote monitoring change OSA management and CPAP adherence? *Respirology* **2017**, *22*, 1508–1517. [CrossRef]

14. Shamim-Uzzaman, Q.A.; Bae, C.J.; Ehsan, Z.; Setty, A.R.; Devine, M.; Dhankikar, S.; Donskoy, I.; Fields, B.; Hearn, H.; Hwang, D.; et al. The use of telemedicine for the diagnosis and treatment of sleep disorders: An American Academy of Sleep Medicine update. *J. Clin. Sleep Med.* **2021**, *17*, 1103–1107. [CrossRef]
15. Garmendia, O.; Monasterio, C.; Guzmán, J.; Saura, L.; Ruiz, C.; Salord, N.; Negrín, M.A.; Izquierdo Sanchez, C.; Suarez-Girón, M.; Montserrat, J.M.; et al. Telemedicine Strategy for CPAP Titration and Early Follow-up for Sleep Apnea During COVID-19 and Post-Pandemic Future. *Arch. Bronconeumol.* **2021**, *57* (Suppl. 2), 56–58. [CrossRef]
16. Kuna, S.T. Optimizing Chronic Management of Adults with Obstructive Sleep Apnea. *Ann. Am. Thorac. Soc.* **2020**, *17*, 280–281. [CrossRef]
17. Lugo, V.; Villanueva, J.A.; Garmendia, O.; Montserrat, J.M. The role of telemedicine in obstructive sleep apnea management. *Expert Rev. Respir. Med.* **2017**, *11*, 699–709. [CrossRef]
18. Hwang, D.; Chang, J.W.; Benjafield, A.V.; Crocker, M.E.; Kelly, C.; Becker, K.A.; Kim, J.B.; Woodrum, R.R.; Liang, J.; Derose, S.F. Effect of Telemedicine Education and Telemonitoring on Continuous Positive Airway Pressure Adherence. The Tele-OSA Randomized Trial. *Am. J. Respir. Crit. Care Med.* **2018**, *197*, 117–126. [CrossRef]
19. Fietze, I.; Herberger, S.; Wewer, G.; Woehrle, H.; Lederer, K.; Lips, A.; Willes, L.; Penzel, T. Initiation of therapy for obstructive sleep apnea syndrome: A randomized comparison of outcomes of telemetry-supported home-based vs. sleep lab-based therapy initiation. *Sleep Breath.* **2021**, in press. [CrossRef]
20. Frasnelli, M.; Baty, F.; Niedermann, J.; Brutsche, M.H.; Schoch, O.D. Effect of telemetric monitoring in the first 30 days of continuous positive airway pressure adaptation for obstructive sleep apnoea syndrome—A controlled pilot study. *J. Telemed. Telecare* **2016**, *22*, 209–214. [CrossRef]
21. Aardoom, J.J.; Loheide-Niesmann, L.; Ossebaard, H.C.; Riper, H. Effectiveness of eHealth Interventions in Improving Treatment Adherence for Adults With Obstructive Sleep Apnea: Meta-Analytic Review. *J. Med. Internet Res.* **2020**, *22*, e16972. [CrossRef] [PubMed]
22. Pépin, J.L.; Bailly, S.; Rinder, P.; Adler, D.; Szeftel, D.; Malhotra, A.; Cistulli, P.A.; Benjafield, A.; Lavergne, F.; Josseran, A.; et al. CPAP Therapy Termination Rates by OSA Phenotype: A French Nationwide Database Analysis. *J. Clin. Med.* **2021**, *10*, 936. [CrossRef] [PubMed]
23. Peker, Y.; Glantz, H.; Eulenburg, C.; Wegscheider, K.; Herlitz, J.; Thunström, E. Effect of Positive Airway Pressure on Cardiovascular Outcomes in Coronary Artery Disease Patients with Nonsleepy Obstructive Sleep Apnea. The RICCADSA Randomized Controlled Trial. *Am. J. Respir. Crit. Care Med.* **2016**, *194*, 613–620. [CrossRef] [PubMed]
24. Bakker, J.P.; Weaver, T.E.; Parthasarathy, S.; Aloia, M.S. Adherence to CPAP: What Should We Be Aiming For, and How Can We Get There? *Chest* **2019**, *155*, 1272–1287. [CrossRef] [PubMed]
25. Murase, K.; Tanizawa, K.; Minami, T.; Matsumoto, T.; Tachikawa, R.; Takahashi, N.; Tsuda, T.; Toyama, Y.; Ohi, M.; Akahoshi, T.; et al. A Randomized Controlled Trial of Telemedicine for Long-Term Sleep Apnea Continuous Positive Airway Pressure Management. *Ann. Am. Thorac. Soc.* **2020**, *17*, 329–337. [CrossRef] [PubMed]
26. Rossi, V.A.; Stoewhas, A.C.; Camen, G.; Steffel, J.; Bloch, K.E.; Stradling, J.R.; Kohler, M. The effects of continuous positive airway pressure therapy withdrawal on cardiac repolarization: Data from a randomized controlled trial. *Eur. Heart J.* **2012**, *33*, 2206–2212. [CrossRef] [PubMed]
27. Guest, J.F.; Helter, M.T.; Morga, A.; Stradling, J.R. Cost effectiveness of using continuous positive airway pressure in the treatment of severe obstructive sleep apnoea/hypopnoea syndrome in the UK. *Thorax* **2008**, *63*, 860–865. [CrossRef]
28. Kapur, V.; Blough, D.K.; Sandblom, R.E.; Hert, R.; de Maine, J.B.; Sullivan, S.D.; Psaty, B.M. The medical cost of undiagnosed sleep apnoea. *Sleep* **1999**, *22*, 749–755. [CrossRef]
29. Knauert, M.; Naik, S.; Gillespie, M.B.; Kryer, M. Clinical consequences and economic costs of untreated obstructive sleep apnea syndrome. *World J. Otorhinolaryngol. Head Neck Surg.* **2015**, *1*, 17–27. [CrossRef]
30. Farré, R.; Navajas, D.; Montserrat, J.M. Is Telemedicine a Key Tool for Improving Continuous Positive Airway Pressure Adherence in Patients with Sleep Apnea? *Am. J. Respir. Crit. Care Med.* **2018**, *197*, 12–14. [CrossRef]

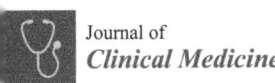

Article

A Pharyngoplasty with a Dorsal Palatal Flap Expansion: The Evaluation of a Modified Surgical Treatment Method for Obstructive Sleep Apnea Syndrome—A Preliminary Report

Ewa Olszewska [1,*], Piotr Fiedorczuk [2], Adam Stróżyński [3], Agnieszka Polecka [3], Ewa Roszkowska [4] and B. Tucker Woodson [5]

1. Department of Otolaryngology, Medical University of Bialystok, 15-328 Bialystok, Poland
2. Doctoral School of the Medical University of Bialystok, 15-328 Bialystok, Poland; piotr.fiedorczuk@umb.edu.pl
3. Medical University of Bialystok, 15-328 Bialystok, Poland; ad.strozynski@gmail.com (A.S.); polecka.aga@gmail.com (A.P.)
4. Faculty of Economics and Finance, University of Bialystok, 15-062 Bialystok, Poland; e.roszkowska@uwb.edu.pl
5. Department of Otolaryngology Medical, Division of Sleep Medicine and Upper Airway Reconstructive Surgery, Medical College Wisconsin, Milwaukee, WI 53226, USA; bwoodson@mcw.edu
* Correspondence: Ewa.Olszewska@umb.edu.pl; Tel.: +48-858318696

Abstract: Surgical techniques for obstructive sleep apnea syndrome (OSAS) constantly evolve. This study aims to assess the effectiveness and safety of a new surgical approach for an OSAS pharyngoplasty with a dorsal palatal flap expansion (PDPFEx). A total of 21 participants (mean age 49.9; mean BMI 32.5) underwent a type III sleep study, an endoscopy of the upper airways, a filled medical history, a visual analog scale for snoring loudness, an Epworth Sleepiness Scale, and a Short Form Health Survey-36 questionnaire. A follow-up re-evaluation was performed 11 ± 4.9 months post-operatively. The study group (4 with moderate, 17 with severe OSAS) showed an improvement in all measured sleep study characteristics ($p < 0.05$), apnea-hypopnea index (pre-median 45.7 to 29.3 post-operatively, $p = 0.009$, $r = 0.394$), oxygen desaturation index (pre-median 47.7 and 23.3 post-operatively, $p = 0.0005$, $r = 0.812$), mean oxygen saturation (median 92% pre-operatively and median 94% post-operatively, $p = 0.0002$, $r = 0.812$), lowest oxygen saturation ($p = 0.0001$, $r = 0.540$) and time of sleep spent with blood oxygen saturation less than 90% ($p = 0.0001$, $r = 0.485$). The most commonly reported complications were throat dryness (11 patients) and minor difficulties in swallowing (5 patients transient, 3 patients constant). We conclude that a PDPFEx is a promising new surgical method; however, further controlled studies are needed to demonstrate its safety and efficacy for OSAS treatment in adults.

Keywords: obstructive sleep apnea; sleep surgery; pharyngoplasty; dorsal palatal flap expansion

1. Introduction

Obstructive sleep apnea syndrome (OSAS) is a nocturnal disorder of multifactorial causes characterized by recurrent episodes of upper airway obstruction during sleep associated with oxygen desaturation and sleep fragmentation with a variety of methods to diagnose and treat. As a frequent and increasingly prevalent condition associated with serious comorbidities, it poses a great impact on public health [1].

1.1. Importance of OSAS

OSAS is a highly prevalent disorder estimated to be 9–38% in the general adult population; 13–33% in men and 6–19% in women [2]. Patients with untreated OSAS are at an increased risk of obesity, hypertension, diabetes mellitus, cardiovascular disease, heart failure, metabolic dysregulation, daytime sleepiness, depression, accidents, strokes, and death [3–6]. Obesity is also one of the major risk factors for OSAS and there has been a colossal increase in rates of obesity over the past decades around the world; therefore, the prevalence of OSAS could increase further in the coming years [7–9]. Therefore, it is important to identify and treat nocturnal breathing disorders early and effectively.

1.2. Management Options

The suspicion of OSAS arises from the symptoms of patients, such as snoring and apnea events observed by a bed partner, and frequent arousals assessed by a medical examination and by various questionnaires that measure daytime sleepiness, snoring, and the quality of life. OSAS is diagnosed with a sleep study that measures sleep parameters such as the apnea-hypopnea index (AHI), mean oxygen saturation, and the percentage of time spent with oxygen saturation below specified thresholds [3].

All the treatment methods aim to decrease the obstructive events, to improve the blood oxygen saturation of the patients during sleep, and to enhance the quality of life of both patients and their partners [10].

Treatment of OSAS includes non-surgical and surgical methods. The first-line management is a non-surgical approach involving the education of patients, which is the cornerstone of treatment for any medical condition. This should include a discussion of the pathophysiology, risk factors, and clinical consequences. The patient should be informed of the benefits of weight loss and behavior modification such as avoiding modifiable risk factors (e.g., tobacco smoking, drinking alcohol, sleeping pill administration). Conservative treatment is not successful for a large percentage of patients [11]. The primary treatment modality for OSAS is positive airway pressure therapy (PAP). Alternative or adjunct non-invasive methods that modify the position of the mandible, move the tongue forward, and widen the retrolingual airway, such as oral appliances including mandibular advancement devices, may be offered as per the anatomy, type, and severity of the OSAS of the patient as well as patient preferences. Additional, less established, non-operative management strategies include positional therapy (PT), transcutaneous electrical stimulation (TES), and drug therapy with steroids and leukotriene receptor antagonists [12].

In patients who are not compliant with or fail the PAP therapy, a variety of surgical methods have been used in the past decades. Of those, several surgical approaches are currently being utilized for the most common site of obstruction—the soft palate. Surgical techniques that aim to alter the lateral pharyngeal wall and soft palate at the level of the velopharynx and oropharynx include an expansion sphincter pharyngoplasty, a lateral pharyngoplasty, a relocation pharyngoplasty, a modified uvulopalatopharyngoplasty with uvula preservation, and a suspension palatoplasty [13].

1.3. Aim of This Study

The aim of this study is to assess the effectiveness and safety of a new technique of a surgical approach for an OSAS treatment pharyngoplasty with a dorsal palatal flap expansion (PDPFEx).

2. Materials and Methods

2.1. Ethical Approval and Informed Consent

The study was approved by the local Bioethics Committee. Participation in the study was voluntary. The participants were informed of the study and the data being collected. A written informed consent form (ICF) was obtained from each participant. The participants could withdraw their consent at any point of the study.

2.2. Study Design

This was a single-center prospective study with a case series study design for a modification of an expansion sphincter pharyngoplasty described by Puccia and Woodson as a pharyngoplasty with a dorsal palatal flap expansion [14].

2.2.1. Study Protocol

The study was conducted at the Department of Otolaryngology in a tertiary care hospital between May 2019 and June 2020. Patients with OSAS were enrolled based on inclusion and exclusion criteria. Surgeries for all cases were performed by the first author (EO).

The inclusion criteria were: (a) adult patients; (b) a moderate or severe OSAS (defined as an apnea-hypopnea index (AHI) of 15–29.9 and $\geq$30 events/h of sleep); (c) a body mass index (BMI) less than 40; (d) significant snoring with a visual analog scale (VAS) for snoring of 1–10 higher than 8 and (e) a failed PAP therapy.

We excluded patients with severe obesity (BMI $\geq$ 40), central sleep apnea syndrome, a sleep apnea treatment within the six months preceding the study, previous surgeries involving the hypopharynx and oropharynx areas, a history of rheumatic diseases, a respiratory infection within the previous four weeks, coagulation disorders, chronic or acute kidney failure (defined as serum creatinine > 2.0 mg/dL), the occurrence of other respiratory disorders including chronic obstructive pulmonary disease (diagnosis based on chest radiography and clinical history) or asthma, systemic inflammatory diseases, severe cardiovascular diseases, diabetes, comorbidities affecting systemic inflammation including cancer and collagen vascular disease, chronic rhinosinusitis or receiving medical treatment such as immune suppressors, hormones, free radical scavengers or cytotoxins.

All patients underwent the same procedures according to the study protocol based on a modified SLEEP-GOAL protocol [4]: a medical history, Epworth Sleepiness Scale (ESS) questionnaire, body mass index (BMI), an endoscopy of the upper airways, a sleep study type III polygraph (PG) and a surgical procedure. ESS is a self-conducted questionnaire consisting of eight questions involving the likelihoods of falling asleep in various situations such as sitting and reading, watching TV, sitting inactive in a public place, riding in a car for an hour without a break as a passenger, lying down in the afternoon to rest, sitting and talking to someone, sitting silently after a lunch without alcohol and sitting in a car stopped for a few minutes in traffic [15]. The patient assesses these options on a scale of 0 to 3 (0: never doze; 3: high chance of dozing). The total score can range from 0 to 24. In healthy adults, the normal range of sleepiness differs from 0 to 10. A higher score is associated with increased sleepiness [16]. Patients were asked to fill in the Short Form Health Survey-36 questionnaire (SF-36), which measures the subjective quality of life in both physical and mental health aspects by eight scales: physical functioning (PF), role physical (RP), bodily pain (BP), general health (GH), vitality (VT), social functioning (SF), role emotional (RE) and mental health (MH). Component analyses have shown that there are two distinct concepts measured by the SF-36 questionnaire: a physical dimension represented by the physical component summary (PCS) and a mental dimension represented by the mental component summary (MCS), all summarized as an SF-36 overall score.

2.2.2. Sleep Study

A PG was performed in each case using a type III sleep study device (SOMNOtouch, SOMNOmed). During the PG, the following parameters were evaluated for this study: mean oxygen saturation (MOS) and lowest oxygen saturation (LSAT), time of sleep spent with blood oxygen saturation less than 90% (SpO2 < 90), and the apnea-hypopnea index (AHI).

The AHI is described as the total number of apnea and hypopnea events per hour of sleep recorded in an overnight sleep study. Apneas are defined as at least a 90% decrease in airflow for at least 10 s and hypopneas as reduction of respiratory signals for at least 10 s associated with a minimum of 3% of oxygen desaturation [17]. MOS is estimated as normal varies between 94% and 98% during sleep [3].

2.3. Description of the Surgical Procedure

The surgical procedure was a further modification of an expansion sphincter pharyngoplasty, which was previously developed by Pang and Woodson to mitigate a fairly low success rate with a traditional uvulopalatopharyngoplasty in OSAS patients [18]. The current modification, hereby referred to as a pharyngoplasty with a dorsal palatal flap expansion (PDPFEx), was first described in print in 2020 by Puccia and Woodson (Figure 1) [14].

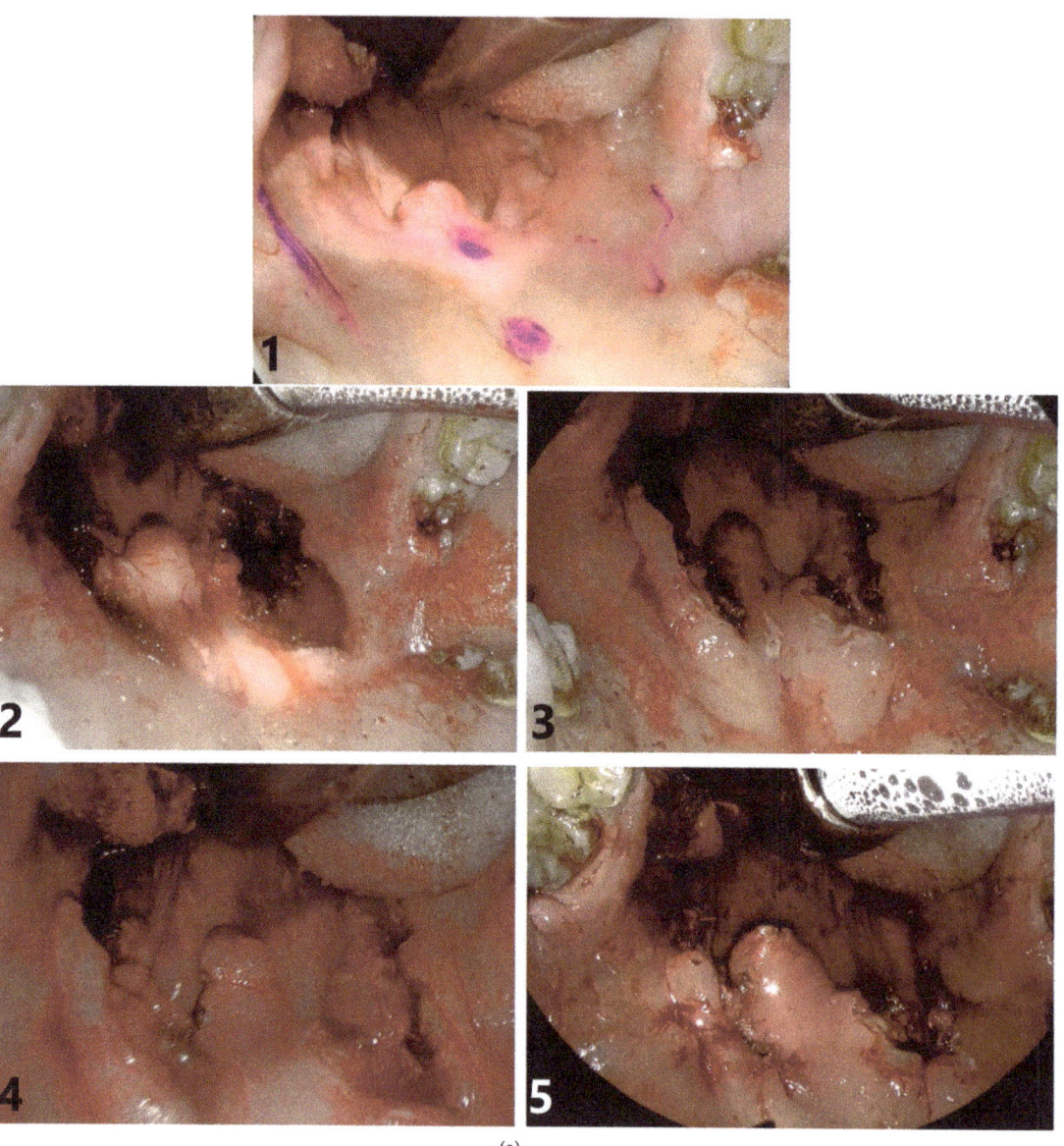

(a)

Figure 1. *Cont.*

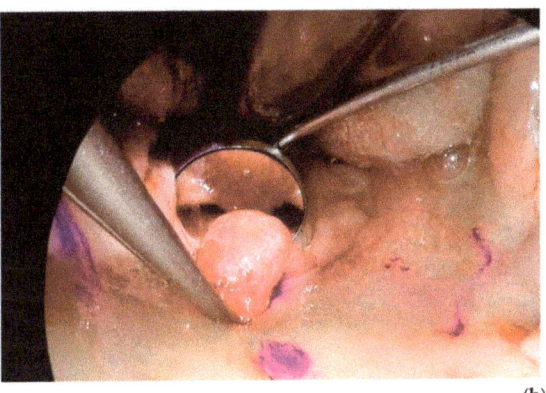
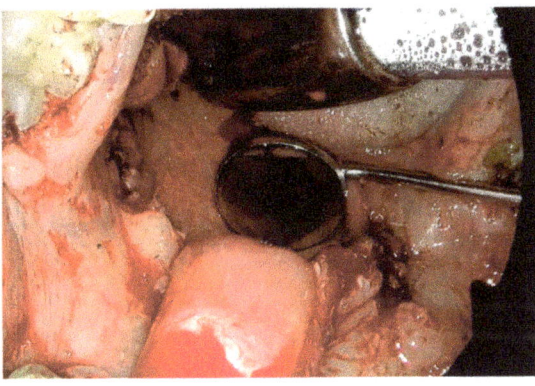

(b)

Figure 1. (a) Endoscopic view. 1: Surgery site with markings at the left and right pterygomandibular raphes, the base of the uvula and the hard palate; 2: palatal tonsils removed and ventral palate triangles of mucosa removed; 3: supratonsillar fat tissue removed and palatopharyngeus muscle dissected from the superior constrictor muscle; 4: dorsal palatal flaps rotated; left flap sutured in place and right flap prepared for suturing and 5: bilateral suturing of the dorsal flaps. (b) On the left: the retropalatal space before the surgery and the assessment of the length of the uvula for excising the tip. On the right: a significantly increased retropalatal space after the surgery and a view after removal of the enlarged uvula.

The surgical steps of a PDPFEx are: (1) the removal of the triangle (base of the triangle at the free edge of the palate on both sides of the uvula with the apex of the triangle extending anteriorly approaching the hard palate) of mucosa at the ventral palate to expose the surgical field; (2) the removal of supratonsillar fat tissue; (3) the dissection, incision and separation of the palatoglossal muscle and to expose the palatopharyngeus muscle; (4) dissection of the freeing of the palatopharyngeus muscle from the superior constrictor muscle; (5) a vertical incision on the dorsal palatal mucosa immediately lateral to the uvula and (6) the anterolateral rotation of this dorsal palatal mucosal flap, suturing it to the lateral edge of the ventral palatal mucosa.

2.4. Study Assessments

After surgery, the subjects were invited to a follow-up visit 4–6 months after the surgery. During the visits, the patients were examined by a medical professional and asked about complications regarding the post-surgery period, given the modified SLEEP-GOAL protocol (patient data, blood pressure, ESS score, snoring VAS, comorbidities, ENT examination results, SF-36 questionnaire). A post-surgery type III sleep study was given to the patients to obtain the sleep parameters.

2.5. Post-Operative Patient Care

The patients were closely monitored in hospital conditions for a median of 2 days after the procedure and were administered intravenous pain medications (paracetamol and metamizole; tramadol when the reported pain VAS was 6 or higher) and dexamethasone (to decrease the soft tissue edema). After they were discharged, the patients were prescribed all three pain medications to be taken orally for as long as the pain persisted.

2.6. Study Outcomes

The primary study outcomes consisted of differences in the AHI, ESS, and blood oxygen saturation characteristics established in sleep studies at the baseline and the follow-up.

2.7. Statistical Analysis

The statistical analysis was performed using GraphPad Prism 9. The results are presented as mean ± SD or a number of patients and a percentage of the whole study group. The categorical variables are presented as percentages. For a comparison of the results, the Wilcoxon signed-rank test was used. p-values < 0.05 were accepted as statistically significant.

3. Results

3.1. Study Group

A total of 21 patients (adult men) with an average age of 49.9 ± 12.2 (range 26–72 years old) were included in the study between May 2019 and June 2020. By polygraphy, 4 moderate OSAS (15 ≤ AHI < 30) and 17 severe OSAS (AHI ≥ 30) patients were identified. The biometrics of the patients (including the mean age (49.9 ± 12.2), mean weight (101.9 ± 10.2), and mean BMI (32.5 ± 3.4)) were taken; the blood pressure was measured and the mean arterial blood pressure was 105.4 ± 8.4. The MAP was calculated using the formula (Systolic+2(Diastolic)/:3. A total of 15 patients had existing comorbidities and cardiovascular complications including 5 patients with more than one comorbidity. The palatal anatomy of patients was assessed during an otorhinolaryngological examination; the Friedman Tongue Scale and the Friedman Palatine Tonsils Scale were used. Most of the patients were classified as Friedman Tongue position 3. The patients were asked to fill in ESS and snoring VAS questionnaires. The baseline group characteristics are provided in Table 1.

Table 1. Baseline characteristics of the study group (n = 21 male subjects).

Characteristic	Mean (SD)/n%	Min	Max
Biometrics			
Age (y)	49.9 (12.2)	26	72
Weight (kg)	101.9 (10.2)	85	120
Body Mass Index (kg/m^2)	32.5 (3.4)	26.3	39.7
BMI group I *	6–28.6%		
BMI group II *	10–47.6%		
BMI group III *	5–23.8%		
Mean Blood Pressure (mmHg)	105.4 (8.4)	90.7	121.3
Comorbidities	15–71.4%		
Hypertension	15–71.4%		
Diabetes Mellitus Type 2	4–19%		
Heart Disease	2–9.5%		
Anatomy and OSAS			
Friedman Tongue Position		2	4
Friedman Tongue Position 2	3–14.3%		
Friedman Tongue Position 3	16–76.2%		
Friedman Tongue Position 4	2–9.5%		
Friedman Palatine Tonsils Scale		1	3
Friedman Palatine Tonsils Scale 1	9–42.9%		
Friedman Palatine Tonsils Scale 2	7–33.3%		
Friedman Palatine Tonsils Scale 3	5–23.8%		
Epworth Sleepiness Scale	10.8 (5.7)	1	22
Apnea–Hypopnea Index	45.2 (15.9)	15.2	71.6
Moderate OSAS (15 ≤ AHI < 30)	4–19%		
Severe OSAS (AHI > 30)	17–81%		
Snoring Visual Analog Scale	9.4 (0.9)	8	10

* BMI range in this study: group I (normal weight or overweight) 18.5 to 29.9, group II (class I obesity) 30 to 34.9, group III (class II obesity) 35 to 39.9. Heart disease included arrhythmias, heart failure, heart valve disease, cardiomyopathy, and congenital heart disease.

3.2. Study Outcomes

The follow-up visits were held between May 2020 and December 2020, with a follow-up period that ranged from 4 to 21 months (median 11 months). All 21 patients completed their follow-up; however, the planned 4–6 month period was elongated by the COVID-19 global pandemic. The biometric characteristics of the study group (body weight, BMI, mean arterial blood pressure) did not change during the post-operative period. (Table 2).

Table 2. Study outcome results.

	Median Pre (IQR)	Median Post (IQR)	Significance	Effect Size r
Biometric Characteristics				
Weight	100.0 (92–111.5)	100.0 (93.5–109)	0.275	0.168
BMI	32.6 (29.7–34.8)	32.3 (30.1–34.1)	0.278	0.167
MAP	103.7 (98–111.4)	101.7 (93–109.7)	0.251	0.177
Questionnaires				
Snoring VAS	10 (8.5–10)	5 (4–6)	<0.0001	0.738
ESS	9.0 (7–17)	7.0 (2.5–9.5)	0.0025	0.442
SF-36	41.0 (27.5–58)	35.0 (19–53.3)	0.715	0.056

IQR: interquartile range; BMI: body mass index; MAP: mean arterial blood pressure; VAS: visual analog scale; ESS: Epworth Sleepiness Scale; SF-36: the Short Form Health Survey-36. The results were compared using the Wilcoxon signed-rank test.

There was an improvement in the subjective daytime sleepiness of patients as ranked by the ESS questionnaire score; there was a change in the ESS from a median of 9.0 (IQR 7–17) to 7.0 (IQR 2.5–9.5). No significant difference was observed in the self-reported quality of life assessed by the SF-36 questionnaire in any of the subscales, in the physical and mental component summary nor the SF-36 overall score (Figure 2).

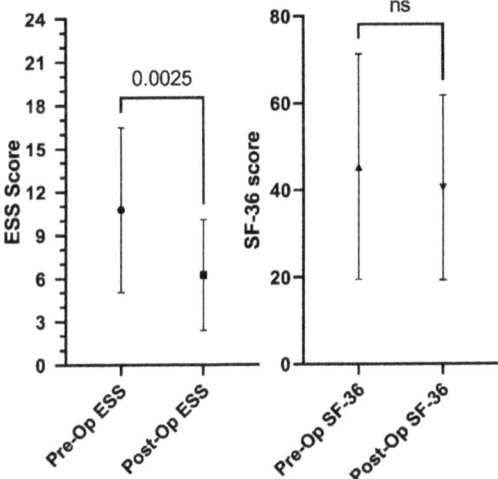

Figure 2. Pre- and post-operative comparison of the Epworth Sleepiness Scale and the SF-36 overall score. The exact *p*-value is shown above the columns.

Most patients in our study group reported a decrease in snoring loudness and inconvenience assessed with the snoring visual analog scale. The snoring VAS changed from a median of 10 (IQR 8.5–10) to 5 (IQR 4–6) (Figure 3).

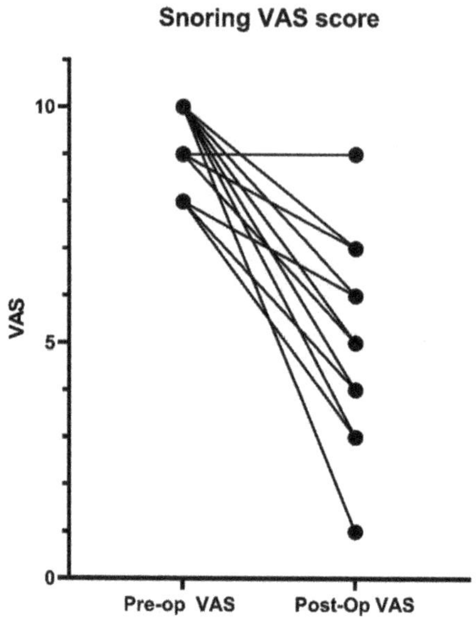

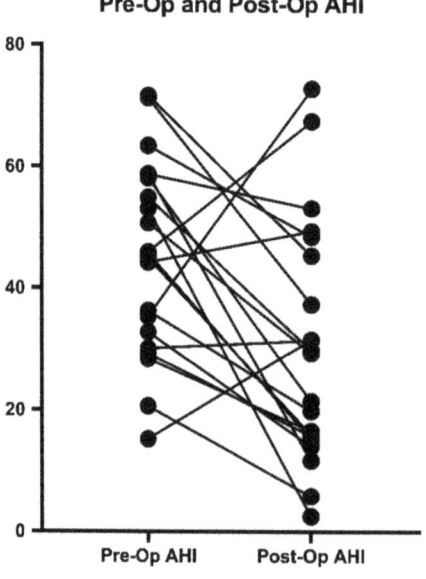

Figure 3. Pre- and post-operative comparison of the reported visual analog scale score for snoring loudness and inconvenience by the patients.

All subjects had a post-operative PG as well. When comparing the pre-operative and post-operative PG characteristics, we observed significant improvements in the AHI from a median of 45.7 (IQR 31.5–58.4) to 29.3 (IQR 15.5–46.9) and in the ODI from a median of 47.7 (IQR 34.7–57.1) to 23.3 (IQR 12.5–44.4) (Figures 4 and 5). There was a decrease in the AHI of 76.1% and a decrease in the ODI in 85.7% of the patients in the study group.

Figure 4. Individual pre- and post-operative AHI distribution. AHI: apnea-hypopnea index.

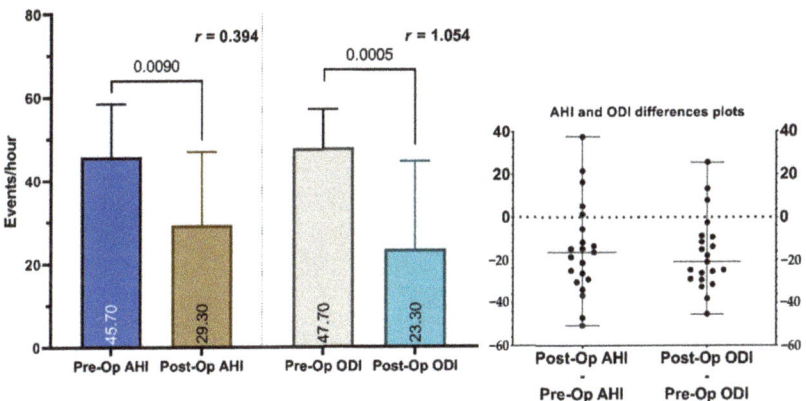

Figure 5. On the left side: a pre- and post-operative comparison of the apnea-hypopnea index and the oxygen desaturation index median and interquartile range values. The median values are shown inside the columns and the *p*-value is shown above the columns. The effect size (*r*-value) is shown above the columns. On the right side: differences plot for the AHI and ODI of individual patients. AHI: apnea-hypopnea index; ODI: oxygen desaturation index.

Our results showed a lower median of the pre-operative ODI than the pre-operative AHI (45.7 and 47.7, respectively) yet a Wilcoxon signed-rank test gave no statistical difference between the compared values ($p = 0.8986$). We observed a significant correlation between the two variables, as shown in Figure 6.

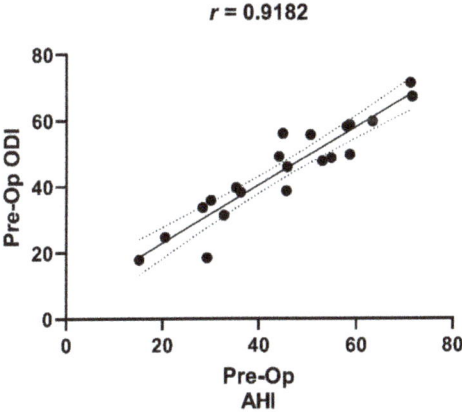

Figure 6. Correlation between the pre-operative AHI and ODI. AHI: apnea–hypopnea index; ODI: oxygen desaturation index; *r*: Spearman's rank correlation coefficient.

Additionally, we observed an improvement in the MOS from a median of 92.0 (IQR 90.3–94.0) to 94.0 (IQR 93.0–95.0), the LSAT from a median of 74.0 (IQR 68.5–81.5) to 82.0 (IQR 74.0–88.0) and the $SpO_2 < 90\%$ from a median of 19.8 (IQR 5.9–45.8) to 4.6 (IQR 0.3–17.3) (Figure 7).

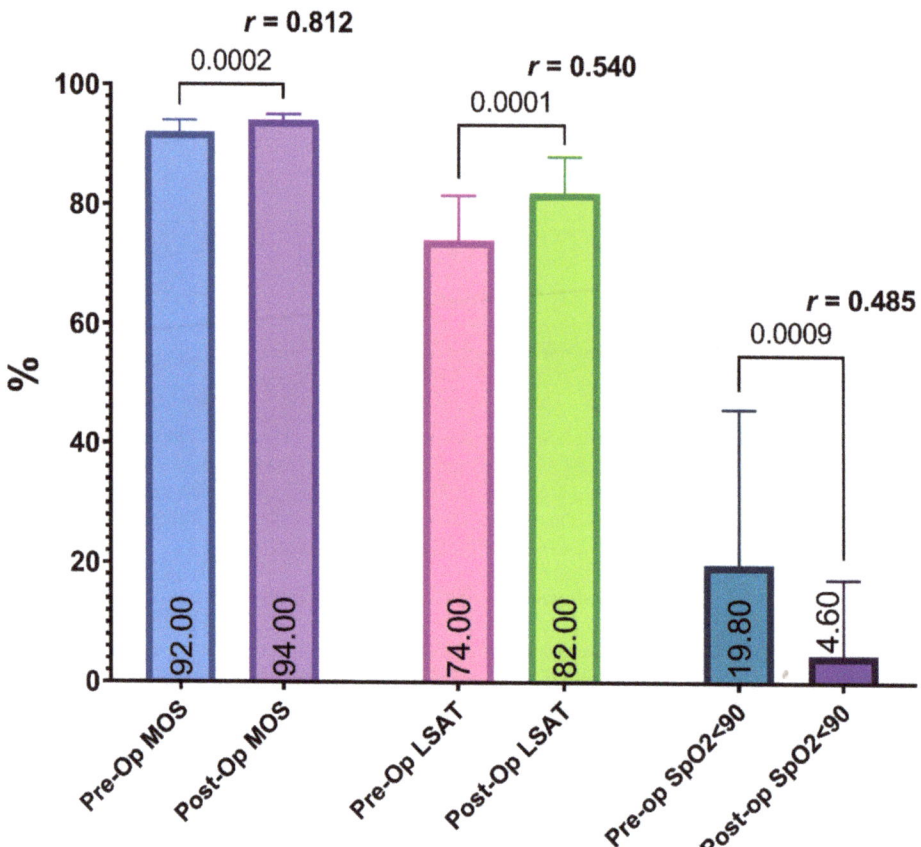

Figure 7. A pre- and post-operative comparison of the median and interquartile range values of the mean oxygen saturation, lowest oxygen saturation, and time of sleep spent with blood oxygen saturation less than 90%. The median values are shown inside the columns and the p-value is shown above the columns. The effect size (r-value) is shown above the columns.

3.3. Post-Operative Complications

After the hospital stay, patients were asked about post-operative pain (duration of pain in days, pain level described on the VAS scale, painkiller intake with a total of three recommended drugs and usage duration) and other symptoms such as throat dryness (prevalence, time of symptom onset and duration), palate hematoma (prevalence, time of symptom onset and duration), post-operative secondary hemorrhage (early (less than 10 days post-operative) and late (10 days or more post-operative)), difficulty in swallowing (prevalence, time of symptom onset and duration), impaired taste (prevalence, time of symptom onset and duration) and other post-operative remarks.

The post-operative pain persisted for a median of 14 days (IQR 10–21) with a median VAS of 8 (IQR 6–9). A total of 18 patients took all 3 medications and for 3 patients the pain was manageable without the opioid. The median drug use duration of the patients was a total of 14 days (IQR 14–21). In 63.2% of cases, the pain lasted for less than 14 days.

The most commonly reported complications were throat dryness and minor difficulties in swallowing. Figure 8 shows a graph of the occurrence of reported complications.

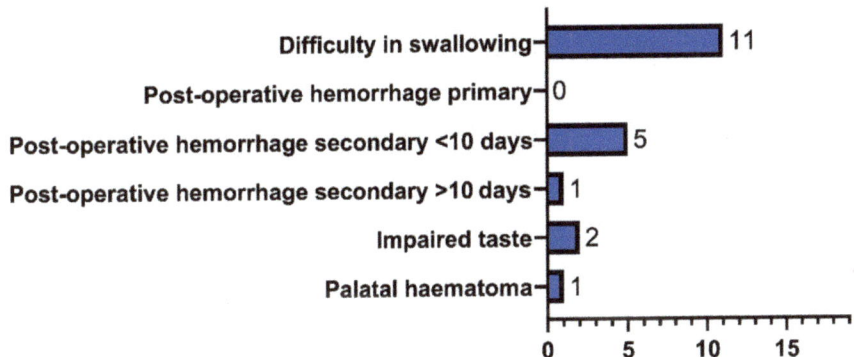

Figure 8. Post-operative symptom occurrence graph showing the number of patients with a post-operative complication.

Throat dryness was reported by 11 patients. In 9 cases, the symptom appeared immediately after the surgery, and 2 patients noticed the dryness a few days after. A total of 7 patients complained about the symptom for more than three months, 1 up to three months, 2 up to three weeks, and in 1 case the dryness lasted three days. Only 1 patient reported a palatal hematoma that appeared two days after the surgery and persisted for two weeks. No primary post-operative hemorrhage was observed but secondary bleeding occurred in 6 cases. A total of 8 patients described a difficulty in swallowing that appeared immediately after the surgery. Of those, 3 patients reported the difficulty for more than three months after; in 2 patients it lasted up to two months, 1 up to one month, and in 2 cases it lasted for two weeks. An impaired taste was noted by 2 patients and, in both cases, it lasted for more than three months. Other mentioned symptoms included a sense of thick mucus in the throat (3 cases), tongue numbness (2 cases), small amounts of blood in nasal discharge (1 case), cough (1 case), a sense of foreign body in the throat (1 case) and a gag reflex (1 case). No major post-operative complications, e.g., major bleeding or palatopharyngeal insufficiency, were noted.

4. Discussion

The goal for all pharyngoplasties is to widen the retropalatal airspace in both the anterior-posterior dimension and between the lateral pharyngeal walls and stiffen the tissues. Interrupting and re-directing the sphincteric action of palatopharyngeal muscles contributes to the widening of the space between the palate and the posterior pharyngeal wall and the lateral dimension of the pharynx. A pharyngoplasty with a dorsal palatal flap expansion has distinct steps that are contributory to each other. Each step is necessary for and facilitates the next. The removal of the anterior triangle of mucosa exposes the surgical field to remove the supratonsillar fat tissue, which exposes the palatoglossus and palatopharyngeus muscles and facilitates their dissection and manipulation. The removal and relocation of these intravelar tissues expose the mirror image of the anterior palatal mucosal triangle at the dorsal palatal mucosa. This dorsal palatal mucosal triangle is freed up by cutting at the medial limit to freely rotate anterolaterally along the axis of the lateral edge of this triangle to cover the lateral palatal space.

This new modification (PDPFEx) has distinct differences compared to the previous technique (ESP): (1) there is enhanced dissection and mobilization of the palatopharyngeus muscle to facilitate (provide space) for the creation and rotation of the dorsal palatal flap; (2) the preservation of the mucosa of the nasopharyngeal surface of the soft palate; (3) the use of this mucosa to cover the anterolateral raw surgical dissection field; (4) the shortening of the medial portion of the soft palate lateral to the uvula resulting in an increased anteroposterior dimension of the nasopharynx; (5) the repositioning of the uvula slightly more anteriorly; (6) the shortening of the elongated uvula due to the medial cuts for the dorsal palatal flap; (7) as a result of these same cuts lateral to the uvula that form the dorsal palatal flap, there is a reduction of the sphincter function of the transverse bundle of the palatopharyngeus muscle.

The success of pharyngoplasties depends on an accurate diagnostic assessment, good patient selection, a well-performed surgical technique, and an uncomplicated post-operative period. Here, we presented our experience with the new modification of the expansion sphincter pharyngoplasty technique for OSA treatment described by Woodson [14]. Having followed the described surgical protocol, we assessed the effectiveness and reported the promising outcomes as improvements in sleep parameters such as the AHI, ODI, MOS, LOS, and T < 90%. This correlation is consistent with the available literature, e.g., as reported by Hussain Basheer et al. who reported a similarly strong correlation between the ODI and AHI [19]. In all assessed sleep parameters, a significant improvement was observed at the final follow-up visit. Although our results were generally similar to those obtained by other authors, we observed a higher degree of improvement compared to the literature in several parameters such as the change in the percentage of lowest oxygen saturation post-operatively [10,20]. Our study may be limited by the number of patients; however, it was adequately powered to establish efficacy and statistical differences. On the other hand, this could partly be a sign of the "regression to the mean" or by random due to the small study sample. Plaza et al. conducted a prospective non-comparative multicenter study of patients who underwent an expansion sphincter pharyngoplasty procedure as a treatment for OSAS and showed a significant improvement in the AHI and ESS post-operatively; however, other sleep parameters were not presented [21]. El-Ahl and El-Anwar described that the lowest oxygen saturation increased significantly in a group of 24 patients with Friedman stage II and III of OSAS [22], which was consistent with our study. In all three publications mentioned above, there was no statistical difference between BMI before and after the surgery, which was similar to our results [10,20,21].

In our study, we compared the mean arterial pressure before and at the final follow-up visit and observed no change. Blood pressure also remained unchanged in the MacKay study [20]. Another parameter evaluated in our study group was the snoring loudness that changed after the surgical treatment. The VAS scale for snoring loudness showed a statistically significant difference. It may mean that this modified technique results in a decrease in pharyngeal tissue vibration.

Our results showed a relatively high percentage of pain on day 14 post-operatively. However, this was in part due to the patients who did not follow the pain management protocol strictly. Moreover, improved sleep parameters and favorable patient satisfaction outcomes may justify the relatively prolonged pain experience.

Pang et al. in their meta-analysis on the effectiveness of palatal surgery showed the superiority of more innovative, anatomically targeted surgical procedures over a traditional uvulopalatopharyngoplasty [23]. This conclusion was consistent with the research conducted by El-Ahl and El-Anwar [22]. Other studies have also shown good results after expansion techniques as a treatment for OSA but more information is needed to modify and improve the sleep surgery methods [24].

Although this current study was not controlled, comparing it to other techniques, we are in the process of expanding our series and designing future controlled studies with additional pre-and post-operative assessments to test the effectiveness of this technique. When the COVID-19 pandemic started in March 2020, several patients refused to submit to a post-operative follow-up in the scheduled time, which further increased the mean group follow-up period. Second, this study included a select population of individuals of white European origin only. Third, primal differences in the characteristics among patients—especially age, with the youngest participant at age 27—could affect the regeneration process and thus have an impact on the progress. Additionally, women were underrepresented in the trial. Therefore, the generalization of findings to sex, populations with a low prevalence of obesity, or people from other ethnic backgrounds was limited. Although the study was limited by the number of patients, it did establish efficacy and statistical differences in several variables. Another limitation involved the diagnosis of OSAS. In this case, we used study type III. We are aware of the limitations that this type of sleep study creates in quantifying the AHI and identifying arousals and in its inability to assess the sleep structure. However, in all participants, we conducted two-night sleep studies, which have advantages compared to one-night polysomnography (PSG). The first-night effect of the sleep study may be a limitation in the single-night PSGs. To reduce the negative impact of home sleep studies, the participants enrolled in our study were thoroughly instructed on how to put them on and how to use the device. Any individuals with comorbidities were excluded from the study. The Academy of Sleep Apnea approves the performance of a sleep study type III when the patient is free from significant comorbid conditions and for a pre-operative clinical evaluation [3,25]. Other studies have indicated that a home portable monitoring device showed a high level of diagnostic agreement between the home diagnostic sleep studies and a simultaneous PSG, especially when manually scored [26]. The difference between the home study and the AHI from the reference PSG as demonstrated by the authors was similar to the difference between the PSGs. Bibbins-Domingo et al. demonstrate that a home sleep study is recommended for the diagnosis of OSAS in uncomplicated patients with an increased risk of moderate-to-severe OSAS as a viable alternative to a PSG in selected circumstances [27]. In the current study, the sleep study was read manually by the first author.

Based on our previous experience and outcomes, we believe that the technique allowed for better control of the muscle tension and sphincteric activity of the palatopharyngeal muscle. Single-arm studies on a specific surgical technique may show better outcomes in a few variables compared to other techniques [18]. However, many potential variables related to the subject characteristics in these studies avoid the comparison of the outcomes between the techniques to draw conclusions. Randomized clinical trials that stratify the important subject factors facilitate such comparisons [10,28,29]. More studies are needed with larger sample sizes and control groups to better demonstrate the differences between the expansion techniques as well as to compare the effectiveness of a PDPFEx and nonsurgical treatment for OSA. Preliminary case series such as this may provide outcome data that may serve to assess the magnitude of the effect and the sample size calculation for a randomized clinical trial. On the other hand, comparing a PDPFEx to another technique with a similarly favorable outcome may not be feasible due to the required large sample size.

5. Conclusions

A better understanding of the palatal anatomy has been applied to reconstructive palatal surgery for the treatment of OSAS. The palatopharyngeus muscle is a major defining element of the palate and lateral pharyngeal wall. This muscle is the key to many current reconstructive pharyngoplasty techniques. This prospective single-center work on a new modification of a pharyngoplasty—a pharyngoplasty with dorsal palatal flap expansion—shows that this technique can provide good outcomes in patients with OSAS. This modification in the technique appears to have advantages in not only changing palatal muscle vectors and reducing the mass of tissues that vibrate and/or collapse but also by expanding the retropalatal space. However, this presumed mechanism remains speculative in the absence of objective measurements such as an MRI or DISE. Further studies should be conducted to adequately compare a PDPFEx with other surgical approaches regarding an improvement in sleep study characteristics and an increase in the quality of life and safety of patients.

Author Contributions: Conceptualization, E.O.; methodology, E.O.; software, P.F. and E.R.; validation, E.O.; formal analysis, E.O., E.R. and P.F.; investigation, E.O., P.F., A.S. and A.P.; resources, E.O., P.F.; data curation, E.O., P.F., A.S. and A.P.; writing—original draft preparation, E.O., P.F., A.S. and A.P.; writing—review and editing, E.O., P.F., A.S., A.P. and B.T.W.; visualization, E.O., P.F.; supervision, E.O.; project administration, E.O. All authors have read and agreed to the published version of the manuscript.

Funding: This research received no external funding.

Institutional Review Board Statement: The study was conducted according to the guidelines of the Declaration of Helsinki and approved by the Ethics Committee of Medical University of Bialystok (no. R-I002/535/2017).

Informed Consent Statement: Informed consent was obtained from all subjects involved in the study.

Data Availability Statement: The data presented in this study are available on request from the corresponding author. The data are not publicly available.

Conflicts of Interest: The authors declare no conflict of interest.

References

1. Morsy, N.E.; Farrag, N.S.; Zaki, N.F.W.; Badawy, A.Y.; Abdelhafez, S.A.; El-Gilany, A.-H.; El Shafey, M.M.; Pandi-Perumal, S.R.; Spence, D.W.; BaHammam, A.S. Obstructive sleep apnea: Personal, societal, public health, and legal implications. *Rev. Environ. Health* **2019**, *34*, 153–169. [CrossRef]
2. Senaratna, C.V.; Perret, J.L.; Lodge, C.J.; Lowe, A.J.; Campbell, B.E.; Matheson, M.C.; Hamilton, G.S.; Dharmage, S.C. Prevalence of obstructive sleep apnea in the general population: A systematic review. *Sleep Med. Rev.* **2017**, *34*, 70–81. [CrossRef]
3. Kapur, V.K.; Auckley, D.H.; Chowdhuri, S.; Kuhlmann, D.C.; Mehra, R.; Ramar, K.; Harrod, C.G. Clinical Practice Guideline for Diagnostic Testing for Adult Obstructive Sleep Apnea: An American Academy of Sleep Medicine Clinical Practice Guideline. *J. Clin. Sleep Med.* **2017**, *13*, 479–504. [CrossRef]
4. Pang, K.P.; Baptista, P.M.J.; Olszewska, E.; Braverman, I.; Carrasco-Llatas, M.; Kishore, S.; Chandra, S.; Yang, H.C.; Chan, Y.H.; Pang, K.A.; et al. SLEEP-GOAL: A multicenter success criteria outcome study on 302 obstructive sleep apnoea (OSA) patients. *Med. J. Malaysia* **2020**, *75*, 117–123. [PubMed]
5. Redline, S.; Yenokyan, G.; Gottlieb, D.J.; Shahar, E.; O'Connor, G.T.; Resnick, H.E.; Diener-West, M.; Sanders, M.H.; Wolf, P.A.; Geraghty, E.M.; et al. Obstructive sleep apnea–hypopnea and incident stroke: The sleep heart health study. *Am. J. Respir. Crit. Care Med.* **2010**, *182*, 269–277. [CrossRef] [PubMed]
6. Olszewska, E.; Panek, J.; O'Day, J.; Rogowski, M. Usefulness of snoreplasty in the treatment of simple snoring and mild obstructive sleep apnea/hypopnea syndrome—Preliminary report. *Otolaryngol. Polska* **2014**, *68*, 184–188. [CrossRef] [PubMed]
7. Benjafield, A.V.; Ayas, N.T.; Eastwood, P.R.; Heinzer, R.; Ip, M.S.M.; Morrell, M.J.; Nunez, C.M.; Patel, S.R.; Penzel, T.; Pépin, J.-L.D.; et al. Estimation of the global prevalence and burden of obstructive sleep apnoea: A literature-based analysis. *Lancet Respir. Med.* **2019**, *7*, 687–698. [CrossRef]
8. Young, T.; Peppard, P.E.; Taheri, S. Excess weight and sleep-disordered breathing. *J. Appl. Physiol.* **2005**, *99*, 1592–1599. [CrossRef] [PubMed]
9. Peppard, P.E.; Young, T.; Palta, M.; Dempsey, J.; Skatrud, J. Longitudinal study of moderate weight change and sleep-disordered breathing. *JAMA* **2000**, *284*, 3015–3021. [CrossRef]
10. MacKay, S.; Carney, A.S.; Catcheside, P.G.; Chai-Coetzer, C.L.; Chia, M.; Cistulli, P.A.; Hodge, J.-C.; Jones, A.; Kaambwa, B.; Lewis, R.; et al. Effect of multilevel upper airway surgery vs medical management on the apnea-hypopnea index and patient-reported daytime sleepiness among patients with moderate or severe obstructive sleep apnea. The SAMS randomized clinical trial. *JAMA* **2020**, *324*, 1168–1179. [CrossRef]
11. Friedman, M.; Ibrahim, H.; Bass, L. Clinical staging for sleep-disordered breathing. *Otolaryngol. Head Neck Surg.* **2002**, *127*, 13–21. [CrossRef] [PubMed]
12. Tingting, X.; Danming, Y.; Xin, C. Non-surgical treatment of obstructive sleep apnea syndrome. *Eur. Arch. Oto Rhino Laryngol.* **2018**, *275*, 335–346. [CrossRef] [PubMed]
13. Olszewska, E.; Woodson, B.T. Palatal anatomy for sleep apnea surgery. *Laryngoscope Investig. Otolaryngol.* **2019**, *4*, 181–187. [CrossRef]
14. Puccia, R.; Woodson, B.T. Palatopharyngoplasty and Palatal Anatomy and Phenotypes for Treatment of Sleep Apnea in the Twenty-first Century. *Otolaryngol. Clin. N. Am.* **2020**, *53*, 421–429. [CrossRef] [PubMed]
15. Johns, M.W. A New Method for measuring daytime sleepiness: The epworth sleepiness scale. *Sleep* **1991**, *14*, 540–545. [CrossRef] [PubMed]
16. Johns, M.W. Reliability and factor analysis of the epworth sleepiness scale. *Sleep* **1992**, *15*, 376–381. [CrossRef] [PubMed]
17. Pevernagie, D.A.; Gnidovec-Strazisar, B.; Grote, L.; Heinzer, R.; McNicholas, W.T.; Penzel, T.; Randerath, W.; Schiza, S.; Verbraecken, J.; Arnardottir, E.S. On the rise and fall of the apnea-hypopnea index: A historical review and critical appraisal. *J. Sleep Res.* **2020**, *29*. [CrossRef] [PubMed]
18. Pang, K.P.; Woodson, B.T. Expansion sphincter pharyngoplasty: A new technique for the treatment of obstructive sleep apnea. *Otolaryngol. Head Neck Surg.* **2007**, *137*, 110–114. [CrossRef] [PubMed]
19. Basheer, H.; Sharma, S.; Patel, M. Can we use the oxygen desaturation index alone to reliably diagnose obstructive sleep apnoea in obese patients? *Eur. Respir. J.* **2016**, *48*. [CrossRef]

20. Mackay, S.G.; Carney, A.S.; Woods, C.P.D.; Antic, N.P.D.; McEvoy, R.D.; Chia, M.; Sands, T.; Jones, A.; Hobson, J.; Robinson, S. Modified Uvulopalatopharyngoplasty and Coblation Channeling of the Tongue for Obstructive Sleep Apnea: A Multi-Centre Australian Trial. *J. Clin. Sleep Med.* **2013**, *9*, 117–124. [CrossRef] [PubMed]
21. Plaza, G.; Baptista, P.; O'Connor-Reina, C.; Bosco, G.; Pérez-Martín, N.; Pang, K.P. Prospective multi-center study on expansion sphincter pharyngoplasty. *Acta Otolaryngol.* **2019**, *139*, 219–222. [CrossRef]
22. El-Ahl, M.A.S.; El-Anwar, M.W. Expansion Pharyngoplasty by New Simple Suspension Sutures without Tonsillectomy. *Otolaryngol. Head Neck Surg.* **2016**, *155*, 1065–1068. [CrossRef]
23. Pang, K.P.; Plaza, G.; Baptista, P.M.; O'Connor-Reina, C.; Chan, Y.H.; Pang, K.A.; Pang, E.B.; Wang, C.M.Z.; Rotenberg, B. Palate surgery for obstructive sleep apnea: A 17-year meta-analysis. *Eur. Arch. Oto Rhino Laryngol.* **2018**, *275*, 1697–1707. [CrossRef]
24. Despeghel, A.-S.; Mus, L.; Dick, C.; Vlaminck, S.; Kuhweide, R.; Lerut, B.; Speleman, K.; Vinck, A.-S.; Vauterin, T. Long-term results of a modified expansion sphincter pharyngoplasty for sleep-disordered breathing. *Eur. Arch. Oto Rhino Laryngol.* **2017**, *274*, 1665–1670. [CrossRef]
25. Nilius, G.; Domanski, U.; Schroeder, M.; Franke, K.-J.; Hogrebe, A.; Margarit, L.; Stoica, M.; D'Ortho, M.-P. A randomized controlled trial to validate the Alice PDX ambulatory device. *Nat. Sci. Sleep* **2017**, *9*, 171–180. [CrossRef] [PubMed]
26. Chesson, A.L.; Berry, R.B.; Pack, A. Practice parameters for the use of portable monitoring devices in the investigation of suspected obstructive sleep apnea in adults. *Sleep* **2003**, *26*, 907–913. [CrossRef]
27. Bibbins-Domingo, K.; Grossman, D.C.; Curry, S.J.; Davidson, K.W.; Epling, J.W.; Garcia, F.A.R.; Herzstein, J.; Kemper, A.R.; Krist, A.H.; Kurth, A.E.; et al. Screening for obstructive sleep apnea in adults. US preventive services task force recommendation statement. *JAMA* **2017**, *317*, 407–414. [CrossRef]
28. Browaldh, N.; Nerfeldt, P.; Lysdahl, M.; Bring, J.; Friberg, D. SKUP3randomised controlled trial: Polysomnographic results after uvulopalatopharyngoplasty in selected patients with obstructive sleep apnoea. *Thorax* **2013**, *68*, 846–853. [CrossRef] [PubMed]
29. Sundman, J.; Friberg, D.; Bring, J.; Lowden, A.; Nagai, R.; Browaldh, N. Sleep Quality after Modified Uvulopalatopharyngoplasty: Results from the SKUP3 Randomized Controlled Trial. *Sleep* **2018**, *41*. [CrossRef] [PubMed]

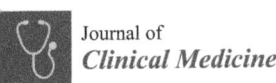

Article

Combined Transoral Robotic Tongue Base Surgery and Palate Surgery in Obstructive Sleep Apnea Syndrome: Modified Uvulopalatopharyngoplasty versus Barbed Reposition Pharyngoplasty

Yung-An Tsou [1,2,3], Chun-Chieh Hsu [1], Liang-Chun Shih [1,4], Tze-Chieh Lin [1], Chien-Jen Chiu [1], Vincent Hui-Chi Tien [1,3], Ming-Hsui Tsai [1,2,3] and Wen-Dien Chang [5,*]

[1] Department of Otolaryngology Head and Neck Surgery, China Medical University Hospital, Taichung 40402, Taiwan; d22052121@gmail.com (Y.-A.T.); jayhsu0522@gmail.com (C.-C.H.); entdrshih7111@gmail.com (L.-C.S.); drofarmyhospital@yahoo.com.tw (T.-C.L.); blueness1103@hotmail.com (C.-J.C.); vincenttien0623@asia.edu.tw (V.H.-C.T.); minghsui5121@gmail.com (M.-H.T.)
[2] School of Medicine, China Medical University, Taichung 40402, Taiwan
[3] Department of Audiology and Speech-Language Pathology, Asia University, Taichung 41354, Taiwan
[4] Graduate Institute of Biomedical Sciences, China Medical University, Taichung 40402, Taiwan
[5] Department of Sport Performance, National Taiwan University of Sport, Taichung 404401, Taiwan
* Correspondence: changwendien@ntus.edu.tw; Tel.: +886-4-22213108

Abstract: Background: Successful surgery outcomes are limited to moderate to severe obstructive sleep apnea (OSA) syndrome. Multilevel collapse at retropalatal and retroglossal areas is often found during the drug-induced sleep endoscopy (DISE). Therefore, multilevel surgery is considered for these patients. The aim of our study was to survey surgical outcomes by modified uvulopalatoplasty (UPPP) plus transoral robotic surgery tongue base reduction (TORSTBR) versus barbed repositioning pharyngoplasty (BRP) plus TORSTBR. Methods: The retrospective cohort study was performed at a tertiary referral center. We collected moderate to severe OSA patients who were not tolerant to positive pressure assistant PAP from September 2016 to September 2019; pre-operative–operative Muller tests all showed retropalatal and retroglossal collapse; pre-operative Friedman Tongue Position (FTP) > III, with the tonsils grade at grade II minimum, with simultaneous velum (V > 1) and tongue base (T > 1), collapsed by drug-induced sleep endoscopy (DISE) under the VOTE grading system. The UPPP plus TORSTBR ($n = 31$) and BRP plus TORSTBR ($n = 31$) techniques were offered. We compare the outcomes using an Epworth sleepiness scale (ESS) questionnaire, and measure the patients' apnea–hypopnea index (AHI), lowest O_2 saturation, cumulative time spent below 90% (CT90), and arousal index (AI) by polysomnography six months after surgery; we also measure their length of hospital stay and complications between these two groups. Results: Comparing BRP plus TORSTBR with UPPP plus TORSTBR, the surgical success rate is 67.74% and 38.71%, respectively. The significantly higher surgical success rate in the BRP plus TORSTBR group was noted. The surgical time is shorter in the BRP plus TORSTBR group. The complication rate is not significant in pain, bleeding, dysgeusia, dysphagia, globus sensation, and prolonged suture stay, even though the BRP plus TORSTBR rendered a higher percentage of globus sensation during swallowing and a more prevalent requirement of suture removal one month after surgery. The length of hospital stay is not significantly different between the two groups. Conclusion: In conclusion, BRP plus TORSTBR is a considerable therapy for moderate to severe OSA patients with DISE showing a multi-level collapse in velum and tongue base area. The BRP technique might offer a better anterior–posterior suspension vector for palate level obstruction.

Keywords: obstructive sleep apnea; uvulopalatoplasty; barbed repositioning pharyngoplasty; transoral robotic surgery tongue base reduction

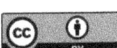

1. Introduction

Patients with obstructive sleep apnea (OSA) often have breathing problems in their sleep due to partial or complete upper airway obstruction. In clinical research, the incidence of symptomatic OSA in male patients was higher than that in females, and the male to female prevalence ratio of OSA was 8:1 [1]. OSA often accompanied circulatory system diseases, such as coronary heart disease, hypertension, and heart failure [2]. There were also reported correlations of OSA to diabetes, Parkinsonism, Alzheimer's disease, or dementia [3–6]. In fact, olfactory disorders were demonstrated as being associated with OSAS, with a significant linear correlation of threshold, discrimination, and identification (TDI) parameters and apnea–hypopnea index (AHI) [7]. Sleep surgery is important to improve life quality and decrease the symptoms of OSA patients [8]. Surgical treatment is one strategy to reduce the obstruction in OSA. Sleep surgery removes the obstructive tissue and enhances the cross-sectional airway area [8]. Surgeries for OSA focus on the management of the tongue base, which is an anatomic target, and remove the retroglossal airway and oropharyngeal obstructions in OSA patients [9]. Transoral robotic surgery (TORS) is a novel surgical technique for OSA patients and provides a visual assistant in targeted tissue operation for surgeons [10]. In addition, it also provides access to the retrolingual area, allowing the removal of the results of recurrent lingual tonsillitis, which, in patients who previously underwent tonsillectomies, can considerably reduce the air space [11].

Uvulopalatopharyngoplasty (UPPP) is a commonly performed surgery for OSA. Undergoing UPPP, the OSA patients had their tonsils resected and their uvula and soft palate removed [12]. A previous study presented that UPPP with transoral robotic tongue base reduction (TORSTBR) had the same rate of success as other surgical techniques, i.e., coblation tongue base resection and upper airway stimulation, and had clinical effects on the improvements in AHI, lowest O_2 saturation, and the Epworth sleepiness scale (ESS) for OSA [13]. Lan et al. recommended that TORSTBR combined with UPPP could effectively reduce disease severity in patients with moderate to severe OSA [14]. However, UPPP demonstrated important fibrotic and stenotic complications secondary to the method; therefore, the procedure should be considered carefully for OSAS treatment. The tongue base is currently a crucial factor for moderate and severe OSA and could be effectively treated by TORSTBR. TORSTBR combined palatal surgery is also widely accepted by sleep surgeons all around the world, which provides better surgical results [15,16]. The barbed repositioning pharyngoplasty (BRP) is a recent surgical technique, and using a barbed suture allows for uninterruption of the muscular and mucosal structures [17]. BRP is a quick surgical procedure and is considered safe, feasible, and effective for OSA [17]. However, the surgical outcome is limited in moderate to severe OSA patients, since most of them have multilevel obstructions, including simultaneous retropalatal and retrolingual obstructions [18]. The appropriate surgical treatment should be multilevel, and there is still a lack of suitable surgical techniques for UPPP or BRP with TORSTBR in moderate to severe OSA patients. Therefore, we performed two kinds of multilevel surgery for moderate to severe OSA patients, including transoral robotic tongue base reduction with simultaneous different palatal surgeries by BRP or UPPP plus TORSTBR, and we compared the functional outcome and success rate in the patients with moderate to severe OSA.

2. Methods

2.1. Study Procedures

We conducted a retrospective case series with two comparative groups (UPPP plus TORSTRB, BRP plus TORSTBR) to survey these two surgical outcomes for patients with moderate to severe sleep apnea syndrome. This study was registered with the Research Ethics Committee of China Medical University and Hospital. Clinically, all of the patients were enrolled because of sleep apnea with loud snoring and symptoms of daytime sleepiness. Patients included in the study were 20 years or older, had an AHI over 15, and had more than three months postoperative polysomnography to diagnose their OSA as moderate to severe. All the PSG was performed overnight in a CMUH sleep center (Level I sleep study). Physical examinations revealed at least grade II enlarged tonsils, Grade III Mallampati score, and a thick soft palate with an elongated uvula [19]. Drug-induced sleep endoscopy was performed for all the patients. All patients revealed vellum anterior–posterior collapse over 50% and oropharyngeal lateral 50% collapse, reaching the Friedman grade II of lingual tonsils hypertrophy without epiglottic collapse by drug-induced sleep endoscopy (DISE) under the VOTE grading system [20]. In addition, all patients underwent PSG, which revealed at least moderate and severe OSA. The patients without a bulky tongue or those who were diagnosed to have mild sleep apnea were excluded from our study. Following diagnosis, all patients underwent multilevel surgery for managing multilevel obstruction by TORSTBR surgery with simultaneous palatal surgery by barbed suspension pharyngoplasty or modified UPPP in CMUH from September 2016 to September 2019. All patients who underwent either UPPP plus TORSTBR or BRP plus TORSTBR were enrolled. Informed consent for surgery was signed by both the sleep surgeon and patients.

2.2. Participants

The 109 charts of OSA patients undergoing BRP or UPPP plus TORSTBR from September 2016 to September 2019 were reviewed. The included participants ($n = 62$) were informed of the study process, and informed consent for a retrospective review of their medical records was obtained before the study. We retrospectively reviewed patients who underwent BRP plus TORSTBR ($n = 31$) and UPPP plus TORSTBR ($n = 31$) groups. All of the tongue base volume resected was at least over 3 mL in both groups. (Figure 1). All participants and one researcher, a statistician, who analyzed the outcomes data, were unaware of the two surgical methods in this study.

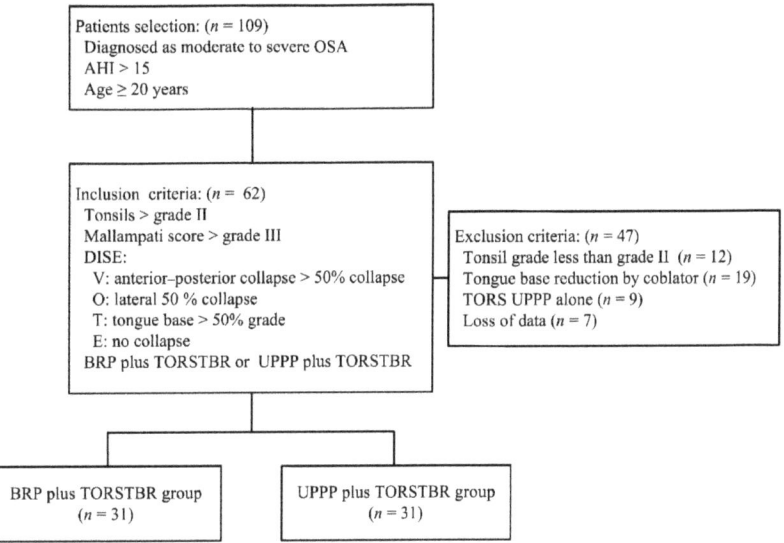

Figure 1. The flow chart of the current study. OSA, obstructive sleep apnea; AHI, apnea–hypopnea index; BRP, barbed repositioning pharyngoplasty; TORSTBR, transoral robotic tongue base reduction; UPPP, uvulopalatopharyngoplasty.

2.3. Surgical Technique of BRP and UPPP

In the BRP plus TORSTBR group (Figure 2A,B), barbed suspension pharyngoplasty was performed using a barbed suture V-Loc™ wound closure device in the soft palate for increasing anterior–posterior and lateral space velum and stiffness of the soft palate. We used two V-Loc sutures and started bidirectional suturing after tonsillectomy from the posterior nasal spine (midline of the junction of the soft palate and hard palate) through to the posterior pillar and back to the soft palate, reintroducing the needle close to the point of exit toward to pterygomandibular raphe near maxillary tuberosity, and then the lateral pharyngeal wall, and repeatedly anchoring to the pterygomandibular raphe [17]. The procedure was repeated on the other side. The palatopharyngeal muscle was neither divided nor repositioned.

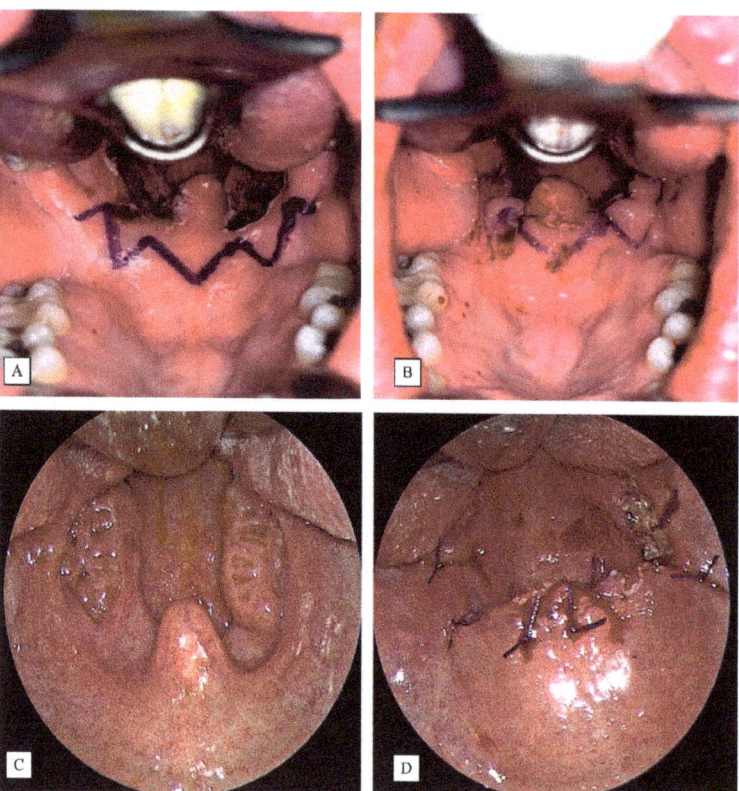

Figure 2. Before (**A**) and after (**B**) barbed suspension pharyngoplasty in the BRP plus TORSTBR group; before (**C**) and after (**D**) modified UPPP in the UPPP plus TORSTBR group.

In the UPPP plus TORSTBR group (Figure 2C,D), the surgery was under general anesthesia, and the patient was put in a supine position with a shoulder roll for neck extension. The Crowe–Davis mouth gag was applied for mouth opening. After a good surgical view is gained, the same was secured for the bilateral. Tonsillectomy was performed first by incising a 1 cm anterior tonsillar pillar cut above the upper pole of the palatine tonsil using a #15 blade and then dissecting the tonsillar capsule off the underlying palatal pharyngeal muscles [21]. A cold knife instrument was used, and the bleeder was stopped by bipolar electrocautery. Then, we preserved the posterior tonsillar pillar for less tension by suturing the posterior tonsillar pillar to the anterior tonsillar pillar by 3-0 vicryls sutures interruptedly from the upper tonsillar fossa towards the tongue. The uvulectomy was not routinely performed, except in instances where there was a longer uvula that was redundant to the tongue base. Most of the uvulas were not resected and preserved in our UPPP group patients.

2.4. TORSTBR

All patients underwent TORSTBR under general anesthesia by nasotracheal intubation [22,23]. The tongue base was exposed by a laryngeal advanced retractor system (Fentex, Tuttlingen, Germany) using the proper size of tongue blade in order to expose the tongue base. Then, the lingual tonsillectomy, including partial trimming of the tongue base musculature, was performed under a 30-degree 3D camera endoscope by the monopolar electrode. The resection area was 1.5 cm posterior to the foramen cecum. The width of resection was 3 cm (1.5 cm apart from mid-line tongue base bilaterally), and the depth of resection was 1.5 cm from the surface of the tongue base. The resection was performed until the epiglottis was visible, without injury to the epiglottis mucosa.

2.5. Assessments

Following the normal medical care process, all OSA patients were assessed using polysomnography (PSG) and ESS by the same otolaryngologist before and after the operations. The assessments were conducted in a sleep medicine center of CMUH.

2.5.1. Polysomnography

The standard PSG was used to analyze the patients in accordance with the American Academy of Sleep Medicine (AASM) guidelines [24]. All OSA patients were assessed using PSG and ESS by the same otolaryngologist before and at least six months after surgery. The AHI, minimum $SpO_2\%$, cumulative time spent below 90% (CT90), and arousal index (AI) were analyzed. AHI was calculated using the sum of apneas and hypopneas by sleep hours and classified as mild (AHI = 5–15), moderate (AHI = 16–29), and severe (AHI $\geq$ 30) [25]. Surgical success has been traditionally defined as a reduction in the AHI by 50% and AHI < 20 after surgery. The criteria for a treatment cure are defined as an AHI < 5 after treatment.

2.5.2. Epworth Sleepiness Scale

The ESS is a self-administered questionnaire with eight items. A 4-point scale was used to measure the falling asleep probability. The total score of ESS was a range from 0 to 24, and a higher ESS represented the higher daytime sleepiness [26].

2.5.3. Follow-Up Assessments

In the follow-up of clinical care, the patients in both BRP plus TORSTBR and UPPP plus TORSTBR groups were monitored for adverse events, such as post-surgical pain, complications, and removal suture after the surgeries. At the 3-day and 14-day postoperative visits, the post-surgical pain was measured by the Visual Analogue Scale (VAS), scoring from 0 (no pain) to 10 (severe pain) [27]. The records of removal suture 1 month after surgery were collected. The complications of bleeding, dysgeusia, dysphagia, and globus were monitored within one month by one physician.

2.6. Statistical Analysis

Statistical analyses were performed using SPSS 25 software (SPSS Inc., Chicago, IL, USA). Data were expressed as mean ± standard deviation. The categorical variables were analyzed by the chi-square test, and continuous variables were compared using the t-test. For comparisons of variables before and after interventions, the paired t-test was used for analysis. Effect size (d) was calculated in both groups and was classified according to the study of Cohen et al. into very small (d < 0.2), small (0.2 $\leq$ d < 0.5), medium (0.5 $\leq$ d < 0.8), and large (d $\geq$ 0.8) [28]. A p < 0.05 was considered statistically significant.

3. Results

Among the 62 patients in this analysis, 31 patients received the surgery of BRP plus TORSTBR and 31 patients received the surgery of UPPP plus TORSTBR. There were no significant differences in demographic data between the two groups before the surgery (all $p > 0.05$, Table 1).

Table 1. Demographic data of the two groups.

	BRP Plus TORSTBR Group ($n = 31$)	UPPP Plus TORSTBR Group ($n = 31$)	p
Age	37.51 ± 9.42	39.61 ± 11.63	0.59
Male/female	26/5	24/7	0.52
Body mass index	28.22 ± 3.19	28.20 ± 3.62	0.88
Preop ESS	9.02 ± 4.57	11.02 ± 4.58	0.28
Tonsil grade	1.93 ± 1.14	2.11 ± 1.38	0.55
FTP	2.92 ± 0.66	3.01 ± 0.55	0.22
Preop AHI	46.35 ± 21.76	48.24 ± 21.18	0.69

UPPP, uvulopalatoplasty; BRP, barbed repositioning pharyngoplasty; TORSTBR, transoral robotic surgery tongue base reduction; FTP, Friedman Tongue Position; AHI, apnea–hypopnea index.

In Table 2, after undergoing the operation of BRP plus TORSTBR, the BRP plus TORSTBR group had significantly improved the outcomes of ESS, AHI, minimum $SpO_2\%$, CT90, and AI (all $p < 0.05$, effect size d = 0.68–1.12). Similarly, in the UPPP plus TORSTBR group, significant improvements in all variables were found after the operation (all $p < 0.05$, effect size d = 0.52–0.97).

Table 2. Within-group comparison of the treatment outcomes.

	BRP Plus TORSTBR Group ($n = 31$)				UPPP Plus TORSTBR Group ($n = 31$)			
	Pre-Op	Post-Op	p	Effect Size	Pre-Op	Post-Op	p	Effect Size
ESS	9.03 ± 4.52	6.60 ± 3.82	0.02 *	0.58	11.01 ± 4.52	7.82 ± 3.45	0.01 *	0.79
AHI	46.21 ± 22.03	21.60 ± 21.54	0.001 *	1.12	45.13 ± 19.31	28.75 ± 23.09	0.04 *	0.76
Minimum $SpO_2\%$	76.44 ± 7.63	80.51 ± 7.33	0.02 *	0.54	75.12 ± 7.66	82.56 ± 7.64	0.02 *	0.97
CT90	16.32 ± 17.13	6.95 ± 10.46	0.001 *	0.66	14.24 ± 14.65	7.54 ± 10.37	0.03 *	0.52
AI	31.66 ± 23.53	14.39 ± 18.34	0.001 *	0.81	33.3 ± 19.24	16.5 ± 17.57	0.01 *	0.91

* $p < 0.05$. CT90, cumulative time spent below 90%; AI, arousal index; UPPP, uvulopalatoplasty; BRP, barbed repositioning pharyngoplasty; TORSTBR, transoral robotic surgery tongue base reduction; AHI, apnea–hypopnea index.

Before the operations, there were no significant differences in the patients with different levels of AHI ($p > 0.05$, Table 3). The numbers of patients with normal and abnormal AHI also did not show a significant difference ($p > 0.05$). Compared to the UPPP plus TORSTBR group, the higher increases in AHI reduction, AHI reduction rate, and surgical success were noted in the BRP plus TORSTBR group (all $p < 0.05$). However, there was no significant difference in cure after the operation between the two groups.

For postoperative visits, there were no significant differences in pain VAS between the BRP plus TORSTBR and UPPP plus TORSTBR groups at the 3-day (5.31 ± 3.76 versus 5.74 ± 4.21, $p = 0.67$) and 14-day marks (3.78 ± 2.87 versus 4.32 ± 3.56, $p = 0.51$). The length of hospital stay was not significantly different between the two groups. Within one month, one patient had bleeding (3.22%), one patient had dysgeusia (3.22%), five patients (16.12%) had dysphagia, and seven patients had globus (22.58%) in the BRP plus TORS group. In the UPPP plus TORSTBR group, two patients had bleeding (6.45%), one patient had dysgeusia (3.22%), six patients (19.35%) had dysphagia, and three patients had globus (9.67%). However, there were no significant differences in symptoms of bleeding, dysgeusia, and globus between the two groups (all $p > 0.05$). The records of removal suture after one month were found that eleven patients (35.48%) in BRP plus TORSTBR were needed, and three patients (9.67%) in UPPP plus TORSTBR were needed. No significant difference in records of removal sutures between the two groups was noted ($p = 0.07$).

Table 3. Between-group comparison of the treatment outcomes.

	BRP Plus TORSTBR Group (n = 31)	UPPP Plus TORSTBR Group (n = 31)	p
Pre-op AHI			
Mild (AHI 5–15) (n, %)	0 (0%)	0(0%)	0.75
Moderate (AHI 16–30)(n, %)	11 (35.48%)	10 (32.25%)	
Severe (AHI > 30)(n, %)	20 (64.51%)	21 (67.74%)	
Postop AHI			
Normal (AHI < 5)(n, %)	6 (19.35%)	8 (25.80%)	0.54
Abnormal(AHI ≥ 5) (n, %)	25 (80.64%)	23 (74.19%)	
AHI reduction	24.73 ± 10.46	17.34 ± 14.82	0.04 *
AHI reduction rate (%)	62.01 ± 3.03	43.07 ± 9.06	0.01 *
Outcome			
Cure (n, %)	6 (19.35%)	5 (16.12%)	0.69
Surgical success (n, %)	21 (67.74%)	12 (38.71%)	0.02 *
Comorbidities			
Bleeding (n, %)	1 (3.22%)	2 (6.45%)	0.55
Dysgeusia (n, %)	1 (3.22%)	1 (3.22%)	1.00
Dysphagia (n, %)	5 (16.12%)	6 (19.35%)	0.73
Globus (n, %)	7 (22.58%)	3 (9.67%)	0.16

* $p < 0.05$. UPPP, uvulopalatoplasty; BRP, barbed repositioning pharyngoplasty; TORSTBR, transoral robotic surgery tongue base reduction; AHI.

4. Discussion

The incidences of OSA syndrome have increased threefold in the last 20 years [29]. Single-level surgery had a limited number of successful surgical results in the last two decades [29]. UPPP with or without tonsillectomy could not only improve the respiratory events during night sleep but also improve sleep quality, depression, sexual function, ventricular function, and promote safe driving in OSA patients [30]. However, the surgery for moderate and severe OSA by UPPP base therapy produced a limited successful outcome. The BMI, AHI severity, age of patient, pattern of airway collapse, experience of the surgeon, and even the patient's choice all affect the treatment outcome [31]. In addition, the tongue base is addressed more by sleep physicians in moderate and severe OSA patients in the practice of drug-induced sleep endoscopy. Therefore, managing the tongue base could result in further treatment for surgical failure by palatal surgery only. Vicini et al. applied the robotic tongue base surgery combined with ESP to treat OSA patients and reported a higher surgical success rate [15]. Besides, various palatal surgeries that are combined with TORS produce a higher surgical success rate, as found by Cammaroto et al. [16].

Managing the tongue is not only a diagnostic issue, it also affects the surgical treatment strategy. The unresolved sleep apnea forces the sleep physicians to apply the drug-induced sleep endoscopy to find out the anatomic obstruction site of the upper airway to surgically solve the OSA. In the current study, we compared the effects on ESS, AHI, minimum SpO$_2$%, CT90, and AI in BRP plus TORSTBR and UPPP plus TORSTBR treatment groups. Significant improvements after BRP or UPPP plus TORSTBR were found in the patients with moderate to severe OSA, and medium to large effect sizes in the BRP plus TORSTBR group (d = 0.54–0.81) and UPPP plus TORSTBR group (d = 0.52–0.97) were revealed. In the recent literature, simultaneous retropalatal and retroglossal collapse or obstruction are frequently found in 25–33% of OSA cases [32–34]. Therefore, multilevel surgery for patients with OSA should be considered to achieve more effective outcomes than single-level surgery. Multilevel surgery rendered a 66% surgical success rate offered by Lin et al. [35]. Our results revealed that the surgery of BRP plus TORSTBR had a better AHI reduction rate and surgical success rate on moderate to severe OSA than the operation of UPPP plus TORSTBR, although outcomes were not significantly different since both methods reduced disease severity in ESS, AHI, minimum SpO$_2$%, CT90, and AI, measured by post-operation PSG. Concerning palatal surgery as a part of the multilevel surgery, there was still residual obstruction at the retropalatal level, even after palatal surgery. Thus, plenty of crucial innovations for palatal surgery are offered as relocation pharyngoplasty, expansion sphincter palatoplasty, and suspension palatoplasty in order to achieve higher surgical success [36,37]. The number of palatal surgeries performed with barbed suture has been rising recently due to the innovation in suture stitches by v-loc sutures. The barbed suture in pharyngoplasty was demonstrated by Mantovani et al. in 2013 [38] and Salamanca et al. in 2014 [39], and following this, pharyngoplasty performed with barbed suture increased and became more widely recommended. Barbed reposition pharyngoplasty in multilevel surgery was noted by Vicini et al., as it could conduct a widening of the oropharyngeal lateral wall and forward sustaining of the soft palate; it was also faster, easier, and more feasible within the robotic surgery framework [40].

Barbed reposition pharyngoplasty has had the same effect as expansion sphincter pharyngoplasty combined with anterior palatoplasty in terms of enlarging both the lateral and anteroposterior direction of retropalatal space in the study by Babademez et al. [41]. Barbed suspension pharyngoplasty was shown in a 2019 study by Barbieri et al., and the study compared barbed reposition pharyngoplasty and barbed suspension pharyngoplasty [42]. Both surgeries had the same excellent result. The BRP was the less invasive procedure for preserving palatopharyngeal muscle than barbed reposition pharyngoplasty, and the comparisons of cured rates between BRP and BRP were not statically significant [42]. In our study, we selected patients with moderate to severe OSA and proved multilevel collapse (retropalatal and retroglossal spaces collapse) for multilevel surgery by DISE. After enrolling these patients, we completed multilevel surgery, including the palatal surgery with TORSTBR to compare its effects in different palatal surgeries (BRP versus modified UPPP). We analyzed the pre-operative and postoperative polysomnography data, Epworth sleepiness scale, tonsil grade, and the Friedman tongue position between the BRP and UPPP groups.

Figure 3 illustrates the difference in palatal suture mechanism of BRP plus TORSTBR and UPPP plus TORSTBR techniques. The barbed palatal suture offered a good quality of posterior tonsillar pillar suspension and lateralization vector to increase not only anterior–posterior diameter but also to widen the lateral space of the retropalatal area [43]. In addition, the palatoglossus muscle suture being fixed to the pterygo-mandible-raphy offered the opportunity for the suspension vector to keep the tongue base from dropping. Therefore, we were able to not only widen the retropalatal space but also increase the anterior–posterior diameter of the retroglossal area [44]. Our findings were similar to the results of Cammaroto et al., and the effect of the barbed palatal suture mechanism was proven [16].

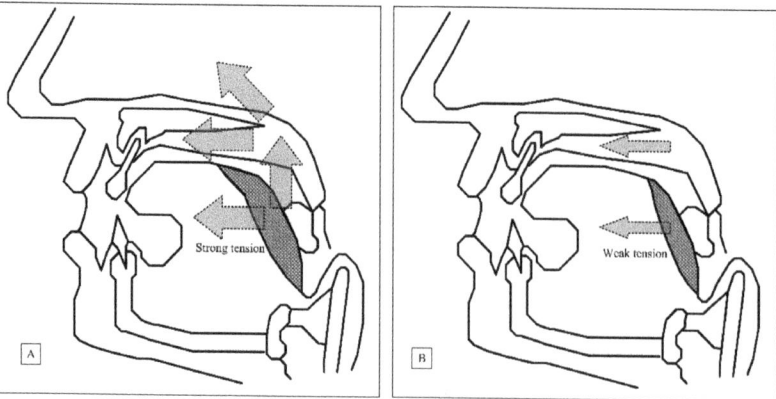

Figure 3. The palatal suture mechanism of BRP plus TORSTBR (**A**) and UPPP plus TORSTBR (**B**) techniques.

The pre-operative data between the two groups were not significantly different. The postoperative AHI and ESS were significantly decreased in both groups, and multilevel surgery was considered to be effective. The surgical success rate of the BRP plus TORSTBR group (67.74%) was significantly superior to UPPP plus TORSTBR group (38.71%), and it indicated that the different palatal surgery performed in multilevel OSA surgery had a different effect on surgical success. BRP is superior to modified UPPP in multilevel surgery for moderate to severe OSA patients. The results of our study are similar to the outcomes of Cammaroto et al. [16]. Modified UPPP with TORSTBR had a poor success rate of 38.71%. In our patient data, the Friedman tongue position in the UPPP group is not significantly severe compared to those in the BRP group. However, a higher surgical success rate is obtained in the BRP group. Therefore, we consider BRP to be more suitable as a part of multilevel surgery for moderate and severe OSA in managing the retroglossal space narrowing related OSA.

Barbed surgery had an advantage in terms of reduced operative time (less knot time), less knot rupture, more stiffness of the soft palate, and fewer minor complications, such as extruded thread, bleeding, suture rupture, and pharyngoplasty dehiscence [45]. Barbed suspension pharyngoplasty in multilevel surgery is the more feasible, faster, and less invasive method [46]. However, further study is warranted for comparing BRP to lateral pharyngoplasty and extension sphincter pharyngoplasty to treat moderate and severe OSA. In the current study, the complications included post-operational pain, bleeding, dysgeusia, transient dysphagia, throat globus sensation, and the need to remove prolonged stitches after one month; all showed no significant differences between the BRP plus TORSTBR versus UPPP plus TORSTBR groups ($p > 0.05$). Although there was a higher rate of prolonged stitches that needed to be removed one month after surgery, no significance could be found. Thus, we need to care for the prolonged stitches in patients who receive barbed suspension palatoplasty.

There are some limitations to the current study. The small sample size is one of the main limits of our study, and the non-parametric approach means that we were unable to adjust for potential confounders. Long-term results of barbed suspension pharyngoplasty in multilevel surgery are warranted. In the future, prospective, randomized, and controlled trials that incorporate similar surgical techniques will be needed to evaluate the efficacy of different palatal surgeries in multilevel surgery.

5. Conclusions

In our study, BRP with TORSTBR was a feasible, faster, and effective multilevel surgery for moderate to severe OSA. Modified UPPP might be less effective compared to BRP as a part of multilevel surgery for moderate to severe OSA.

Author Contributions: Y.-A.T. and W.-D.C. contributed to designing the method and wrote the first draft of the report, with input from the other authors. C.-C.H., L.-C.S., T.-C.L., C.-J.C., V.H.-C.T., and M.-H.T. collected data and conducted the data analyses. All authors have read and agreed to the published version of the manuscript.

Funding: This research received no funding.

Institutional Review Board Statement: The study protocol was approved by the Internal Review Board of China Medical University Hospital (No. CMUH106-REC2-027, approved on 23 March 2017).

Informed Consent Statement: All participants provided written informed consent before study.

Data Availability Statement: Data is contained within the article.

Acknowledgments: The authors are grateful to the support from Ministry of Science and Technology (No. 109-2410-H-028 -002 and 108-2410-H-028 -007) in Taiwan.

Conflicts of Interest: The authors declare no conflict of interests regarding the publication of this paper.

Abbreviations

OSA	obstructive sleep apnea
TDI	threshold, discrimination, and identification
FTP	Friedman Tongue Position
CT90	cumulative time spent below 90%
AI	arousal index
DISE	drug-induced sleep endoscopy
UPPP	uvulopalatoplasty
BRP	barbed repositioning pharyngoplasty
TORS	transoral robotic surgery
TORSTBR	transoral robotic surgery tongue base reduction
AHI	apnea–hypopnea index
PSG	polysomnography
AASM	American Academy of Sleep Medicine
VAS	Visual Analogue Scale

References

1. Bozkurt, M.K.; Öy, A.; Aydın, D.; Bilen, S.H.; Ertürk, I.Ö.; Saydam, L.; Özgen, F. Gender differences in polysomnographic findings in Turkish patients with obstructive sleep apnea syndrome. *Eur. Arch. Otorhinolaryngol.* **2008**, *265*, 821–824. [CrossRef]
2. Hao, W.; Wang, X.; Fan, J.; Zeng, Y.; Ai, H.; Nie, S.; Wei, Y. Association between apnea-hypopnea index and coronary artery calcification: A systematic review and meta-analysis. *Ann. Med.* **2021**, *53*, 302–317. [CrossRef] [PubMed]
3. Reutrakul, S.; Mokhlesi, B. Obstructive sleep apnea and diabetes: A state of the art review. *Chest* **2017**, *152*, 1070–1086. [CrossRef] [PubMed]
4. Chen, J.C.; Tsai, T.Y.; Li, C.Y.; Hwang, J.H. Obstructive sleep apnea and risk of Parkinson's disease: A population-based cohort study. *J. Sleep Res.* **2015**, *24*, 432–437. [CrossRef] [PubMed]
5. Andrade, A.G.; Bubu, O.M.; Varga, A.W.; Osorio, R.S. The relationship between obstructive sleep apnea and Alzheimer's disease. *J. Alzheimer's Dis.* **2018**, *64*, 255–270. [CrossRef] [PubMed]
6. Dzierzewski, J.M.; Dautovich, N.; Ravyts, S. Sleep and Cognition in Older Adults. *Sleep Med. Clin.* **2018**, *13*, 93–106. [CrossRef]
7. Iannella, G.; Magliulo, G.; Maniaci, A.; Meccariello, G.; Cocuzza, S.; Cammaroto, G.; Gobbi, R.; Sgarzani, R.; Firinu, E.; Corso, R.M.; et al. Olfactory function in patients with obstructive sleep apnea: A meta-analysis study. *Eur. Arch. Otorhinolaryngol.* **2021**, *278*, 883–891. [CrossRef]
8. Seet, E.; Nagappa, M.; Wong, D.T. Airway Management in Surgical Patients with Obstructive Sleep Apnea. *Anesth. Analg.* **2021**, *132*, 1321–1327. [CrossRef]
9. Cho, H.-J.; Park, D.-Y.; Min, H.J.; Chung, H.J.; Lee, J.-G.; Kim, C.-H. Endoscope-guided coblator tongue base resection using an endoscope-holding system for obstructive sleep apnea. *Head Neck* **2015**, *38*, 635–639. [CrossRef]
10. Vicini, C.; Dallan, I.; Canzi, P.; Frassineti, S.; Nacci, A.; Seccia, V.; Panicucci, E.; Grazia La Pietra, M.; Montevecchi, F.; Tschabitscher, M. Transoral robotic surgery of the tongue base in obstructive sleep apnea-hypopnea syndrome: Anatomic considerations and clinical experience. *Head Neck* **2012**, *34*, 15–22. [CrossRef]
11. Di Luca, M.; Iannella, G.; Montevecchi, F.; Magliulo, G.; De Vito, A.; Cocuzza, S.; Maniaci, A.; Meccariello, G.; Cammaroto, G.; Sgarzani, R.; et al. Use of the transoral robotic surgery to treat patients with recurrent lingual tonsillitis. *Int. J. Med. Robot. Comput. Assist. Surg.* **2020**, *16*. [CrossRef] [PubMed]
12. Sheen, D.; Abdulateef, S. Uvulopalatopharyngoplasty. *Oral Maxillofac. Surg. Clin. N. Am.* **2021**, *33*, 295–303. [CrossRef] [PubMed]
13. Tsou, Y.-A.; Chang, W.-D. Comparison of transoral robotic surgery with other surgeries for obstructive sleep apnea. *Sci. Rep.* **2020**, *10*, 18163. [CrossRef] [PubMed]
14. Lan, W.C.; Chang, W.D.; Tsai, M.H.; Tsou, Y.A. Trans-oral robotic surgery versus coblation tongue base reduction for obstructive sleep apnea syndrome. *Peer J.* **2019**, *7*, 7812. [CrossRef]
15. Vicini, C.; Montevecchi, F.; Pang, K.; Bahgat, A.; Dallan, I.; Frassineti, S.; Campanini, A. Combined transoral robotic tongue base surgery and palate surgery in obstructive sleep apnea-hypopnea syndrome: Expansion sphincter pharyngoplasty versus uvulopalatopharyngoplasty. *Head Neck* **2014**, *36*, 77–83. [CrossRef]
16. Cammaroto, G.; Montevecchi, F.; D'Agostino, G.; Zeccardo, E.; Bellini, C.; Meccariello, G.; Vicini, C. Palatal surgery in a transoral robotic setting (TORS): Preliminary results of a retrospective comparison between uvulopalatopharyngoplasty (UPPP), expansion sphincter pharyngoplasty (ESP) and barbed repositioning pharyngoplasty (BRP). *Acta Otorhinolaryngol. Ital.* **2017**, *37*, 406–409. [CrossRef] [PubMed]
17. Vicini, C.; Hendawy, E.; Campanini, A.; Eesa, M.; Bahgat, A.; Alghamdi, S.; Meccariello, G.; DeVito, A.; Montevecchi, F.; Mantovani, M. Barbed reposition pharyngoplasty (BRP) for OSAHS: A feasibility, safety, efficacy and teachability pilot study. "We are on the giant's shoulders". *Eur. Arch. Otorhinolaryngol.* **2015**, *272*, 3065–3070. [CrossRef] [PubMed]

18. Meccariello, G.; Cammaroto, G.; Montevecchi, F.; Hoff, P.T.; Spector, M.E.; Negm, H.; Shams, M.; Bellini, C.; Zeccardo, E.; Vicini, C. Transoral robotic surgery for the management of obstructive sleep apnea: A systematic review and meta-analysis. *Eur. Arch. Otorhinolaryngol.* **2016**, *274*, 647–653. [CrossRef]
19. Friedman, M.; Hamilton, C.; Samuelson, C.G.; Lundgren, M.E.; Pott, T. Diagnostic value of the Friedman tongue position and Mallampati classification for obstructive sleep apnea: A meta-analysis. *Otolaryngol. Head Neck Surg.* **2013**, *148*, 540–547. [CrossRef]
20. Berg, L.M.; Ankjell, T.K.S.; Sun, Y.-Q.; Trovik, T.A.; Sjögren, A.; Rikardsen, O.G.; Moen, K.; Hellem, S.; Bugten, V. Friedman Score in Relation to Compliance and Treatment Response in Nonsevere Obstructive Sleep Apnea. *Int. J. Otolaryngol.* **2020**, *2020*, 6459276. [CrossRef] [PubMed]
21. Fairbanks, D.N. Operative techniques of uvulopalatopharyngoplasty. *Ear Nose Throat J.* **1999**, *78*, 846–850. [CrossRef]
22. Vicini, C.; Dallan, I.; Canzi, P.; Frassineti, S.; La Pietra, M.G.; Montevecchi, F. Transoral robotic tongue base resection in obstructive sleep apnoea-hypopnoea syndrome: A preliminary report. *ORL J. Otorhinolaryngol. Relat. Spec.* **2010**, *72*, 22–27. [CrossRef]
23. Friedman, M.; Hamilton, C.; Samuelson, C.G.; Kelley, K.; Taylor, D.; Pearson-Chauhan, K.; Maley, A.; Taylor, R.; Venkatesan, T.K. Transoral Robotic Glossectomy for the Treatment of Obstructive Sleep Apnea-Hypopnea Syndrome. *Otolaryngol. Neck Surg.* **2012**, *146*, 854–862. [CrossRef]
24. Berry, R.B.; Budhiraja, R.; Gottlieb, D.J.; Gozal, D.; Iber, C.; Kapur, V.K.; Marcus, C.L.; Mehra, R.; Parthasarathy, S.; Quan, S.F.; et al. Rules for Scoring Respiratory Events in Sleep: Update of the 2007 AASM Manual for the Scoring of Sleep and Associated Events. Deliberations of the Sleep Apnea Definitions Task Force of the American Academy of Sleep Medicine. *J. Clin. Sleep Med.* **2012**, *8*, 597–619. [CrossRef] [PubMed]
25. Cirignotta, F. Classification and definition of respiratory disorders during sleep. *Minerva Med.* **2004**, *95*, 177–185.
26. Johns, M.W. A New Method for Measuring Daytime Sleepiness: The Epworth Sleepiness Scale. *Sleep* **1991**, *14*, 540–545. [CrossRef] [PubMed]
27. Rhee, J.S.; Sullivan, C.D.; Frank, D.O.; Kimbell, J.S.; Garcia, G.J. A systematic review of patient-reported nasal obstruction scores: Defining normative and symptomatic ranges in surgical patients. *JAMA Facial Plast. Surg.* **2014**, *16*, 219–225. [CrossRef]
28. Cohen, J. *Statistical Power Analysis for the Behavioral Sciences*, 2nd ed.; Lawrence Erlbaum Associates: Hillsdale, NJ, USA, 1988.
29. Lechien, J.R.; Chiesa-Estomba, M.C.; Fakhry, N.; Saussez, S.; Badr, I.; Ayad, T.; Chekkoury-Idrissi, Y.; Melkane, A.E.; Bahgat, A.; Crevier-Buchman, L.; et al. Surgical, clinical, and functional outcomes of transoral robotic surgery used in sleep surgery for obstructive sleep apnea syndrome: A systematic review and meta-analysis. *Head Neck* **2021**, *43*, 2216–2239. [CrossRef] [PubMed]
30. Stuck, B.A.; Ravesloot, M.J.; Eschenhagen, T.; de Vet, H.; Sommer, J.U. Uvulopalatopharyngoplasty with or without tonsillectomy in the treatment of adult obstructive sleep apnea—A systematic review. *Sleep Med.* **2018**, *50*, 152–165. [CrossRef]
31. Alcaraz, M.; Bosco, G.; Pérez-Martín, N.; Morato, M.; Navarro, A.; Plaza, G. Advanced Palate Surgery: What Works? *Curr. Otorhinolaryngol. Rep.* **2021**, 1–14. [CrossRef]
32. Mittal, R.; Lee, L.-A.; Lin, C.H.; Hsin, L.-J.; Bhusri, N.; Li, H.-Y. Prediction of tongue obstruction observed from drug induced sleep computed tomography by cephalometric parameters. *Auris Nasus Larynx* **2019**, *46*, 384–389. [CrossRef]
33. Kim, J.-W.; Ahn, J.-C.; Choi, Y.-S.; Rhee, C.-S.; Jung, H.J. Correlation between short-time and whole-night obstruction level tests for patients with obstructive sleep apnea. *Sci. Rep.* **2021**, *11*, 1509. [CrossRef] [PubMed]
34. Turhan, M.; Bostanci, A. Robotic Tongue-Base Resection Combined with Tongue-Base Suspension for Obstructive Sleep Apnea. *Laryngoscope* **2019**, *130*, 2285–2291. [CrossRef] [PubMed]
35. Lin, H.-C.; Friedman, M.; Chang, H.-W.; Gurpinar, B. The Efficacy of Multilevel Surgery of the Upper Airway in Adults with Obstructive Sleep Apnea/Hypopnea Syndrome. *Laryngoscope* **2008**, *118*, 902–908. [CrossRef]
36. Puccia, R.; Woodson, B.T. Palatopharyngoplasty and Palatal Anatomy and Phenotypes for Treatment of Sleep Apnea in the Twenty-first Century. *Otolaryngol. Clin. N. Am.* **2020**, *53*, 421–429. [CrossRef]
37. Mandavia, R.; Mehta, N.; Veer, V. Guidelines on the surgical management of sleep disorders: A systematic review. *Laryngoscope* **2020**, *130*, 1070–1084. [CrossRef]
38. Mantovani, M.; Minetti, A.; Torretta, S.; Pincherle, A.; Tassone, G.; Pignataro, L. The "Barbed Roman Blinds" technique: A step forward. *Acta Otorhinolaryngol. Ital.* **2013**, *33*, 128. [PubMed]
39. Salamanca, F.; Costantini, F.; Mantovani, M.; Bianchi, A.; Amaina, T.; Colombo, E.; Zibordi, F. Barbed anterior pharyngoplasty: An evolution of anterior palatoplasty. *Acta Otorhinolaryngol. Ital.* **2014**, *34*, 434–438. [PubMed]
40. Vicini, C.; Meccariello, G.; Cammaroto, G.; Rashwan, G.; Montevecchi, F. Barbed reposition pharyngoplasty in multilevel robotic surgery for obstructive sleep apnoea. *Acta Otorhinolaryngol. Ital.* **2017**, *37*, 214–217. [CrossRef]
41. Babademez, M.A.; Gul, F.; Teleke, Y.C. Barbed palatoplasty vs. expansion sphincter pharyngoplasty with anterior palatoplasty. *Laryngoscope* **2020**, *130*, E275–E279. [CrossRef]
42. Barbieri, M.; Missale, F.; Incandela, F.; Fragale, M.; Barbieri, A.; Roustan, V.; Canevari, F.R.; Peretti, G. Barbed suspension pharyngoplasty for treatment of lateral pharyngeal wall and palatal collapse in patients affected by OSAHS. *Eur. Arch. Otorhinolaryngol.* **2019**, *276*, 1829–1835. [CrossRef] [PubMed]
43. Vicini, C.; Meccariello, G.; Montevecchi, F.; De Vito, A.; Frassineti, S.; Gobbi, R.; Pelucchi, S.; Iannella, G.; Magliulo, G.; Cammaroto, G. Effectiveness of barbed repositioning pharyngoplasty for the treatment of obstructive sleep apnea (OSA): A prospective randomized trial. *Sleep Breath.* **2019**, *24*, 687–694. [CrossRef] [PubMed]
44. Neruntarat, C.; Khuancharee, K.; Saengthong, P. Barbed reposition pharyngoplasty versus expansion sphincter pharyngoplasty: A meta-analysis. *Laryngoscope* **2021**, *131*, 1420–1428. [CrossRef] [PubMed]

45. Moffa, A.; Rinaldi, V.; Mantovani, M.; Pierri, M.; Fiore, V.; Costantino, A.; Pignataro, L.; Baptista, P.; Cassano, M.; Casale, M. Different barbed pharyngoplasty techniques for retropalatal collapse in obstructive sleep apnea patients: A systematic review. *Sleep Breath* **2020**, *24*, 1115–1127. [CrossRef]
46. Missale, F.; Fragale, M.; Incandela, F.; Roustan, V.; Arceri, C.; Barbieri, A.; Canevari, F.R.; Peretti, G.; Barbieri, M. Outcome predictors for non-resective pharyngoplasty alone or as a part of multilevel surgery, in obstructive sleep apnea-hypopnea syndrome. *Sleep Breath* **2020**, *24*, 1397–1406. [CrossRef] [PubMed]

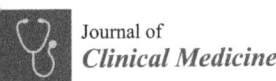

Article

Effect of Upper Airway Stimulation in Patients with Obstructive Sleep Apnea (EFFECT): A Randomized Controlled Crossover Trial

Clemens Heiser [1,*,†], Armin Steffen [2,†], Benedikt Hofauer [1], Reena Mehra [3], Patrick J. Strollo, Jr. [4], Olivier M. Vanderveken [5] and Joachim T. Maurer [6,7]

1. Department of Otorhinolaryngology/Head and Neck Surgery, Klinikum Rechts der Isar, Technical University of Munich, 81675 München, Germany; b.hofauer@tum.de
2. Department of Otorhinolaryngology/Head and Neck Surgery, University of Luebeck, 23562 Luebeck, Germany; Armin.Steffen@uksh.de
3. Department of Sleep Medicine, Cleveland Clinic Foundation, Cleveland, OH 44195, USA; MEHRAR@ccf.org
4. Department of Pulmonary, Allergy and Critical Care Medicine, University of Pittsburgh, Pittsburgh, PA 15261, USA; strollopj@upmc.edu
5. Multidisciplinary Sleep Disorders Centre, Antwerp University Hospital, 2650 Edegem, Antwerp, Belgium; Olivier@ovanderveken.be
6. Department of ORL-HNS, Division of Sleep Medicine, University Medical Centre Mannheim, University Heidelberg, 68167 Mannheim, Germany; joachim.maurer@umm.de
7. Department of Information Technology, University of Applied Sciences, 68163 Mannheim, Germany
* Correspondence: hno@heiser-online.com
† Shared first authorship.

Abstract: Background: Several single-arm prospective studies have demonstrated the safety and effectiveness of upper airway stimulation (UAS) for obstructive sleep apnea. There is limited evidence from randomized, controlled trials of the therapy benefit in terms of OSA burden and its symptoms. Methods: We conducted a multicenter, double-blinded, randomized, sham-controlled, crossover trial to examine the effect of therapeutic stimulation (*Stim*) versus sham stimulation (*Sham*) on the apnea-hypopnea index (AHI) and the Epworth Sleepiness Scale (ESS). We also examined the Functional Outcomes of Sleep Questionnaire (FOSQ) on sleep architecture. We analyzed crossover outcome measures after two weeks using repeated measures models controlling for treatment order. Results: The study randomized 89 participants 1:1 to *Stim* (45) versus *Sham* (44). After one week, the AHI response rate was 76.7% with *Stim* and 29.5% with *Sham*, a difference of 47.2% (95% CI: 24.4 to 64.9, $p < 0.001$) between the two groups. Similarly, ESS was 7.5 ± 4.9 with *Stim* and 12.0 ± 4.3 with *Sham*, with a significant difference of 4.6 (95% CI: 3.1 to 6.1) between the two groups. The crossover phase showed no carryover effect. Among 86 participants who completed both phases, the treatment difference between *Stim* vs. *Sham* for AHI was −15.5 (95% CI −18.3 to −12.8), for ESS it was −3.3 (95% CI −4.4 to −2.2), and for FOSQ it was 2.1 (95% CI 1.4 to 2.8). UAS effectively treated both REM and NREM sleep disordered breathing. Conclusions: In comparison with sham stimulation, therapeutic UAS reduced OSA severity, sleepiness symptoms, and improved quality of life among participants with moderate-to-severe OSA.

Keywords: hypoglossal nerve stimulation; obstructive sleep apnea; upper airway stimulation; surgical treatments; randomized trial

1. Introduction

Obstructive sleep apnea (OSA) is a common and under-recognized disease in western industrialized countries. In the United States, the estimated prevalence of moderate-to-severe OSA in those 30–70 years old is 6% in women and 13% in men [1]. In the HypnoLaus study from Switzerland, Heinzer et al. reported mild OSA in nearly 40% of men under

60 years of age [2]. The Wisconsin Sleep Cohort Study, established over two decades ago, demonstrated a relationship between OSA and obesity, thus, as obesity increases globally, the incidence of OSA is expected to increase as well [3]. The standard treatment for OSA is continuous positive airway pressure (CPAP), which is effective but fraught with challenges of maintaining adherence [4]. Other treatment options include mandibular advancement devices (MAD), weight loss, behavior modifications, and surgical options [4,5].

Breathing-cycle-synchronized selective upper airway stimulation (UAS) has evolved as a viable treatment for OSA patients intolerant of CPAP [6,7]. UAS targets the loss of upper airway muscle tone during sleep, mainly in the genioglossus muscle [6,8,9]. Several multicenter prospective clinical trials have demonstrated the effectiveness of UAS in participants with moderate-to-severe OSA [10–17]. The initial multicenter Stimulation Therapy for Apnea Reduction (STAR) trial in 2014 demonstrated a decrease in the apnea–hypopnea index (AHI) from 32.0/h at baseline to 15.3/h after 12 months ($p < 0.001$) [10]. Additional data from this cohort showed a sustained AHI reduction after 5 years [15]. Several additional multicenter international prospective studies subsequent to the STAR trial have reported the consistent effectiveness of UAS as well as a favorable safety profile and patient receptivity [16–19].

The STAR trial included a randomized withdrawal study arm performed after 12 months. By protocol, the first 46 successfully treated participants were randomized to either therapy maintenance (therapy remained active) or therapy withdrawal. After one week, participants were then reassessed with an in-lab polysomnography (PSG) [20]. The AHI in the therapy withdrawal group increased to the levels observed before surgery, while the AHI in the therapy maintenance group remained stable. The trial's main limitation was only including participants who were responders to therapy. To address this limitation, we designed a randomized control trial to prospectively enroll UAS recipients regardless of their therapy response. The primary endpoints were the improvement in sleep disordered breathing measured by the AHI and self-reported daytime sleepiness assessed by the Epworth Sleepiness Scale (ESS). Secondary endpoints included the change in sleep-related quality of life using the Functional Outcomes of Sleep Questionnaire (FOSQ) and the Clinical Global Impression of Improvement (CGI-I) by the treating investigators, as well as the differential impact of UAS on sleep-disordered breathing in NREM versus REM sleep.

2. Materials and Methods

Trial design and participants The effect of Upper Airway Stimulation in patients with OSA (EFFECT) trial was a multicenter, double-blinded, randomized, sham-controlled, crossover study. All participants were recruited from three clinical centers in Germany (Mannheim, Munich, and Luebeck). Klinikum rechts der Isar, Technical University of Munich, coordinated and managed the trial. The relevant regulatory authorities and ethics committees at each participating site approved the protocol. The crossover study design assessed the treatment effect of UAS at two different time points with two therapy settings. The study flow chart is depicted in Figure 1. The study was registered at clinicaltrials.gov (NCT03760328).

Participants received implantation of UAS (Inspire Medical Systems, Golden Valley, MN, USA) at least six months prior to enrollment. The main inclusion criteria for UAS were moderate-to-severe OSA (AHI $\geq$ 15), CPAP intolerance, and the absence of complete concentric retropalatal collapse during drug-induced sleep endoscopy. All recipients of UAS between 2014 to 2019 were eligible for recruitment and were *consecutively* recruited regardless of whether they were responders or non-responders to therapy according to the Sher criteria [21]. All participants gave written informed consent.

Randomization and masking Upon completion of the baseline PSG with therapy ON, each participant was randomized 1:1 to one of two groups: therapeutic stimulation (*Stim*) or sham stimulation (*Sham*) using a centralized, computer-generated, password-protected system. The UAS devices implanted in the participants were then programmed to the setting assigned to their respective groups, i.e., *Stim* (continued therapeutic stimulation, average amplitude 1.6 V ± 0.7) and *Sham* (stimulation voltage set at 0.1 V as a subtherapeutic stimulation level and a deception for the patient).

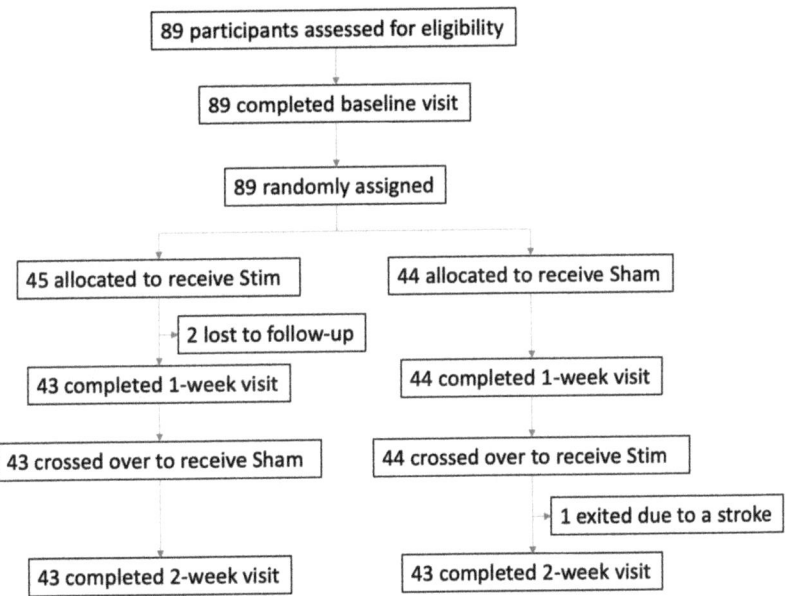

Figure 1. Flow diagram of the EFFECT randomized sham-controlled crossover trial.

The sleep technician at each center randomized the sequence of the intervention participants were exposed to and programmed their devices without the knowledge of the participant or physician investigator, who remained blinded to the randomization status. The PSGs were analyzed and scored by another sleep technician, who was blinded during all procedures.

Procedures The crossover design of the EFFECT study included three separate visits at intervals of one week. All participants received therapeutic stimulation during the first visit (baseline visit). After receiving randomized assignment, the *Stim–Sham* group received therapeutic stimulation while the *Sham–Stim* group received sham stimulation for one week. During the second week, the *Stim–Sham* group received sham stimulation while the *Sham–Stim* group received therapeutic stimulation. At each of the three study visits, participants underwent PSG. AHI and oxygen desaturation index (ODI) were scored using standard 2017 scoring criteria of the AASM, with hypopnea scored according to 30% airflow reduction and 4% oxygen desaturation [22]. At each visit, participants completed a standard medical history and demographic survey that documented body mass index (BMI), sex, blood pressure, race, current medications, alcohol use, a functional tongue exam, snoring history, and a Clinical Global Impression-Improvement (CGI-I) assessment. Participants also completed two questionnaires, ESS and FOSQ, and a Patient Satisfaction Survey (PSS) [23,24].

Study Outcome Measures The study had two co-primary endpoints. The first was the proportion of AHI responders between parallel randomized groups at the 1-week visit. AHI responder was defined as AHI ≤ 15/h. The second co-primary endpoint was the self-reported sleepiness measure using the ESS questionnaire at the 1-week visit. If the primary efficacy endpoints were met, the endpoints were then analyzed according to the crossover design. For additional outcome measures, participants completed the FOSQ, a quality-of-life questionnaire designed specifically to evaluate the impact of excessive sleepiness on activities of daily living, at every visit. Clinicians assessed participants using the CGI-I scale to measure the severity of participants' overall improvement with the intervention. The 7-point CGI-I scale requires the clinician to assess how much a participant's illness has improved or worsened relative to a baseline state at the beginning of the intervention. Finally, sleep data on each participant was collected at every visit using an in-lab PSG. The recorded data was converted and scored for analysis by a blinded independent sleep technician at each site.

Statistical analysis Sample size was conservatively estimated for the parallel group comparisons of the 1-week endpoints. For the primary endpoints, a one-sided chi-square test of superiority with a superiority margin of 10% was used with the following assumptions: one-sided Type I error of 0.25, power of $\geq 80\%$, expected response rates of 70% with continued therapeutic stimulation and 30% with sham stimulation with a superiority margin Δ of 10%. Under these assumptions, the required minimum sample size was 84 participants (42 per group). The significance level of 0.025 was based on a two-sided Type I error rate of 5%. A one-sided test was performed because we were testing the expected response rate with a superiority margin. For the co-primary endpoint, self-reported sleepiness, the test was a one-sided test of null improvement of 2 points using a t-test under the following assumptions: overall one-sided Type I error of 0.025 and power $\geq 80\%$. Under these assumptions, the required minimum sample size was 24 participants (12 per group). The required minimum sample size was based on the observed improvement in the STAR trial, assuming the same means and standard deviations of ESS of 5.6 ± 3.9 with therapy ON and 10.0 ± 6.0 with therapy OFF [10,20].

We analyzed crossover outcome measures after 2 weeks using repeated measures models controlling for treatment order. To compare the PSG characteristics, ESS and FOSQ between Stim versus Sham, we used a random effects model including the baseline value as a covariate and controlling for testing order. P-values shown reflect the test of difference between Stim and Sham in changes from baseline.

3. Results

A total of 89 participants were assessed for eligibility and randomized between December 2018 and November 2019 (Figure 1). After the baseline visit with therapy, 45 participants were randomized to the Stim–Sham group and 44 participants to the Sham–Stim group. Three participants did not complete the study: two participants from the Stim–Sham group were lost to follow-up prior to the 1-week visit. One participant from the Sham–Stim group exited the study prior to the 2-week visit due to a stroke that was deemed unrelated to UAS. Baseline characteristics of the study cohort revealed that the two groups were well-balanced in baseline characteristics (Table 1). The participants were middle-aged and mildly obese with moderate-to-severe OSA. The average UAS use in the Stim–Sham group was 33.9 ± 22.6 months versus 26.4 ± 15.4 in the Sham–Stim group ($p = 0.07$).

Table 1. Baseline Characteristics by Randomization Group.

	All $n = 89$	Stim–Sham $n = 45$	Sham–Stim $n = 44$
Age, years	57.5 ± 9.8	58.3 ± 9.4	56.6 ± 10.4
BMI, kg/m^2	29.2 ± 4.4	28.6 ± 3.7	29.5 ± 3.9
Male sex, %	81.0	82.2	79.5
Race, % Caucasian	100	100	100
Baseline ESS	7.0 ± 4.4	7.0 ± 4.2	7.0 ± 4.6
Baseline ESS before implantation	10.6 ± 3.8	10.0 ± 4.7	10.0 ± 4.7
Baseline AHI	8.3 ± 8.9	9.7 ± 8.5	6.9 ± 9.2
Baseline AHI before implantation	32.3 ± 11.4	32.1 ± 9.8	31.9 ± 11.4

Values are presented as mean $\pm$ standard deviation or % (*n*). AHI = apnea–hypopnea index, BMI = body mass index, ESS = Epworth Sleepiness Scale.

Stimulation versus *Sham Stimulation* One week after the randomization, there was a statistically significantly difference in the *Stim–Sham* group (73.3%) regarding AHI-responders compared to the *Sham–Stim* group (29.5%), a difference of 43.8% (95% CI 25.1–62.5, $p < 0.001$) between the parallel randomized groups based on intention-to-treat analysis, i.e., the two participants in the *Stim–Sham* lost to follow-up were treated as AHI non-responders (see Table 2). The effect size of the treatment difference measured by Crohn's h was 0.99, showing a large effect size.

Table 2. Primary Endpoint 1: ITT comparison of proportions with AHI $\leq$ 15 by randomization group at visit 2.

Endpoint	Treatment 1	Treatment 2	Difference (95% CI) p-Value
AHI $\leq$ 15 (ITT)	73.3% (33/45)	29.5% (13/44)	43.8% (25.1, 62.5) < 0.001

For sensitivity analysis of AHI $\leq$ 10, the response rate was 51.1% versus 15.9% and for AHI $\leq$ 5, 35.6% versus 0% between the Stim–Sham and *Sham–Stim* group (see Table 3). The average ESS change from the *Stim–Sham* group was 0.4 $\pm$ 2.3 and from the *Sham–Stim* group was 5.0 $\pm$ 4.6, with a significant difference of 4.6 (95% CI of 3.1 to 6.1, p = 0.001) between the two groups, exceeding the two point superiority margin. The effect size of the treatment difference measured by Cohen's d was 1.07, showing a large effect size. The EFFECT study met both co-primary endpoints.

Table 3. Primary Endpoint 1 Sensitivity: Comparison of proportions with AHI $\leq$ 10 and 5 by randomization group at visit 2.

Endpoint	Treatment 1	Treatment 2
AHI $\leq$ 10 (ITT)	51.1% (23/45)	15.9% (7/44)
AHI $\leq$ 5 (ITT)	35.6% (16/45)	0.0% (0/44)

AHI changes over time showed a significant decrease in AHI with *Stim* compared to *Sham* during the baseline, 1-week and 2-week visits (see Figure 2A). Similarly, participants reported a lower ESS with Stim as opposed to Sham during all visits (Figure 2B).

Crossover Analysis We assessed the change of AHI and ESS from the baseline to the 1-week and 2-week visits between the Stim–Sham and Sham–Stim groups and found no statistical evidence of a carryover effect for AHI (p = 0.55) or ESS (p = 0.23). Table 4 compares outcome measures between *Stim* and *Sham* from all complete participants under the crossover design.

Table 4 also shows other PSG parameters, highlighting the differential impact of Stim versus Sham on OSA as well as NREM versus REM sleep over the entire monitoring period. There were significant treatment differences between *Stim* and *Sham* in AHI, the apnea index, AHI in both supine and non-supine position, and AHI in both REM and non-REM (N1, N2, N3) sleep. The central and mixed apnea index did not differ between groups. The oxygen desaturation index, minimal measured oxygen saturation, and total time oxygen saturation <90% were lower with *Stim*, while mean oxygen saturation showed no difference (See Supplement for Complete PSG Data).

FOSQ improved with *Stim* compared to *Sham* (17.0 $\pm$ 3.2 versus 14.9 $\pm$ 3.6 points; $p < 0.001$). The CGI-I in the *Stim* group revealed that 76% of physician investigators rated syndromic improvement. A much stronger effect was detected in the *Sham* stimulation group, where 95% of physician investigators rated syndromic worsening (See Supplement Table S2).

For patient and physician assessment of study arm allocation at the 1-week and 2-week visits after randomization, participants and physicians were asked to guess whether the participants were in the therapeutic stimulation group or in the sham stimulation group. Among participants, 92% guessed correctly, 3.5% guessed incorrectly, and the remaining

3.5% did not guess. Of physicians, 90% guessed correctly, 1.3% guessed wrong, and the remaining 8.7% did not guess.

The only serious adverse event in this trial was a stroke suffered by one participant in the *Sham–Stim* group during the time period of stimulation ON. He completely recovered from this event. No other adverse and severe adverse events were detected.

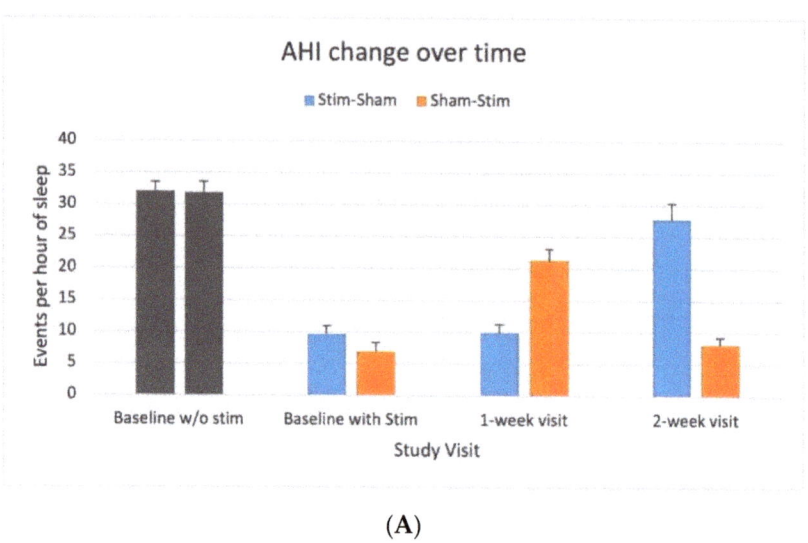

(A)

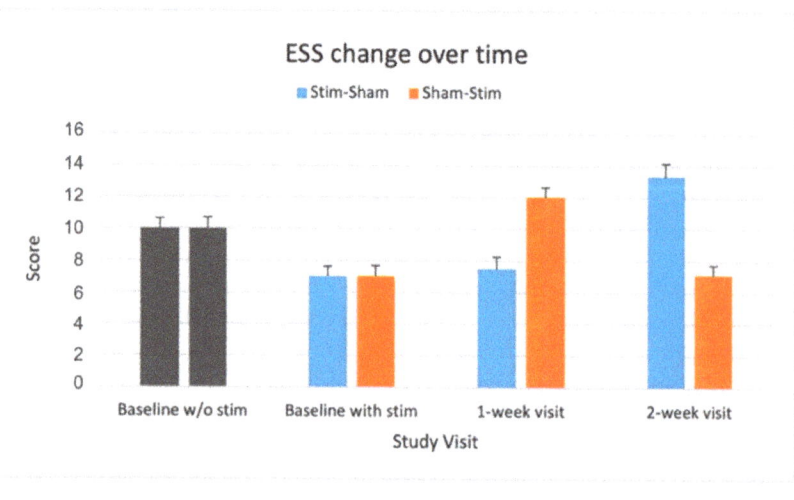

(B)

Figure 2. (**A**) OSA severity measured by apnea–hypopnea index (AHI) in response to upper airway stimulation versus sham. AHI values (mean and standard error bar) without stimulation before implantation and with stimulation at baseline, 1-week and 2-week visits for *stim–sham* and *sham–stim* groups. AHI values <15 events per hour of sleep considered as free of moderate-to-severe OSA [22]. (**B**). Subjective sleep propensity by Epworth Sleepiness Scale (ESS) in response to upper airway stimulation versus sham. ESS values <10 considered as free of excessive of daytime sleepiness [23].

Table 4. Change from baseline between Stim versus Sham in all participants with moderate to severe OSA.

Parameter	Stim (n = 86)	Sham (n = 86)	Treatment Difference	p-Value
PSG Parameters				
AHI (events/h)	0.6 (−1.8, 2.9)	16.1 (13.7, 18.4)	−15.5 (−18.3, −12.8)	<0.001
ODI (events/h)	0.6 (−1.9, 3.0)	12.7 (10.3, 15.2)	−12.2 (−14.8, −9.6)	<0.001
Apnea index (events/h)	0.5 (−1.2, 2.3)	8.9 (7.2, 10.7)	−8.4 (−10.6, −6.2)	<0.001
AHI in supine position (events/h)	2.2 (−2.3, 6.6)	23.8 (19.4, 28.2)	−21.6 (−27.2, −16.0)	<0.001
AHI in non-supine position (events/h)	−0.1 (−3.2, 2.9)	3.1 (0.1, 6.1)	−3.3 (−6.4, −0.1)	0.044
AHI in REM sleep (events/h)	2.0 (−1.6, 5.6)	17.1 (13.5, 20.6)	−15.1 (−19.7, −10.5)	<0.001
AHI in non-REM sleep (events/h)	0.0 (−2.4, 2.5)	15.7 (13.3, 18.2)	−15.7 (−18.5, −12.8)	<0.001
Central Apnea Index (events/h)	0.1 (−0.1, 0.4)	0.3 (0.0, 0.5)	−0.1 (−0.4, 0.1)	0.285
Mixed Apnea Index (events/h)	0.1 (−0.3, 0.4)	0.3 (−0.1, 0.6)	−0.2 (−0.6, 0.2)	0.355
Central Mixed Apnea Index (events/h)	−0.0 (−0.8, 0.7)	0.4 (−0.3, 1.1)	−0.4 (−1.2, 0.4)	0.283
Hypopnea Index (events/h)	0.0 (−1.6, 1.6)	7.0 (5.4, 8.6)	−7.0 (−8.9, −5.1)	<0.001
Minimal measured SaO2 (%)	−0.9 (−1.9, 0.2)	−4.0 (−5.0, −3.0)	3.1 (2.1, 4.2)	<0.001
Mean SaO2 (%)	−0.2 (−0.9, 0.4)	−0.5 (−1.2, 0.1)	0.3 (−0.5, 1.1)	0.493
Total time SaO2 <90%	2.4 (−1.7, 6.4)	9.0 (4.9, 13.0)	−6.6 (−11.2, −2.0)	0.005
Quality of life measures				
ESS (points)	0.2 (−0.7, 1.1)	3.5 (2.6, 4.4)	−3.3 (−4.4, −2.2)	<0.001
FOSQ (points)	0.2 (−0.5, 0.9)	−1.9 (−2.6, −1.2)	2.1 (1.4, 2.8)	<0.001

4. Discussion

The main findings of this study are that therapeutic stimulation of the hypoglossal nerve effectively treated 76.7% of participants with moderate-to-severe OSA and reduced self-reported daytime sleepiness, as compared to those with sham stimulation. After the initial sham-controlled comparison, the second crossover phase of the study showed no carryover effect. Therapeutic stimulation significantly reduced AHI, ODI and ESS and improved FOSQ. Sham stimulation led to a recurrence of OSA after one week and a return of subjective sleepiness. In addition, REM and NREM related sleep-disordered breathing were effectively treated with therapeutic stimulation versus sham stimulation.

Several multicenter single arm prospective trials have demonstrated UAS to be highly effective [13,15,18,19,25,26]. Adequately powered, double-blinded, randomized, controlled trials are the gold standard for intervention studies eliminating the influence of unknown or immeasurable confounding variables that may otherwise lead to biased and incorrect estimates of treatment effect. Previously, only the STAR trial had included a randomized therapy withdrawal arm among therapy responders of 46 participants. The EFFECT trial provides additional support the efficacy of UAS with a randomized, sham-controlled crossover study of 89 participants. Both RCTs demonstrate consistent UAS treatment benefits in terms of OSA burden and severity, quality of life indices, and favorable sleep architectural features.

Many patients may suffer from high cardiovascular risk if their OSA remains untreated or suboptimally treated [27]. If patients fail standard treatment with CPAP, UAS is a suitable intervention to treat sleepiness and impaired quality of life related to OSA. Because the study period was short, we did not measure any cardiovascular outcome parameters. However, it is biologically plausible that a decreased AHI and daytime sleepiness over the longer-term should be associated with improvement of cardiovascular outcomes [28].

Our observation that UAS effectively treats both NREM- and REM-related OSA is important. REM sleep is physiologically distinct from NREM sleep. REM-related sleep-disordered breathing is complicated by decreased lung volumes, increased upper airway collapsibility, increased sympathetic tone, and decreased respiratory drive that result in longer obstructive events, greater desaturation, and an increased rise in blood pressure at the end of an obstructive apnea [29]. Reports indicate that REM-related OSA has been independently associated with cardiovascular, neurocognitive, and metabolic risk [30]. For any treatment to be considered completely successful, OSA in REM, as well as NREM sleep, must be addressed [30].

4.1. Strengths of the Study

The strengths of the study include the randomized design, the use of a crossover approach, enhanced study efficiency, and increased power, allowing for the use of a smaller sample size because participants served as their own control. This trial had a low dropout rate despite the use of a crossover design that prolonged the length of the study. To the greatest possible extent, we also attempted to minimize bias by ensuring all participants and the research team were blinded to randomization assignment.

4.2. Limitations of the Study

This study had several limitations. The study population was predominately male (81%) and exclusively Caucasian. Our findings therefore may not be generalizable to women or the non-Caucasian population. Most participants randomized to sham stimulation became aware of the group allocation, and this may have affected subjective outcomes [31]. Because of ethical concerns and ethic committee requirements, the withdrawal period was one week. The limited withdrawal period precluded evaluating long-term consequences of subtherapeutic UAS, e.g., cardiovascular events and increased mortality associated with untreated OSA.

5. Conclusions

Therapeutic UAS reduced OSA severity among participants with moderate-to-severe OSA who did not tolerate CPAP. However, subtherapeutic UAS leads to the return of OSA severity within the first week of therapy withdrawal and is associated with an increase in self-reported sleepiness and a negative impact on sleep-related quality of life.

Supplementary Materials: The following are available online at https://www.mdpi.com/article/10.3390/jcm10132880/s1, Figure S1: Study flow of participants from baseline through completion after the 2-week visit, Table S1: Sleep Architectural Differences in Response to Upper Airway Stimulation versus Sham. Table S2: Sleep Architectural Differences in Response to Upper Airway Stimulation versus Sham.

Author Contributions: Conceptualization: C.H., A.S., B.H., J.T.M.; methodology: C.H., A.S., B.H., J.T.M. Validation: C.H., A.S., B.H., J.T.M., R.M., P.J.S.J., O.M.V.; formal analysis: C.H., A.S., B.H., J.T.M., R.M., P.J.S.J., O.M.V.; investigation: C.H., A.S., B.H., J.T.M., R.M., P.J.S.J., O.M.V.; writing—original draft preparation: C.H., A.S., B.H., J.T.M., R.M., P.J.S.J., O.M.V.; writing—review and editing: C.H., A.S., B.H., J.T.M., R.M., P.J.S.J., O.M.V.; visualization: C.H., A.S., B.H., J.T.M., R.M., P.J.S.J., O.M.V. All authors have read and agreed to the published version of the manuscript.

Funding: This research was funded by Inspire Medical Systems, Inc.

Institutional Review Board Statement: The study was conducted according to the guidelines of the Declaration of Helsinki, and approved by the Ethics Committee of Klinikum rechts der Isar, Technical University of Munich (364/18 S-AS on the 6 December 2018).

Informed Consent Statement: Informed consent was obtained from all participants involved in the study.

Data Availability Statement: All the individual patient data collected during the trial will be shared. In addition, the study protocol and statistical analysis plan will be available as well. The data will be made available within 12 months of publication. All available data can be obtained by contacting the corresponding author (clemens.heiser@tum.de). It will be necessary to provide a detailed protocol for the proposed study, to provide the approval of an ethics committee, to supply information about the funding and resources one has to carry out the study, and to consider inviting the original authors to participate in the re-analysis.

Acknowledgments: We acknowledge Quan Ni from Inspire Medical Systems for technical support. Furthermore, we acknowledge Katharina Eckbauer (Technical University Munich), Nicole Behm (University Schleswig-Holstein) and Oliver Schmitt (University Heidelberg).

Conflicts of Interest: Clemens Heiser was a consultant for Inspire Medical Systems (USA), received personal fees from Neuwirth Medical Products (Germany), and research grants from Sutter Medizintechnik (Germany), Löwenstein Medical (Germany), Nyxoah (Belgium) and Inspire Medical Systems (USA). Armin Steffen received grants from the Department of Otorhinolaryngology/Technical University of Munich during the conduct of the study. Armin Steffen received grants, personal fees and non-financial support from Inspire Medical Systems (USA), Respicardia (USA) Intersect, Merz (Germany), Onyx/Clinigen (USA) and Proveca. Benedikt Hofauer received personal fees and research grants from Inspire Medical Systems (USA) outside the submitted work. Oliver Vanderveken received support from Inspire Medical Systems (USA), grants from SomnoMed (Germany), grants from Philips (Netherlands), support from Nyxoah (Belgium), and support from Zephyr Sleep (USA) outside the submitted work. Patrick Strollo received grants and personal fees from Inspire Medical Systems (USA), personal fees from Philips-Respironics (Netherlands), grants and personal fees from Philips (Netherlands), and personal fees from Itamar (Israel) outside the submitted work. Reena Mehra reports being a site principal investigator of the Inspire ADHERE registry and post-approval study at the Cleveland Clinic. Joachim Maurer received grants from the Department of Otorhinolaryngology/Technical University of Munich during the conduct of the study, grants and personal fees from Imthera/LivaNova (USA), grants and personal fees from Nyxoah (Belgium), grants and personal fees from Revent (USA), grants and personal fees from Inspire Medical Systems (USA), grants and personal fees from Medel (Austria), and personal fees from Neuwirth Medical (Germany) outside the submitted work.

References

1. Peppard, P.E.; Young, T.; Barnet, J.H.; Palta, M.; Hagen, E.W.; Hla, K.M. Increased prevalence of sleep-disordered breathing in adults. *Am. J. Epidemiol.* **2013**, *177*, 1006–1014. [CrossRef] [PubMed]
2. Heinzer, R.; Vat, S.; Marques-Vidal, P.; Marti-Soler, H.; Andries, D.; Tobback, N.; Mooser, V.; Preisig, M.; Malhotra, A.; Waeber, G.; et al. Prevalence of sleep-disordered breathing in the general population: The HypnoLaus study. *Lancet Respir. Med.* **2015**, *3*, 310–318. [CrossRef]
3. Garvey, J.F.; Pengo, M.F.; Drakatos, P.; Kent, B.D. Epidemiological aspects of obstructive sleep apnea. *J. Thorac. Dis.* **2015**, *7*, 920–929. [PubMed]
4. Verse, T.; Dreher, A.; Heiser, C.; Herzog, M.; Maurer, J.T.; Pirsig, W.; Rohde, K.; Rothmeier, N.; Sauter, A.; Steffen, A.; et al. ENT-specific therapy of obstructive sleep apnoea in adults: A revised version of the previously published German S2e guideline. *Sleep Breath* **2016**, *20*, 1301–1311. [CrossRef]
5. Randerath, W.J.; Verbraecken, J.; Andreas, S.; Bettega, G.; Boudewyns, A.; Hamans, E.; Jalbert, F.; Paoli, J.R.; Sanner, B.; Smith, I.; et al. European Respiratory Society task force on non Ctisa. Non-CPAP therapies in obstructive sleep apnoea. *Eur. Respir. J.* **2011**, *37*, 1000–1028. [CrossRef]
6. Heiser, C.; Hofauer, B. Hypoglossal nerve stimulation in patients with CPAP failure: Evolution of an alternative treatment for patients with obstructive sleep apnea. *HNO* **2017**, *65*, 99–106. [CrossRef]
7. Schwartz, A.R.; Bennett, M.L.; Smith, P.L.; De Backer, W.; Hedner, J.; Boudewyns, A.; Van de Heyning, P.; Ejnell, H.; Hochban, W.; Knaack, L.; et al. Therapeutic Electrical Stimulation of the Hypoglossal Nerve in Obstructive Sleep Apnea. *Arch. Otolaryngol. Head Neck Surg.* **2001**, *127*, 1216–1223. [CrossRef]
8. Heiser, C.; Steffen, A.; Randerath, W.; Penzel, T. Hypoglossal nerve stimulation in obstructive sleep apnea. *Somnologie* **2017**, *21*, 140–148. [CrossRef]
9. Heiser, C.; Hofauer, B. Addressing the Tone and Synchrony Issue during Sleep: Pacing the Hypoglossal Nerve. *Sleep Med. Clin.* **2019**, *14*, 91–97. [CrossRef]

10. Strollo, P.J.; Soose, R.J.; Maurer, J.T.; de Vries, N.; Cornelius, J.; Froymovich, O.; Hanson, R.D.; Padhya, T.A.; Steward, D.L.; Gillespie, M.B.; et al. Upper-Airway Stimulation for Obstructive Sleep Apnea. *N. Engl. J. Med.* **2014**, *370*, 139–149. [CrossRef]
11. Stimulation Therapy for Apnea Reduction (STAR) Trial Group; Strollo, P.J.; Gillespie, M.B.; Soose, R.J.; Maurer, J.T.; de Vries, N.; Cornelius, J.; Hanson, R.D.; Padhya, T.A.; Steward, D.L.; et al. Upper Airway Stimulation for Obstructive Sleep Apnea: Durability of the Treatment Effect at 18 Months. *Sleep* **2015**, *38*, 1593–1598.
12. Soose, R.J.; Woodson, B.T.; Gillespie, M.B.; Maurer, J.T.; de Vries, N.; Steward, D.L.; Strohl, K.P.; Baskin, J.Z.; Padhya, T.A.; Badr, M.S.; et al. Upper Airway Stimulation for Obstructive Sleep Apnea: Self-Reported Outcomes at 24 Months. *J. Clin. Sleep Med.* **2016**, *12*, 43–48. [CrossRef]
13. Woodson, B.T.; Soose, R.J.; Gillespie, M.B.; Strohl, K.P.; Maurer, J.T.; de Vries, N.; Steward, D.L.; Baskin, J.Z.; Badr, M.S.; Lin, H.S.; et al. Three-Year Outcomes of Cranial Nerve Stimulation for Obstructive Sleep Apnea: The STAR Trial. *Otolaryngol. Head Neck Surg.* **2016**, *154*, 181–188. [CrossRef]
14. Gillespie, M.B.; Soose, R.J.; Woodson, B.T.; Strohl, K.P.; Maurer, J.T.; de Vries, N.; Steward, D.L.; Baskin, J.Z.; Badr, M.S.; Lin, H.-S.; et al. Upper Airway Stimulation for Obstructive Sleep Apnea: Patient-Reported Outcomes after 48 Months of Follow-up. *Otolaryngol. Neck Surg.* **2017**, *156*, 765–771. [CrossRef]
15. Woodson, B.T.; Strohl, K.P.; Soose, R.J.; Gillespie, M.B.; Maurer, J.T.; de Vries, N.; Padhya, T.A.; Badr, M.S.; Lin, H.-S.; Vanderveken, O.M.; et al. Upper Airway Stimulation for Obstructive Sleep Apnea: 5-Year Outcomes. *Otolaryngol. Neck Surg.* **2018**, *159*, 194–202. [CrossRef]
16. Heiser, C.; Maurer, J.T.; Hofauer, B.; Sommer, J.U.; Seitz, A.; Steffen, A. Outcomes of Upper Airway Stimulation for Obstructive Sleep Apnea in a Multicenter German Postmarket Study. *Otolaryngol. Neck Surg.* **2016**, *156*, 378–384. [CrossRef]
17. Steffen, A.; Sommer, J.U.; Hofauer, B.; Maurer, J.T.; Hasselbacher, K.; Heiser, C. Outcome after one year of upper airway stimulation for obstructive sleep apnea in a multicenter German post-market study. *Laryngoscope* **2018**, *128*, 509–515. [CrossRef]
18. Heiser, C.; Steffen, A.; Boon, M.; Hofauer, B.; Doghramji, K.; Maurer, J.T.; Sommer, J.U.; Soose, R.; Strollo, P.J.; Schwab, R.; et al. Post-approval upper airway stimulation predictors of treatment effectiveness in the ADHERE registry. *Eur. Respir. J.* **2019**, *53*, 1801405. [CrossRef]
19. Thaler, E.; Schwab, R.; Maurer, J.; Soose, R.; Larsen, C.; Stevens, S.; Stevens, D.; Boon, M.; Huntley, C.; Doghramji, K.; et al. Results of the ADHERE upper airway stimulation registry and predictors of therapy efficacy. *Laryngoscope* **2020**, *130*, 1333–1338. [CrossRef]
20. Woodson, B.T.; Gillespie, M.B.; Soose, R.J.; Maurer, J.T.; de Vries, N.; Steward, D.L.; Baskin, J.Z.; Padhya, T.A.; Lin, H.S.; Mickelson, S.; et al. Randomized controlled withdrawal study of upper airway stimulation on OSA: Short- and long-term effect. *Otolaryngol. Head Neck Surg.* **2014**, *151*, 880–887. [CrossRef]
21. Sher, A.E.; Schechtman, K.B.; Piccirillo, J.F. The Efficacy of Surgical Modifications of the Upper Airway in Adults with Obstructive Sleep Apnea Syndrome. *Sleep* **1996**, *19*, 156–177. [CrossRef]
22. Berry, R.B.; Brooks, R.; Gamaldo, C.; Harding, S.M.; Lloyd, R.M.; Quan, S.F.; Troester, M.T.; Vaughn, B.V. AASM Scoring Manual Updates for 2017 (Version 2.4). *J. Clin. Sleep Med.* **2017**, *13*, 665–666. [CrossRef]
23. Weaver, T.E.; Laizner, A.M.; Evans, L.K.; Maislin, G.; Chugh, D.K.; Lyon, K.; Smith, P.L.; Schwartz, A.R.; Redline, S.; Pack, A.; et al. An Instrument to Measure Functional Status Outcomes for Disorders of Excessive Sleepiness. *Sleep* **1997**, *20*, 835–843.
24. Johns, M.; Hocking, B. Daytime Sleepiness and Sleep Habits of Australian Workers. *Sleep* **1997**, *20*, 844–847. [CrossRef]
25. Heiser, C.; Knopf, A.; Bas, M.; Gahleitner, C.; Hofauer, B. Selective upper airway stimulation for obstructive sleep apnea: A single center clinical experience. *Eur. Arch. Oto Rhino Laryngol.* **2016**, *274*, 1727–1734. [CrossRef]
26. Steffen, A.; Sommer, U.J.; Maurer, J.T.; Abrams, N.; Hofauer, B.; Heiser, C. Long-term follow-up of the German post-market study for upper airway stimulation for obstructive sleep apnea. *Sleep Breath.* **2019**, *24*, 979–984. [CrossRef]
27. Bradley, T.D.; Floras, J.S. Obstructive sleep apnoea and its cardiovascular consequences. *Lancet* **2009**, *373*, 82–93. [CrossRef]
28. Zinchuk, A.; Yaggi, H.K. Sleep Apnea Heterogeneity, Phenotypes, and Cardiovascular Risk. Implications for Trial Design and Precision Sleep Medicine. *Am. J. Respir. Crit. Care Med.* **2019**, *200*, 412–413. [CrossRef]
29. Penzel, T.; Kantelhardt, J.W.; Bartsch, R.; Riedl, M.; Kraemer, J.F.; Wessel, N.; Garcia, C.; Glos, M.; Fietze, I.; Schöbel, C. Modulations of Heart Rate, ECG, and Cardio-Respiratory Coupling Observed in Polysomnography. *Front. Physiol.* **2016**, *7*, 460. [CrossRef]
30. Aurora, R.N.; Crainiceanu, C.; Gottlieb, D.J.; Kim, J.S.; Punjabi, N.M. Obstructive Sleep Apnea during REM Sleep and Cardiovascular Disease. *Am. J. Respir. Crit. Care Med.* **2018**, *197*, 653–660. [CrossRef]
31. Mehra, R.; Steffen, A.; Heiser, C.; Hofauer, B.; Withrow, K.; Doghramji, K.; Boon, M.; Huntley, C.; Soose, R.J.; Stevens, S.; et al. Upper Airway Stimulation versus Untreated Comparators in Positive Airway Pressure Treatment–Refractory Obstructive Sleep Apnea. *Ann. Am. Thorac. Soc.* **2020**, *17*, 1610–1619. [CrossRef] [PubMed]

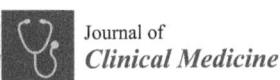

Article

Evaluation of Respiratory Resistance as a Predictor for Oral Appliance Treatment Response in Obstructive Sleep Apnea: A Pilot Study

Hiroyuki Ishiyama [1,2], Masayuki Hideshima [2,*], Shusuke Inukai [3], Meiyo Tamaoka [4], Akira Nishiyama [1,2] and Yasunari Miyazaki [5]

1. Dental Anesthesiology and Orofacial Pain Management, Graduate School of Medical and Dental Sciences, Tokyo Medical and Dental University, Tokyo 113-8549, Japan; h.ishiyama.rpro@tmd.ac.jp (H.I.); anishi.tmj@tmd.ac.jp (A.N.)
2. Dental Clinic for Sleep Disorders (Apnea and Snoring), Oral and Maxillofacial Rehabilitation, Dental Hospital, Tokyo Medical and Dental University, Tokyo 113-8549, Japan
3. Removable Partial Prosthodontics, Oral Health Sciences, Graduate School of Medical and Dental Sciences, Tokyo Medical and Dental University, Tokyo 113-8549, Japan; inurpro@tmd.ac.jp
4. Department of Respiratory Physiology and Sleep Medicine, Graduate School of Medical and Dental Sciences, Tokyo Medical and Dental University, Tokyo 113-8549, Japan; meiyou2.pulm@tmd.ac.jp
5. Department of Respiratory Medicine, Graduate School of Medical and Dental Sciences, Tokyo Medical and Dental University, Tokyo 113-8549, Japan; miyazaki.pilm@tmd.ac.jp
* Correspondence: m.hideshima.rpro@tmd.ac.jp; Tel.: +81-3-5803-4551

Abstract: The aim of this study was to determine the utility of respiratory resistance as a predictor of oral appliance (OA) response in obstructive sleep apnea (OSA). Twenty-seven patients with OSA (mean respiratory event index (REI): 17.5 ± 6.5 events/h) were recruited. At baseline, the respiratory resistance (R20) was measured by impulse oscillometry (IOS) with a fitted nasal mask in the supine position, and cephalometric radiographs were obtained to analyze the pharyngeal airway space (SPAS: superior posterior airway space, MAS: middle airway space, IAS: inferior airway space). The R20 and radiographs after the OA treatment were evaluated, and the changes from the baseline were analyzed. A sleep test with OA was carried out using a portable device. The subjects were divided into Responders and Non-responders based on an REI improvement ≥ 50% from the baseline, or REI < 5 after treatment, and the R20 reduction rate between the two groups were compared. The subjects comprised 20 responders and 7 non-responders. The R20 reduction rate with OA in responders was significantly greater than it was in non-responders (14.4 ± 7.9 % versus 2.4 ± 9.8 %, $p < 0.05$). In responders, SPAS, MAS, and IAS were significantly widened and R20 was significantly decreased with OA ($p < 0.05$). There was no significant difference in non-responders ($p > 0.05$). A logistic multiple regression analysis showed that the R20 reduction rate was predictive for OA treatment responses (2% incremental odds ratio (OR), 24.5; 95% CI, 21.5–28.0; $p = 0.018$). This pilot study confirmed that respiratory resistance may have significant clinical utility in predicting OA treatment responses.

Keywords: obstructive sleep apnea; oral appliance; predictor; respiratory resistance; impulse oscillometry

1. Introduction

Obstructive sleep apnea (OSA) is characterized by intermittent obstruction of the upper airway during sleep and by repeated apnea and hypopnea, which cause intermittent hypoxia and sleep fragmentation, reducing sleep quality [1–3]. Oral appliance (OA) therapy is a treatment option for OSA. An OA widens the upper airway by advancing the mandible; this prevents upper airway obstructions during sleep [4,5]. Although its efficacy is inferior to that of continuous positive airway pressure (CPAP) therapy, OA therapy has high compliance [6,7] and not only improves apnea, hypopnea, and symptoms of OSA, but has recently also been shown to be effective on the cardiovascular comorbidity in OSA, such as hypertension and arrhythmia [8]. The success rate of OA therapy in patients with mild–severe OSA was reported to be 35–64% in a recent review [9] and individual variability in response to OA treatment represented a significant clinical challenge for implementing this therapy [10]. According to the clinical practice guidelines for the treatment of OSA, OA therapy is recommended mainly for patients with mild to moderate OSA, or patients who cannot tolerate CPAP [11]. Therefore, the indication of OA in current OSA treatment is determined based on the severity of the Apnea Hypopnea Index (AHI). However, OA therapy is reported to be effective even in severe cases [12,13], and thus, severity by itself is not considered to accurately indicate the need for OA therapy.

To determine whether it is indicated, it is also necessary to conduct appropriate pretreatment evaluations in addition to the AHI, in order to predict the potential treatment effects. To determine OA therapy indications, evaluating the relationship of morphological changes of the upper airway and an obstruction site during mandibular advancement is highly important. The factors that are affected by changes in the upper airway include breathing sounds, respiratory resistance, and muscular function. However, a method for predicting the treatment effects of OA in a simple and non-invasive procedure using these parameters has not yet been established.

The Impulse Oscillation System (IOS) is a method that assesses breath dynamics while breathing at rest [14], unlike conventional pulmonary function testing (spirometry) that requires forced breathing. The air pressure oscillations are inserted into the oral cavity through a mouthpiece attached to a device, in order to measure respiratory resistance from the differences in the phases between the pressure and airflow, which change depending on the diameter of the airway and its elasticity. The localization of resistance can be inferred using frequency characteristics, and IOSs have been used for the diagnosis and treatment of bronchial asthma and chronic obstructive pulmonary disease (COPD) [15]. Its advantages include the fact that testing can be conducted in a short period of time and that the measuring method is non-invasive and easy to perform. The aim of this study was to measure respiratory resistance using the IOS in the waking state and to examine how the changes in respiratory resistance resulting from mandibular advancement reflect the treatment effects of OA.

2. Materials and Methods

2.1. Subjects

The subjects were adult patients, diagnosed with OSA (AHI $\geq$ 5), and recruited from the Dental Clinic for Sleep Disorders (Apnea and Snoring) from Tokyo Medical and Dental University Dental Hospital. The following patients were excluded: (1) those with fewer than 19 remaining teeth, including the residual anterior teeth; (2) those receiving combined OA and CPAP therapy. (3) Those regularly using a sleep-inducing drug; (4) those with a mandibular advancement <9 mm; (5) those having a medical history of respiratory disease or suffering from a respiratory disease; (6) those allergic to steroids and vasoconstrictors; (7) those with mental illness; (8) those having temporomandibular disorders with pain or trismus; and (9) those having any caries or periodontal diseases that required treatment. All subjects were provided verbal and written information about the study and signed informed consent forms. The study protocol was approved by the Tokyo Medical and Dental University Dental Hospital ethics committee (protocol code D2012-024, 9 March 2016). The study was registered at UMIN-CTR (https://www.umin.ac.jp/ctr/ (accessed on 28 August 2014); UMIN000014984; Development of treatment effect prediction method of oral appliance therapy for obstructive sleep apnea syndrome).

2.2. Sleep Test

In order to assess the efficacy of the OA treatment, an out-of-center sleep test (OCST) was performed before and after the treatment. During testing, we used a Type-3 portable sleep testing device (Pulsleep LS-120S; Fukuda Denshi, Tokyo, Japan), which is capable of measuring the SpO2, pulse rate, airflow, snoring, and posture [16]. Expiratory and inspiratory flow was measured using a nasal cannula, and respiratory conditions during sleep were recorded. The SpO2 and pulse rate were confirmed using a fingertip pulse oximeter.

The sleep test was performed for three consecutive nights, and mean values were used as representative values. When the test data were inconclusive, they were excluded from the analysis. After confirming the original waveforms, data were manually analyzed, and a standardized procedure was applied to score the results [17]. The data were all scored by a single researcher (H.I.), who was blinded to the participants' IOS data. The subjects were asked to keep a sleep diary and to record their sleep duration on the days of testing (including bedtime and the time they woke up), as well as the number and times of nocturnal awakenings, which were used as references for the analyses.

For analysis, the following values of the sleep test results were assessed: the REI (Respiratory Event Index) and the lowest SpO2. REI indicates the number of instances of apnea and hypopnea per hour of measurement. Apnea is defined as a 90% reduction in airflow for at least 10 seconds, and hypopnea is defined as $\geq 30\%$ reduction in airflow for at least 10 seconds, associated with $\geq 3\%$ reduction in oxygen saturation [17]. OSA was defined as a REI ≥ 5, and classified as mild (REI 5.0–14.9), moderate (REI 15.0–29.9), and severe (REI ≥ 30) [18].

2.3. Oral Appliance

A custom-made, monobloc, mandibular advancement oral appliance, made from a 2.0-mm polyethylene plate (Erkodur, Erkodent Inc., Pfalzgrafenweiler, Germany), was prescribed for all participants. The absolute range of the maximum mandibular advancement was measured using the George Gauge (Great Lakes Orthodontics, Ltd., New York, NY, USA) [19]. The amount of mandibular advancement in this study was set at 50–70% of the maximum, considering the discomfort and pain of the temporomandibular joint and masticatory muscles [20].

During follow-up of 2 months after the OA provision, the changes in OSA symptoms and the degrees of side effects that were associated with OA use were evaluated. The appliance was incrementally titrated to either a maximal comfortable protruded position of the mandible or a resolution of snoring and daytime symptoms [21]. Increased advancement of the appliance was facilitated by the separation of the upper and lower components of the appliance, and then repositioning at a more advanced mandibular position.

2.4. Assessment of Treatment Outcome

After the OA was fully adjusted (approximately 2.5 months after baseline), the OCST was performed with the OA in place. In this study, the efficacy of the OA treatment was evaluated using the relative REI improvement rates. The REI improvement rate was calculated using the following formula: [(REI before treatment) − (REI after treatment)]/(REI before treatment) × 100. Subjects with a rate of REI improvement $\geq 50\%$, or REI < 5 after treatment, were defined as responders, and those with a rate < 50% were defined as non-responders [22].

2.5. IOS and Test Task

Master screen IOS-J (Jaeger, Wurzburg, Germany) was used to assess respiratory resistance (Figure 1). This device releases impulse-like acoustic signals (frequency: 0–35 Hz) from a round speaker to detect the intraoral pressure and flow rate during breathing at rest, and then conducts Fourier transformations of the data to analyze respiratory resistance. IOS parameters, such as resistance at 5 Hz (R5) and resistance at 20 Hz (R20), were recorded. R5 and R20 represent the total airway resistance and resistance of the region from the upper airway through to the central airway, respectively (Figure 2) [14]. R20 was used for the analysis in this study, due to its usefulness in the prediction of AHI values [23].

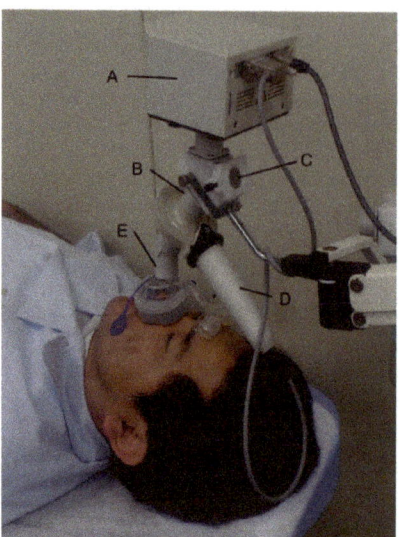

Figure 1. Impulse oscillometry system used in this study: loudspeaker (**A**), screen flap (**B**), Y-adapter (**C**), pnuemochomatograph (**D**), nasal mask (**E**).

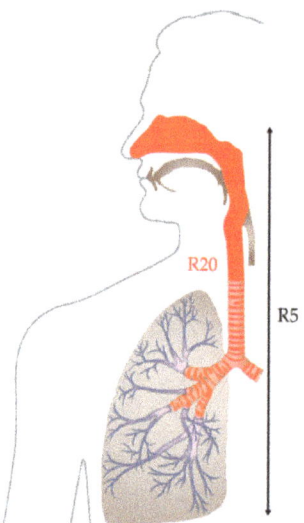

Figure 2. Scheme of Impulse Oscillation System (IOS) values: resistance at 5 Hz (R5); resistance at 20 Hz (R20). R5 and R20 represent the total airway resistance and the resistance of the region from the upper airway through to the central airway, respectively.

A single researcher (S.I.) measured the patients' respiratory resistances in the waking state. The researcher was blinded to the results of sleep test. The subjects were in the supine position and put on a nasal mask without any air leaks during the measurements. Because the measurements took place via the nasal cavity, the congestion in the nasal mucosa tended to occur over time, and accurate measurements of respiratory resistances can be hampered [24]. To prevent this, subjects were instructed to spray a vasoconstrictor nasal drop (cor-tyzine nasal solution; Tetrahydrozoline hydrochloride-prednisolone) into the nasal cavity several times, and measurements were performed 10 minutes later [25].

At the time of measurement, the subject was instructed to breathe while at rest. Respiratory resistance was measured three times under each condition with and without OA, and the mean values were used as the representative values. The measurements without OA were performed in the intercuspal position.

2.6. Cephalogram

In all recruited patients, lateral cephalometric radiographs were obtained in order to evaluate the subjects' maxillofacial morphology at baseline, as well as the changes in the pharyngeal airway space with and without OA. The morphology of the pharyngeal airway on the lateral cephalogram is known to be largely affected by the skeleton, body type, posture, and respiratory phase; the comparative reproducibility of the upper airway morphology cannot be considered to be high [26]. Therefore, the subjects were placed in an upright position with the Frankfurt plane parallel to the floor, and photographed in the end-tidal position [27]. A cephalometric analysis was carried out as previously described (Figure 3) [28]. An analysis was performed by a single researcher (H.I.), and the names of patients were blinded.

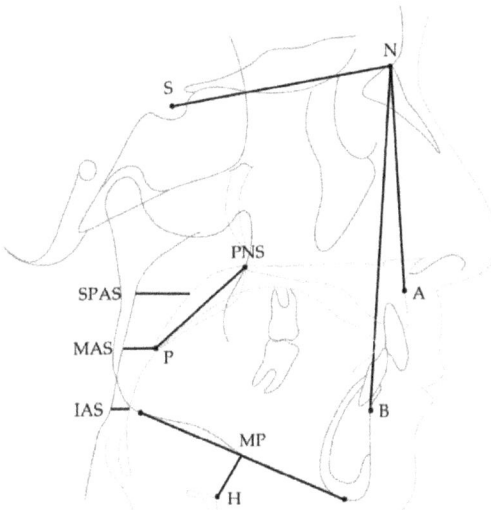

Figure 3. Cephalometric landmarks. The following points were identified on lateral cephalograms. Points: S (sella: the midpoint of the pituitary fossa), N (nasion: the most anterior point on the frontonasal suture), ANS (anterior nasal spine: the tip of the median, sharp bony process of the maxilla at the lower margin of the anterior nasal opening), PNS (posterior nasal spine: the intersection of the continuation of the anterior wall of the pterygopalatine fossa and the floor of the nose, marking the dorsal limit of the maxilla), A (the deepest midline concavity on the anterior maxilla), B (the deepest midline concavity on the mandibular symphysis), P (most inferior tip of the soft palate), H (hyoidale). Planes: MP (mandibular plane according to Steiner: the line through the gonion and gnathion). Linear measurements: PNS-P (linear distance between PNS and P), MP-H (linear distance perpendicular from H to the mandibular plane), SPAS: superior posterior airway space (width of airway behind soft palate along parallel line to gonion (Go)-B line), MAS: middle airway space (width of airway along parallel line to Go-B line through P), IAS: inferior airway space (width of airway along Go-B line).

2.7. Statistical Analysis

Continuous variables were described as mean ± SD for variables with a normal distribution and median (interquartile range) for variables with a non-normal distribution. Normality of distribution was assessed using the Shapiro-Wilk test.

The comparisons between groups were made using Student's t-test for variables with a normal distribution and a Mann-Whitney U test for variables with a non-normal distribution, and Fisher's exact test was used for categorical variables. The within-subject comparisons in each group were made using pared t-test for variables with a normal distribution and Wilcoxon signed-rank test with a non-normal distribution. The effect size (Cohen's d) of the continuous variables was calculated. The R20 reduction rate with OA was calculated using the formula: [(pre-treatment R20) − (post-treatment R20]/(pre-treatment R20) × 100. In order to determine the predictive factors for the efficacy of the OA treatment, a binominal logistic regression (stepwise method) was performed. In the analysis, the explanatory variables were set as the responders and non-responders in the OA treatment, and the objective variables were set as the R20 reduction rates and the conventional predictors (sex, age, BMI, baseline-REI, and MR-H) [29–31]. In addition, to obtain a value that allows the highest discriminability for the prediction of the efficacy of OA therapy, the receiver operating characteristic curve and the area under the curve (AUC) were calculated in order to determine the significant factor in the regression analysis, and the cut-off value was determined using the Youden index. An odds ratio (OR) ≥ 2 or ≤ 0.5 was considered a clinically meaningful predictor. A value of $p < 0.05$ was considered statistically significant. All statistical analyses were performed using the SPSS version 21.0 software (IBM, Inc., Armonk, NY, USA).

3. Results

3.1. Baseline Characteristics of the Subjects

Thirty-five OSA patients were recruited into this study, and eight patients refused to participate in the study. Twenty-seven patients, with mild ($n = 9$), moderate ($n = 17$), and severe ($n = 1$) OSA, completed the full study protocol. The subject characteristics at baseline are shown in Table 1. The majority (81.5%) of patients were men. The median age of all subjects was 65.0 (56.0–70.0) years; their median Body Mass Index (BMI) was 25.1 (22.2–26.8) kg/m². The mean REI of the subjects was 17.5 ± 6.5 events/h. The median Epworth Sleepiness Scale (ESS) of the subjects was 8.0 (6.0–11.0). Of the 27 subjects, 20 subjects were responders and 7 subjects were non-responders. There was a significant difference due to sex at baseline between responders and non-responders, whereas there was no significant difference in age, BMI, ESS, and R20. In addition, there was no significant difference in the ratio of the mandibular advancement after the OA adjustment, nor in any parameters representing maxillofacial morphology (SNA, SNB, ANB, PNS-P, or MP-H) between responders and non-responders. Furthermore, there was no significant difference in the pharyngeal airway space (SPAS, MAS, and IAS) on the cephalogram between the two groups.

Table 1. Patient characteristics of the responders and non-responders receiving oral appliance (OA) therapy.

	All ($n = 27$)	Responders ($n = 20$)	Non-Responders ($n = 7$)	p-Value [a]	ES
Sex (%men)	81.5 (22/27)	66.7 (15/20)	100 (7/7)	<0.01	-
Age (years)	65.0 (56.0–70.0)	65.5 (44.3–70.0)	65.0 (58.0–70.0)	0.50	-
BMI (kg/m²)	25.1 (22.2–26.8)	26.5 (22.1–28.8)	25.1 (22.2–25.5)	0.31	-
Mallampati class	3.0 (3.0–4.0)	3.0 (3.0–3.8)	4.0 (2.0–4.0)	0.53	-
REI (events/hour)	17.5 ± 6.5	16.4 ± 5.9	20.7 ± 7.1	0.22	0.69
REI severity					
Mild-n (%)	9 (33.3)	8 (40.0)	1 (14.3)		

Table 1. Cont.

	All (n = 27)	Responders (n = 20)	Non-Responders (n = 7)	p-Value [a]	ES
Moderate-n (%)	17 (63.0)	11 (55.0)	6 (85.7)		
Severe-n (%)	1 (3.7)	1 (5.0)	0 (0.0)		
LowestSpO2 (%)	83.5 ± 5.8	84.1 ± 5.2	81.7 ± 7.1	0.36	0.42
R20 (kPa/L/s)	0.48 ± 0.15	0.49 ± 0.17	0.47 ± 0.11	0.85	0.13
ESS	8.0 (6.0–11.0)	8.0 (7.0–12.5)	6.0 (4.0–8.0)	0.13	-
OAM/MaxM (%)	59.8 ± 10.4	58.8 ± 10.4	62.6 ± 9.8	0.43	0.37
SNA (°)	83.0 ± 4.2	82.4 ± 4.1	84.6 ± 4.2	0.25	0.54
SNB (°)	78.6 ± 4.5	78.1 ± 5.0	79.8 ± 2.3	0.27	0.38
ANB (°)	4.4 ± 2.7	4.3 ± 2.7	4.7 ± 2.5	0.73	0.15
PNS-P (mm)	41.4 ± 4.7	42.0 ± 7.9	39.6 ± 6.5	0.49	0.32
MP-H (mm)	17.3 ± 7.6	16.9 ± 6.6	18.5 ± 9.8	0.64	0.21
SPAS (mm)	4.5 (0.0–9.0)	5.8 (4.7)	0.0 (0.0–9.0)	0.10	0.76
MAS (mm)	13.4 ± 5.4	13.1 ± 5.6	14.2 ± 4.7	0.65	0.20
IAS (mm)	9.7 ± 4.3	9.5 ± 4.0	10.3 ± 5.7	0.67	0.18

Data expressed as mean ± standard deviation (SD), median, and interquartile range (IQR). [a] Comparison between responders and non-responders. ES: Effect size (Cohen's d). BMI: Body Mass Index, REI: Respiratory Event Index, R20: Respiratory resistance at 20 Hz. ESS: Epworth Sleepiness Scale, OAM: Mandibular advancement with appliance. MaxM: Maximum mandibular advancement, SPAS: Superior posterior airway space. MAS: Middle airway space, IAS: Inferior airway space.

3.2. The Comparison of the Responders and the Non-Responders in OA Therapy

The values of each parameter with and without the OA are shown in Table 2. With respect to within-subject comparisons, the responders showed a significant decrease in REI, R20, and ESS ($p < 0.01$) and a significant increase in LowestSpO2 with OA ($p < 0.05$). In the cephalogram, the responders showed a significant increase in SPAS, MAS, and IAS with OA ($p < 0.05$). In non-responders, the REI was significantly decreased with OA ($p < 0.05$), whereas there were no significant differences in the other parameters ($p > 0.05$). The results from the R20 reduction rate comparison between responders and non-responders are shown in Figure 4. The R20 reduction rate was significantly higher in responders compared to non-responders ($p < 0.01$; Cohen's d = 1.46).

Table 2. Efficacy of oral appliance therapy in the responders and the non-responders.

	Responders (n = 20)			Non-Responders (n = 7)		
	w/o OA	with OA	ES	w/o OA	with OA	ES
REI (events/h)	16.4 ± 5.9	5.3 ± 2.1 *	2.51	20.7 ± 7.1	15.5 ± 4.6 *	0.87
Lowest SpO$_2$ (%)	84.1 ± 5.2	88.7 ± 4.0 *	1.07	81.7 ± 7.1	83.6 ± 4.9	0.31
R20 (kPa/L/s)	0.49 ± 0.17	0.41 ± 0.13 *	0.5	0.47 ± 0.11	0.46 ± 0.1	0.1
ESS	8.0 (7.0–12.5)	6.0 (4.0–11.5) *	-	6.0 (4.0–8.0)	7.0 (4.0–8.0)	-
SPAS (mm)	5.8 ± 4.7	10.1 ± 6.2 *	0.8	2.4 ± 3.6	4.3 ± 5.8	0.39
MAS (mm)	13.1 ± 5.6	15.9 ± 5.7 *	0.5	14.2 ± 4.7	15.8 ± 4.7	0.34
IAS (mm)	9.5 ± 4.0	11.8 ± 4.6 *	0.53	10.3 ± 5.0	9.3 ± 5.6	0.19

Data expressed as mean ± standard deviation (SD), median, and interquartile range (IQR). * $p < 0.05$. ES: Effect size (Cohen's d), REI: Respiratory Event Index, R20: Respiratory resistance at 20 Hz, ESS: Epworth Sleepiness Scale, SPAS: Superior posterior airway space, MAS: Middle airway space, IAS: Inferior airway space.

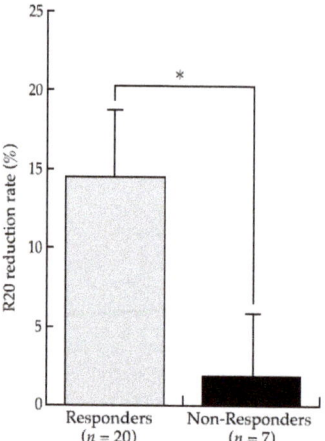

Figure 4. Comparison of responders and non-responders in terms of R20 improvement rates (* $p < 0.05$).

3.3. The Predictors Associated with Oral Appliance Treatment Success

The results of the binary logistic regression are shown in Table 3. The R20 reduction rate was shown to be an independent predictor of OA treatment response (2% incremental OR, 24.5; 95% CI, 21.5–28.0). However, sex, age, BMI, baseline-REI, and MP-H were not significant predictors. The ORs of the R20 improvement rates are presented for 0.1% increments, 1% increments, and 2% increments. The calculated cut-off value of the R20 reduction rate from the Youden index was 8.6% (AUC: 0.839, sensitivity: 0.80, specificity: 0.86) (Figure 5).

Table 3. Logistic regression results for factors associated with oral appliance treatment success.

Variables	β	*p*-Value	Odds Ratio	95% CI
Improvement in R20				
0.1% increments	0.16	0.018	1.17	1.03–1.34
1% increments	0.16	0.018	4.95	4.33–5.66
2% increments	0.16	0.018	24.5	21.5–28.0

95% CI: 95% Confidence Interval. R20: Respiratory resistance at 20 Hz.

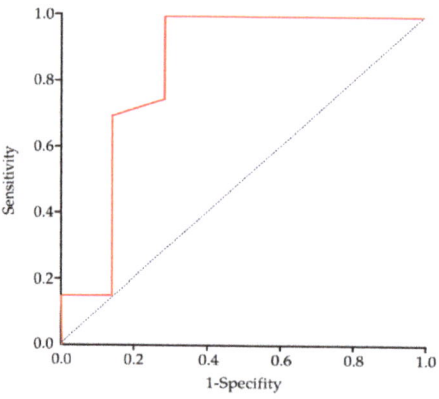

Figure 5. Receiver operating characteristic (ROC) curves of the R20 improvement rates.

4. Discussion

This study demonstrated that the higher the respiratory resistance reduction rates following mandibular advancement, the larger the improvement in REI due to OA. This indicates that the rate of reduction in respiratory resistance is useful for predicting the efficacy of OA therapy. This predictive measure is clinically straightforward, and has good sensitivity and specificity. Although the previous studies have reported that there was a positive correlation between AHI and respiratory resistance [32], and that respiratory resistance was decreased by advancing the mandible [33], the utility of respiratory resistance in the prediction of OA treatment responses has not been shown. The results of this study are the first to demonstrate the clinical utility of respiratory resistance for the prediction of OA treatment response in OSA patients using quantitative methodology. Though various types of OAs are available, OAs are broadly classified into two types: Mono-block and Bi-block types [34]. In Japan, where OA therapy is provided under the National Health Insurance, mono-block OA types are commonly used to balance the costs and the technical simplicity of the treatment procedure. Therefore, a mono-block OA was used in this study.

In this study, there was no significant difference in the R20 at baseline between the responders and non-responders. Similarly, no significant differences were seen between the measurements of the pharyngeal airway spaces and maxillofacial morphology at baseline. Thus, the OA treatment response could not be predicted by the position of the mandible at rest, because there was no difference between anatomical characteristics and the respiratory resistance values between the two groups at baseline. However, despite the fact that the mandibular positions were sufficiently adjusted with the OA in all subjects, the R20 reduction rate according to the mandibular advancement was higher in the responders compared to non-responders. Furthermore, we performed a regression analysis including the conventional predictors (sex, age, BMI, and MR-H) of OA treatment responses in addition to R20. Only the R20 reduction rate was a predictor of OA treatment responses, and no other factors were determined. These results suggested that the reduction rate of respiratory resistance via mandibular advancement was highly correlated with OA treatment effects, and a larger reduction in respiratory resistance was shown to lead to the higher efficacy of OA.

A cephalometric analysis showed that in the responders, the superior/middle/inferior regions of the pharyngeal airway space were all widened by advancing the mandible, with the upper airway widening in a particularly large amount. In the non-responders, widening of the pharyngeal regions with mandibular advancement was not seen. Thus, the reduction of respiratory resistance via mandibular advancement can be expected to result from the widening of the pharyngeal region. In the endoscopy, Sasao et al. [35] reported that there were two types of morphological changes seen in responders to OA therapy: "all-round-type," which is a circumferential widening in the antero-posterior/lateral directions via mandibular advancement, and a "lateral dominant type," which is a widening primarily in the lateral direction. Among the responders in this study, some showed poor widening of the pharynx on the cephalogram, despite the large reductions in respiratory resistance by advancing the mandible. Since the cephalometry is capable of observing only morphological changes in the antero-posterior direction, the corresponding subjects presumably belonged to the lateral dominant-type, in which widening occurred in the lateral direction.

The reported conventional testing methods that predict the efficacy of OA therapy include cephalometry [36], computed tomography (CT) [37], magnetic resonance imaging (MRI) [38], and endoscopy [39]. Concerning the prediction of the efficacy of OA therapy using cephalometry, a shorter soft palate, shorter distance between the soft palate and the posterior pharyngeal wall, larger ANB angle, and smaller SNB angle have all been shown to lead to a higher OA efficacy [36]. Similar to in this study, the efficacy of OA therapy has been shown to be high in CT [37], MRI [38], and endoscopy [39] studies, in which a widening of the upper airway via mandibular advancement was seen. However, although these testing methods are useful to predict the efficacy of OA therapy, they require a special testing room and have several issues, such as exposure at the time of imaging/testing, invasion, and a high cost. The protocol that was used to predict the efficacy of OA using respiratory resistance in this study is a simple, non-invasive, low-cost method, because it can be measured by simply purchasing a test device and wearing a nasal mask. Therefore, this method is considered beneficial for all physicians, dentists, and patients involved with OA therapy.

This study has a number of limitations. In this sleep test, electroencephalography was not conducted, and it was not possible to measure the exact sleep time. Therefore, the REI calculated from the test results may be underestimated. In addition, this test cannot distinguish between obstructive and central events. The study included a small sample size, and the number of subjects with varying OSA severities was uneven. In the present study (n = 27), the number of severe cases was small (mild [n = 10], moderate [n = 16], and severe [n = 1]), and the subjects were unevenly distributed compared to the typical distributions of patients with OSA. By increasing the sample size, an analysis in patients with severe OSA needs to be conducted in the future. Another potential limitation is the relatively lower BMI than other studies. The World Health Organization Expert Consultation has reported that for many Asian populations, trigger points for public health action were identified as $\geq$ 23 kg·m^2, because Asians generally have a higher percentage of body fat than Caucasians of the same BMI [40]. Additionally, the Committee of Japan Society for the Study of Obesity reported that the criteria for obesity disease for Japanese was defined as a BMI $\geq$ 25 kg·m^2 [41]. Therefore, our Japanese sample (mean BMI 25.4 kg·m^2) was considered obese for their standard. To better understand if this study is valid in a Caucasian obese population, further trials with the same methodology are still required. Additionally, there were some cases whose REI reduction rates were not high enough, despite a large reduction in their respiratory resistance via mandibular advancement. Conversely, there were also cases whose REI reduction rates were high, despite small reductions in respiratory resistance. Since we performed comparisons in order to analyze the changes in respiratory resistance while subjects were awake, and measured their respiratory conditions during sleep in the present examination, the differences in environments during the awake state and during sleep may have affected the results. Although the muscles surrounding the pharynx relax during sleep, and the airway is thought to become narrower than while awake, how findings during wakefulness are reflected in the efficacy of OA treatment during sleep remains unclear, and further research is needed. The utility of R20 as a predictor of the success rate of treatment to CPAP was not evaluated in this study; this is necessary to evaluate in a further study. In this study, we prepared a titrated OA and measured the respiratory resistance with and without OA for 2 days. For clinical application, the methods used in this study need to be simpler. As a future prospect, the change in respiratory resistance by advancing the mandibulae will be measured using a George gauge before OA treatment. The response of OA treatment may be predicted by evaluating the change in 1-day measurement and using the cut-off value calculated in this study.

Our study results can be considered to be useful for both physicians seeking OA therapy and dentists responsible for OA therapy. In the current clinical setting, due to difficulty in preoperatively predicting the efficacy of OA therapy, preparing/wearing/adjusting an OA and undergoing a sleep test for the evaluation of efficacy require time and labor. Consequently, when an expected result is not obtained, disadvantages for the patient/dentist/physician are significant, which results in a loss of reliability of OA therapy. In order to avoid such a situation, if suitability of OA therapy can be screened by predicting the efficacy of OA therapy at a medical organization in advance, physicians would then be able to explain the suitability to patients with mild to moderate OSA who desire OA therapy and those who are intolerant to CPAP. In addition, both dentists receiving a request for OA therapy and patients receiving treatment can smoothly proceed with OA therapy based on the prior prediction, and evidence-based medicine (EBM), which is required in modern medicine, can be realized, and accountability can be expected to be fulfilled.

Furthermore, although either CPAP or OA therapy is uniformly chosen using the AHI of sleep testing in the current OSA treatment, tailor-made medicine, which determines diagnosis and optimal therapy depending on each case, can be chosen.

5. Conclusions

With the aim of evaluating OA indications, respiratory resistance in the waking state, as well as examining how changes in respiratory resistance via mandibular advancement affected the efficacy of the OA treatment, were measured. This study showed that the OA treatment was highly efficient in cases with large reductions in respiratory resistance. In addition, the results suggested that the use of a cut-off value for the reduction rate of respiratory resistance analyzed in this study allowed for the diagnosis and selection of patients in whom OA therapy is effective. However, in order to confirm the reliability and universality of the study results, further analyses need to be performed with a larger sample size, and with uniform conditions in the groups.

Author Contributions: Drafting of the manuscript: H.I.; study concept and design: M.H., H.I., S.I., M.T., and Y.M.; data acquisition: M.H., H.I., S.I., and A.N.; analysis and interpretation of data: M.H. and H.I.; critical revision of the manuscript: M.H., H.I., A.N., M.T., and Y.M.; statistical analysis: H.I. and A.N.; study supervision: M.T. and Y.M. All authors have read and agreed to the published version of the manuscript.

Funding: This research was funded by JSPS Grants-in-Aid for Scientific Research (grant numbers 24792064).

Institutional Review Board Statement: The study was conducted according to the guidelines of the Declaration of Helsinki, and approved by the ethics committee at the Tokyo Medical and Dental University Dental Hospital (protocol code D2012-024, 9 March 2016).

Informed Consent Statement: Informed consent was obtained from all subjects involved in the study.

Data Availability Statement: The data presented in this study are available on request from the corresponding author.

Acknowledgments: The authors are most grateful to Tatsu Suzuki for his collaboration in this research.

Conflicts of Interest: The authors declare no conflict of interest.

References

1. Young, T.; Palta, M.; Dempsey, J.; Skatrud, J.; Weber, S.; Badr, S. The occurrence of sleep-disordered breathing among middle-aged adults. *N. Engl. J. Med.* **1993**, *328*, 1230–1235. [CrossRef]
2. Flemons, W.W. Clinical practice. Obstructive sleep apnea. *N. Engl. J. Med.* **2002**, *347*, 498–504. [CrossRef]
3. White, D.P. Pathogenesis of obstructive and central sleep apnea. *Am. J. Respir. Crit. Care Med.* **2005**, *172*, 1363–1370. [CrossRef] [PubMed]
4. Sutherland, K.; Cistulli, P.A. Oral Appliance Therapy for Obstructive Sleep Apnoea: State of the Art. *J. Clin. Med.* **2019**, *8*, 2121. [CrossRef]
5. Ishiyama, H.; Inukai, S.; Nishiyama, A.; Hideshima, M.; Nakamura, S.; Tamaoka, M.; Miyazaki, Y.; Fueki, K.; Wakabayashi, N. Effect of jaw-opening exercise on prevention of temporomandibular disorders pain associated with oral appliance therapy in obstructive sleep apnea patients: A randomized, double-blind, placebo-controlled trial. *J. Prosthodont. Res.* **2017**, *61*, 259–267. [CrossRef] [PubMed]
6. Vanderveken, O.M.; Dieltjens, M.; Wouters, K.; De Backer, W.A.; van de Heyning, P.H.; Braem, M.J. Objective measurement of compliance during oral appliance therapy for sleep-disordered breathing. *Thorax* **2013**, *68*, 91–96. [CrossRef]
7. Dieltjens, M.; Braem, M.J.; Vroegop, A.; Wouters, K.; Verbraecken, J.A.; De Backer, W.A.; van de Heyning, P.H.; Vanderveken, O.M. Objectively measured vs self-reported compliance during oral appliance therapy for sleep-disordered breathing. *Chest* **2013**, *144*, 1495–1502. [CrossRef] [PubMed]
8. Phillips, C.L.; Grunstein, R.R.; Darendeliler, M.A.; Mihailidou, A.S.; Srinivasan, V.K.; Yee, B.J.; Marks, G.B.; Cistulli, P.A. Health outcomes of continuous positive airway pressure versus oral appliance treatment for obstructive sleep apnea: A randomized controlled trial. *Am. J. Respir. Crit. Care Med.* **2013**, *187*, 879–887. [CrossRef] [PubMed]
9. Sutherland, K.; Vanderveken, O.M.; Tsuda, H.; Marklund, M.; Gagnadoux, F.; Kushida, C.A.; Cistulli, P.A. Oral appliance treatment for obstructive sleep apnoea: An update. *J. Clin. Sleep Med.* **2014**, *10*, 215–227. [CrossRef] [PubMed]
10. Sutherland, K.; Takaya, H.; Qian, J.; Petocz, P.; Ng, A.T.; Cistulli, P.A. Oral Appliance Treatment Response and Polysomnographic Phenotypes of Obstructive Sleep Apnea. *J. Clin. Sleep Med.* **2015**, *11*, 861–868. [CrossRef] [PubMed]

11. Kushida, C.A.; Morgenthaler, T.I.; Littner, M.R.; Alessi, C.A.; Bailey, D.; Coleman, J., Jr.; Friedman, L.; Hirshkowitz, M.; Kapen, S.; Kramer, M.; et al. Practice parameters for the treatment of snoring and Obstructive Sleep Apnea with oral appliances: An update for 2005. *Sleep* **2006**, *29*, 240–243. [CrossRef]
12. Blanco, J.; Zamarron, C.; Abeleira Pazos, M.T.; Lamela, C.; Suarez Quintanilla, D. Prospective evaluation of an oral appliance in the treatment of obstructive sleep apnea syndrome. *Sleep Breath.* **2005**, *9*, 20–25. [CrossRef]
13. Hoekema, A.; Stegenga, B.; Wijkstra, P.J.; van der Hoeven, J.H.; Meinesz, A.F.; de Bont, L.G. Obstructive sleep apnea therapy. *J. Dent. Res.* **2008**, *87*, 882–887. [CrossRef]
14. Bednarek, M.; Grabicki, M.; Piorunek, T.; Batura-Gabryel, H. Current place of impulse oscillometry in the assessment of pulmonary diseases. *Respir. Med.* **2020**, *170*, 105952. [CrossRef] [PubMed]
15. Ohishi, J.; Kurosawa, H.; Ogawa, H.; Irokawa, T.; Hida, W.; Kohzuki, M. Application of impulse oscillometry for within-breath analysis in patients with chronic obstructive pulmonary disease: Pilot study. *BMJ Open* **2011**, *1*, e000184. [CrossRef] [PubMed]
16. Mazaki, T.; Kasai, T.; Yokoi, H.; Kuramitsu, S.; Yamaji, K.; Morinaga, T.; Masuda, H.; Shirai, S.; Ando, K. Impact of Sleep-Disordered Breathing on Long Term Outcomes in Patients with Acute Coronary Syndrome Who Have Undergone Primary Percutaneous Coronary Intervention. *J. Am. Heart Assoc.* **2016**, *5*, e003270. [CrossRef] [PubMed]
17. Berry, R.B.; Brooks, R.; Gamaldo, C.E.; Harding, S.M.; Lloyd, R.M.; Marcus, C.L.; Vaughn, B.V. *The AASM Manual for The Scoring of Sleep and Associated Events: Rules, Terminology and Technical Specifications*; Version 2.1; American Academy of Sleep Medicine: Darien, IL, USA, 2014.
18. American Academy of Sleep Medicine. *International Classification of Sleep Disorders*, 3rd ed.; American Academy of Sleep Medicine: Darien, IL, USA, 2014.
19. George, P.T. A new instrument for functional appliance bite registration. *J. Clin. Orthod.* **1992**, *26*, 721–723. [PubMed]
20. Aarab, G.; Lobbezoo, F.; Hamburger, H.L.; Naeije, M. Effects of an oral appliance with different mandibular protrusion positions at a constant vertical dimension on obstructive sleep apnea. *Clin. Oral Investig.* **2010**, *14*, 339–345. [CrossRef] [PubMed]
21. Dieltjens, M.; Vanderveken, O.M.; Heyning, P.H.; Braem, M.J. Current opinions and clinical practice in the titration of oral appliances in the treatment of sleep-disordered breathing. *Sleep Med. Rev.* **2012**, *16*, 177–185. [CrossRef]
22. Ferguson, K.A.; Cartwright, R.; Rogers, R.; Schmidt-Nowara, W. Oral appliances for snoring and obstructive sleep apnea: A review. *Sleep* **2006**, *29*, 244–262. [CrossRef]
23. Aihara, K.; Oga, T.; Harada, Y.; Chihara, Y.; Handa, T.; Tanizawa, K.; Watanabe, K.; Hitomi, T.; Tsuboi, T.; Mishima, M.; et al. Analysis of anatomical and functional determinants of obstructive sleep apnea. *Sleep Breath.* **2012**, *16*, 473–481. [CrossRef] [PubMed]
24. Stroud, R.H.; Wright, S.T.; Calhoun, K.H. Nocturnal nasal congestion and nasal resistance. *Laryngoscope* **1999**, *109*, 1450–1453. [CrossRef]
25. Virkkula, P.; Maasilta, P.; Hytönen, M.; Salmi, T.; Malmberg, H. Nasal obstruction and sleep-disordered breathing: The effect of supine body position on nasal measurements in snorers. *Acta Otolaryngol.* **2003**, *123*, 648–654. [CrossRef] [PubMed]
26. Hellsing, E. Changes in the pharyngeal airway in relation to extension of the head. *Eur. J. Orthod.* **1989**, *11*, 359–365. [CrossRef] [PubMed]
27. Minagi, H.O.; Okuno, K.; Nohara, K.; Sakai, T. Predictors of Side Effects with Long-Term Oral Appliance Therapy for Obstructive Sleep Apnea. *J. Clin. Sleep Med.* **2018**, *14*, 119–125. [CrossRef]
28. Nishio, Y.; Hoshino, T.; Murotani, K.; Furuhashi, A.; Baku, M.; Sasanabe, R.; Kazaoka, Y.; Shiomi, T. Treatment outcome of oral appliance in patients with REM-related obstructive sleep apnea. *Sleep Breath.* **2020**, *24*, 1339–1347. [CrossRef] [PubMed]
29. Ng, A.T.; Darendeliler, M.A.; Petocz, P.; Cistulli, P.A. Cephalometry and prediction of oral appliance treatment outcome. *Sleep Breath.* **2012**, *16*, 47–58. [CrossRef]
30. Liu, Y.; Lowe, A.A.; Fleetham, J.A.; Park, Y.C. Cephalometric and physiologic predictors of the efficacy of an adjustable oral appliance for treating obstructive sleep apnea. *Am. J. Orthod. Dentofac. Orthop.* **2001**, *120*, 639–647. [CrossRef] [PubMed]
31. Sakamoto, Y.; Yanamoto, S.; Rokutanda, S.; Naruse, T.; Imayama, N.; Hashimoto, M.; Nakamura, A.; Yoshida, N.; Tanoue, Y.; Ayuse, T.; et al. Predictors of obstructive sleep apnoea-hypopnea severity and oral appliance therapy efficacy by using lateral cephalometric analysis. *J. Oral Rehabil.* **2016**, *43*, 649–655. [CrossRef] [PubMed]
32. Lorino, A.M.; Maza, M.; d'Ortho, M.P.; Coste, A.; Harf, A.; Lorino, H. Effects of mandibular advancement on respiratory resistance. *Eur. Respir. J.* **2000**, *16*, 928–932. [CrossRef]
33. De Backer, J.W.; Vanderveken, O.M.; Vos, W.G.; Devolder, A.; Verhulst, S.L.; Verbraecken, J.A.; Parizel, P.M.; Braem, M.J.; van de Heyning, P.H.; De Backer, W.A. Functional imaging using computational fluid dynamics to predict treatment success of mandibular advancement devices in sleep-disordered breathing. *J. Biomech.* **2007**, *40*, 3708–3714. [CrossRef]
34. Ishiyama, H.; Hasebe, D.; Sato, K.; Sakamoto, Y.; Furuhashi, A.; Komori, E.; Yuasa, H. The Efficacy of Device Designs (Mono-block or Bi-block) in Oral Appliance Therapy for Obstructive Sleep Apnea Patients: A Systematic Review and Meta-Analysis. *Int. J. Environ. Res. Public Health* **2019**, *16*, 3182. [CrossRef] [PubMed]
35. Sasao, Y.; Nohara, K.; Okuno, K.; Nakamura, Y.; Sakai, T. Videoendoscopic diagnosis for predicting the response to oral appliance therapy in severe obstructive sleep apnea. *Sleep Breath.* **2014**, *18*, 809–815. [CrossRef] [PubMed]
36. Chan, A.S.; Lee, R.W.; Cistulli, P.A. Dental appliance treatment for obstructive sleep apnea. *Chest* **2007**, *132*, 693–699. [CrossRef] [PubMed]

37. Togeiro, S.M.; Chaves, C.M., Jr.; Palombini, L.; Tufik, S.; Hora, F.; Nery, L.E. Evaluation of the upper airway in obstructive sleep apnoea. *Indian J. Med. Res.* **2010**, *131*, 230–235. [PubMed]
38. Gao, X.M.; Zeng, X.L.; Fu, M.K.; Huang, X.Z. Magnetic resonance imaging of the upper airway in obstructive sleep apnea before and after oral appliance therapy. *Chin. J. Dent. Res.* **1999**, *2*, 27–35.
39. Okuno, K.; Sasao, Y.; Nohara, K.; Sakai, T.; Pliska, B.T.; Lowe, A.A.; Ryan, C.F.; Almeida, F.R. Endoscopy evaluation to predict oral appliance outcomes in obstructive sleep apnoea. *Eur. Respir. J.* **2016**, *47*, 1410–1419. [CrossRef] [PubMed]
40. WHO Expert Consultation. Appropriate body-mass index for Asian populations and its implications for policy and intervention strategies. *Lancet* **2004**, *363*, 157–163. [CrossRef]
41. Takahashi, H.; Mori, M. [Characteristics and significance of criteria for obesity disease in Japan 2011]. *Nihon Rinsho* **2013**, *71*, 257–261.

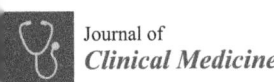

Article

Positive Airway Pressure Therapy Adherence with Mask Resupply: A Propensity-Matched Analysis

Adam V. Benjafield [1], Liesl M. Oldstone [1], Leslee A. Willes [2], Colleen Kelly [3], Carlos M. Nunez [1], Atul Malhotra [4,*] and on behalf of the medXcloud Group [†]

1. ResMed Science Center, San Diego, CA 92123, USA; adam.benjafield@resmed.com.au (A.V.B.); lmoldstone@gmail.com (L.M.O.); carlos.nunez@resmed.com (C.M.N.)
2. Willes Consulting, Encinitas, CA 92024, USA; lesleew@willesconsulting.com
3. Kelly Statistical Consulting, Carlsbad, CA 92011, USA; kstat.consulting@gmail.com
4. Pulmonary, Critical Care and Sleep Medicine, University of California, 9300 Campus Point Drive, La Jolla, San Diego, CA 92037, USA
* Correspondence: amalhotra@ucsd.edu
† Membership of the medXcloud Group is provided at www.medXcloud.org (accessed on 5 February 2021).

Abstract: There are currently few data on the impact of mask resupply on longer-term adherence to positive airway pressure (PAP) therapy. This retrospective analysis investigated the effects of mask/mask cushion resupply on the adherence to PAP versus no resupply. Deidentified patient billing data for PAP supply items were merged with telemonitoring data from Cloud-connected AirSense 10/AirCurve 10 devices via AirView^{TM} (ResMed). Eligible patients started PAP between 1 July 2014 and 17 June 2016, had ≥360 days of PAP device data, and achieved initial U.S. Medicare adherence criteria. Patients who received a resupply of mask systems/cushions (resupply group) were propensity-score-matched with those not receiving any mask/cushion resupply (control group). A total of 100,370 patients were included. From days 91 to 360, the mean device usage was 5.6 and 4.5 h/night in the resupply and control groups, respectively ($p < 0.0001$). The proportion of patients with a mean device usage ≥4 h/night was significantly higher in the resupply group versus the control group (77% vs. 59%; $p < 0.0001$). The therapy termination rate was significantly lower in the resupply group versus the control group (14.7% vs. 31.9%; $p < 0.0001$); there was a trend toward lower therapy termination rates as the number of resupplies increased. The replacement of mask interface components was associated with better longer-term adherence to PAP therapy versus no resupply.

Keywords: positive airway pressure; adherence; leak; patient engagement; sleep apnea; lung

1. Introduction

Obstructive sleep apnea (OSA) is a common disorder with major neurocognitive and cardiometabolic sequelae [1]. Recent estimates suggest that the number of people worldwide with OSA is up to 1 billion [2]. This finding highlights the importance of raising awareness of OSA and emphasizes the need for efficient approaches to large-scale diagnosis and treatment. The use of oral appliances or upper airway surgery are potential options for the treatment of OSA, but are limited by their variable efficacy and a relative lack of outcome data [3–6]. The current treatment of choice for OSA is positive airway pressure (PAP) therapy, which has been shown to improve symptoms, blood pressure, and quality of life in randomized controlled trials [7–10]. However, treatment is often suboptimal due to variable adherence to PAP therapy [11,12]. Adherence with PAP therapy is an important criterion for continuing treatment and is necessary for the benefits of therapy to be realized [11]. Therefore, considerable emphasis has been placed on optimizing adherence to PAP therapy [13,14].

Telemedicine strategies offer the possibility of remotely monitoring PAP therapy adherence and delivering interventions that are designed to improve device usage. We have recently reported that the utilization of new technology might contribute to improved device usage and a higher proportion of patients meeting the U.S. Center for Medicare and Medicaid Services (CMS, Woodlawn, MD, USA) PAP adherence criteria [13]. In our analysis using a propensity matching design, adherence in PAP users provided with a patient engagement tool was significantly higher than that in those managed with usual care monitoring (87% vs. 70%; $p < 0.0001$) [13].

The use of new technology, such as the patient engagement tool in the study described above, is a novel and compelling approach for improving adherence. In addition, basic contributors to good quality care, such as appropriate patient follow-up and supply replenishment, may also play a role in ensuring adherence with PAP therapy. Of note, some providers have advocated for regular changes of masks, hoses, and filters to optimize adherence [15]. Although financial incentives have driven some companies that produce durable medical equipment to provide regular replacement supplies, others might suggest that frequent replacement supplies may not be necessary if the masks are regularly cleaned and maintained. Payers may also limit access to supply items if they do not receive objective confirmation of usage requirements being met as frequently as every 3 months [16]. Patel et al. have reported mask refill rates as a predictor of PAP adherence, but the study used a modest sample size [17]. In clinical practice, many patients forget or lose track of the age of their equipment and supplies, making the optimal timing and approach to resupply unclear.

This study investigated the effects of the resupply of PAP equipment (mask system and/or cushions) on the adherence to PAP therapy compared with no resupply in the first year of therapy. The aim was to test the hypothesis that mask resupply would be associated with improved adherence to PAP therapy versus no resupply.

2. Methods

2.1. Study Design and Participants

This retrospective analysis merged deidentified patient billing data for PAP supply items (Brightree, Peachtree Corners, GA, USA) with telemonitoring data collected from Cloud-connected AirSense 10 and AirCurve 10 (ResMed, San Diego, CA, USA) devices via AirView™ (ResMed, San Diego, CA, USA), a password-protected Cloud-based technology that is compliant with the Health Insurance Portability and Accountability Act. These anonymized data were sent to third-party independent statisticians who assisted with the analyses and presentation of findings. All patients had registered to use AirView™ and provided consent for their data to be used in future analyses. The study protocol was reviewed by the Chesapeake institutional review board (IRB) and was deemed exempt from IRB oversight per the Department of Health and Human Services regulations 45 CFR 46.101(b) (4).

Eligible patients were identified in Brightree as having had initiated PAP therapy between 1 July 2014 and 17 June 2016, had the potential for at least 360 days of AirView™ data available, and had achieved initial CMS adherence (defined as PAP device usage of ≥ 4 h/night on $\geq 70\%$ of nights in a consecutive 30-day period in the first 90 days of therapy) were analyzed. Patients were excluded if they met the following criteria: multiple therapy start dates, use of multiple devices by the same subject, invalid or missing device serial numbers recorded, and the replacement of a patients' continuous positive airway pressure (CPAP) device within 1 year of therapy initiation. Patient data were then merged with the AirView™ data to obtain CPAP daily usage data. Further exclusions were applied as follows: incorrect device serial numbers listed, the same device was used by multiple patients, did not have the potential for 365 days of usage data, did not achieve the CMS 90-day adherence criteria, and date or data entry inconsistencies. These inconsistencies included: the therapy start date was missing or after the first usage date, therapy start date >3 days before the first usage date, and myAir™ registration date >3 days before or >90 days after therapy start date.

Patients were divided into two groups: one including those receiving mask resupply (mask system and/or mask cushion; resupply group) and the other including those who did not receive mask resupply in the first year of therapy (control group) as part of their standard care. To minimize the bias in between-group comparisons, a propensity model was constructed using the following baseline variables to match patients in the resupply and control groups: gender, age at initiation of the PAP therapy, therapy start date, mode of PAP therapy, 95th percentile mask leak on day 1, residual apnea–hypopnea index (AHI) on day 1, and use of a patient engagement strategy (myAir^{TM}). Estimated propensity scores were then used to form 1:1 matched pairs, with the propensity scores being within a window of 5% being matched.

2.2. Endpoints

The primary objective was to compare the adherence with PAP therapy (defined in terms of the average hours of use per day) on days 91–360 in the resupply and control groups. Secondary objectives were the proportion of patients with a mean PAP usage of $\geq$4 h/day, the proportion of patients who stopped using PAP, average unintentional leaks, average residual AHI, and the frequency of resupply distributions in the resupply group. All PAP-related data were obtained from AirView^{TM}.

2.3. Statistical Analysis

The minimum sample size was set at 3800 (1900 per group with 1:1 matching) to provide an 80% probability of detecting a 0.2 h difference in the mean usage between the resupply and control groups, assuming a standard deviation of 2.2 h in each group (as was observed in a pilot study). The required sample size was calculated using the two-sample t-tests assuming equal variance procedure with NCSS Power Analysis Statistical Software, version 14 (Kaysville, UT 84037, USA), based on a two-sided, two-sample t-test. This sample size based on independent groups was expected to be conservative because the two groups were matched for baseline characteristics, reducing the variance of the difference and yielding greater power.

The primary analysis population included all patients fulfilling the inclusion and exclusion criteria and matched in the propensity score procedure. Descriptive statistics were used to present the demographic and therapy characteristics for the primary analysis population, including age, sex, myAir^{TM} use, and device mode. Descriptive statistics were also used to present the mean usage, the proportion of patients with mean usage of $\geq$4 h/night, the proportion of patients with a usage of $\geq$4 h/night on 70% of nights, the mean AHI, the median 95th percentile mask leak between 91 and 360 days after initiation of therapy, and the proportion of patients who terminated therapy (i.e., PAP therapy termination, as studied previously) [18–20]. Continuous parameters were compared between groups using a mixed-effect linear model, with the pair identifier as a random effect and the resupply/control group as a fixed effect. Percentages were compared using the McNemar test. Kaplan–Meier analysis was used to compare survival functions for the resupply and control groups, where survival was defined as remaining adherent to PAP therapy; median adherence times in the two groups were compared using a log-rank test. Patients were considered to have terminated their therapy if their total usage was 0 h during a 30-day window. Kaplan–Meier analyses were also used to investigate the differences in survival probabilities, which was stratified by the number of resupplies received within the first year.

Sensitivity analyses included matching the resupply and control patients using a 0.2 window of the linear propensity scores, as suggested by Rubin [21], and checking the three conditions mentioned therein for regression adjustment methods to be reliable: (1) the means of the propensity scores in the two groups are similar, (2) the standard deviations of the propensity scores in the two groups are similar, and (3) the residual variances of the covariates after adjusting for the propensity score in the two groups are similar.

A piecewise linear model was fit to each of 1000 randomly selected patients' usage data 30 days prior to and 30 days after their first mask resupply following the initial 90 days of usage. Usage data before and after resupply was modeled with separate linear models. A mixed-effect piecewise linear regression model was used to describe daily usage data between 30 days prior and 30 days after the first resupply. The explanatory variables were the random slope and intercepts before resupply (each patient had their own slope and intercept) and the random slope and intercepts after resupply. An AR (1) auto-correlation was assumed for successive daily usage data. The total difference in usage (over 30 days after first resupply) between the predicted usage after resupply and the usage predicted if the before-resupply trend continued was calculated for each subject and then averaged over subjects.

Any p-values < 0.05 were considered statistically significant. All statistical analyses were performed using SAS version 9.3 (Cary, NC 27513, USA) or later. Graphics were generated using SAS software.

3. Results

3.1. Study Sample

The analysis included a total of 100,370 patients (mean age 57 years, 64% male) (Table 1). A flow diagram showing the patient identification and selection is shown in Figure 1.

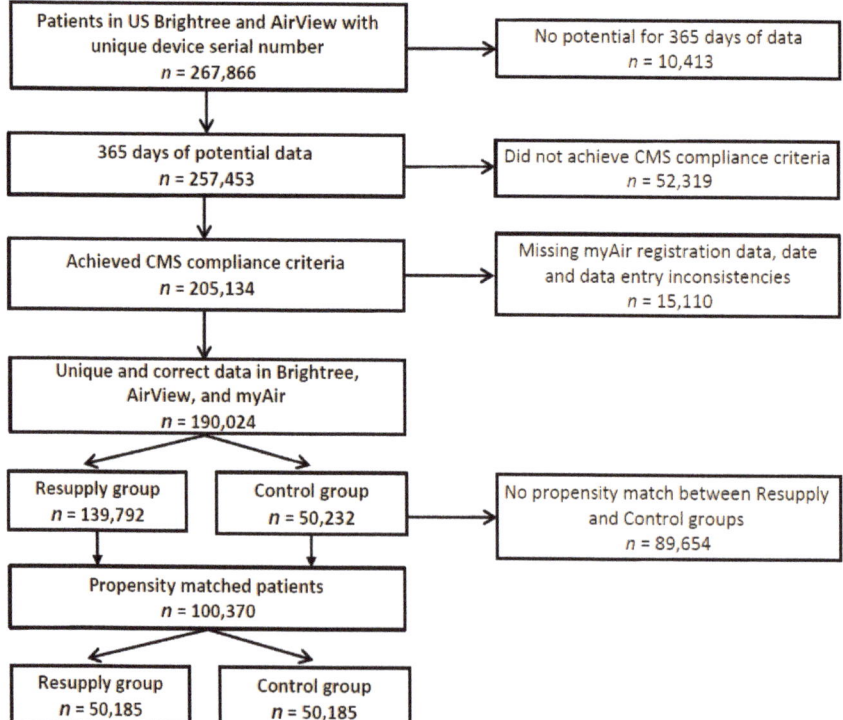

Figure 1. Flow diagram. CMS, Centers for Medicare and Medicaid.

Table 1. Demographics and therapy characteristics for the primary analysis population.

Heading	Control (n = 50,185)	Resupply (n = 50,185)
Age, years		
Mean ± SD	56.9 ± 13.6	57.0 ± 13.5
Median	57.0	57.0
Sex, n (%)		
Female	17,847 (35.6)	17,858 (35.6)
Male	32,312 (64.4)	32,301 (64.4)
Missing	26 (<0.1)	26 (<0.1)
Device/mode, n (%)		
APAP	21,437 (42.7)	21,449 (42.7)
CPAP	23,949 (47.7)	24,022 (47.9)
Bilevel	4272 (8.5)	4187 (8.3)
Missing	527 (1.1)	527 (1.1)
myAir^{TM} use, n (%)	8807 (17.5)	8795 (17.5)
AHI on the first day of therapy, /h		
Mean ± SD	3.9 ± 6.0	3.8 ± 5.7
Median	2.0	2.0
95th percentile leak on the first day of therapy, L/min		
Mean ± SD	23.5 ± 26.3	23.2 ± 25.7
Median	15.6	15.6

AHI, apnea–hypopnea index; APAP, automatically titrating continuous positive airway pressure; CPAP, continuous positive airway pressure; SD, standard deviation.

3.2. Resupply

Patients in the resupply group (n = 50,185) received a mean of 5.0 ± 4.5 (median 3.0) items during the study period (mean 2.1 ± 1.5 (median 2.0) shipments per patient, with a mean of 2.4 ± 1.7 (median 2.0) items per shipment).

3.3. Adherence

Adherence with the PAP therapy from day 91 to day 360 was significantly better in the resupply group versus the control group, including mean daily usage, the proportion of patients with mean usage ≥4 h, and the proportion of patients with daily usage ≥4 h for 70% of nights (all $p < 0.0001$) (Table 2). The overall probability of continuing with the PAP therapy during the study period ("survival" of therapy) was 85.3% in the resupply group and 68.1% in the control group ($p < 0.0001$) (Figure 2), corresponding to therapy termination rates of 14.7% and 31.9%, respectively. This finding was consistent across subgroups based on the number of resupplies shipped (Figure 3).

Table 2. Device usage and respiratory parameters from days 91 to 360 (primary analysis population).

Device Usage	Control (n = 50,185)	Resupply (n = 50,185)	p-Value
Mean usage, h			
Mean (SE)	4.5 (0.1)	5.6 (0.01)	
Median	4.9	6.0	
Mean difference vs. control (95% CI)		1.1 (1.06, 1.13)	<0.0001
Mean usage ≥4 h, %			
Mean (95% CI)	59.2 (58.8, 59.6)	77.0 (76.6, 77.4)	
Mean difference vs. control (95% CI)		17.8 (17.2, 18.3)	<0.0001
Daily usage ≥4 h for 70% of nights, %			
Mean (95% CI)	50.9 (50.5, 51.3)	67.7 (67.3, 68.1)	
Mean difference vs. control (95% CI)		16.8 (16.2, 17.4)	<0.0001

Table 2. Cont.

Device Usage	Control	Resupply	p-Value
	(n = 50,185)	(n = 50,185)	
Respiratory Parameters	(n = 47,373)	(n = 49,359)	
Mean AHI, /h			
Mean (SE)	2.6 (0.02)	2.5 (0.01)	
Median	1.5	1.5	
Mean difference vs. control (95% CI)		−0.2 (−0.21, −0.13)	<0.0001
Median 95% percentile mask leak, L/min			
Mean (SE)	20.4 (0.10)	19.0 (0.09)	
Median	15.0	14.4	
Mean difference vs. control (95% CI)		−1.5 (−1.68, −1.24)	<0.0001

AHI, apnea–hypopnea index; CI, confidence interval; SE, standard error.

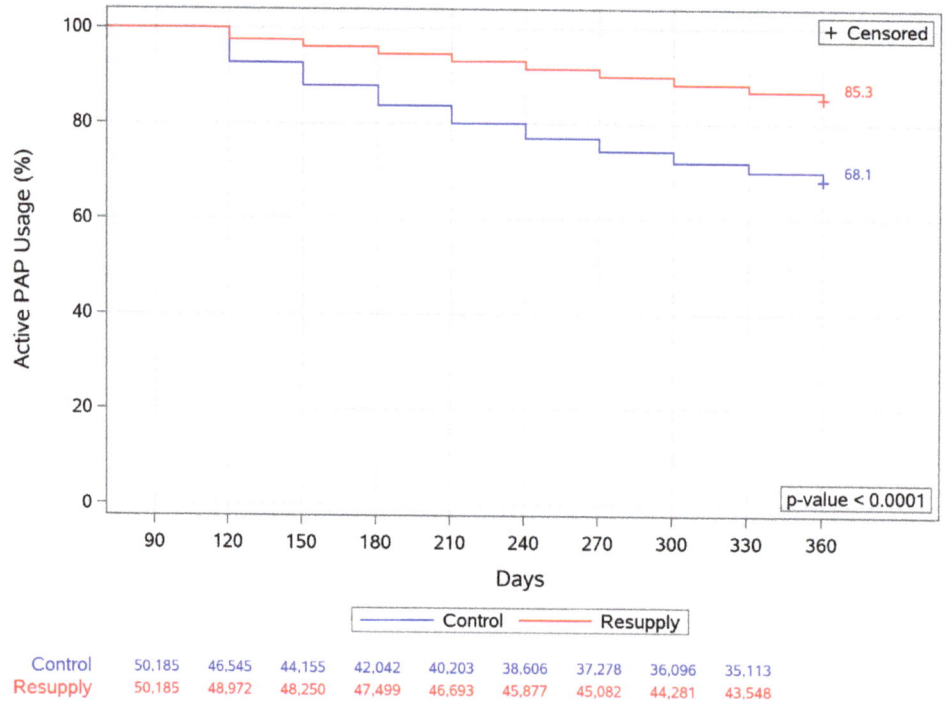

Figure 2. Overall probability of continuing with the positive airway pressure (PAP) therapy ("survival" of therapy) from days 91–360 in the control and resupply groups (primary analysis population). +Censored, patients whose therapy continued after 360 days were censored at the 360 day time point.

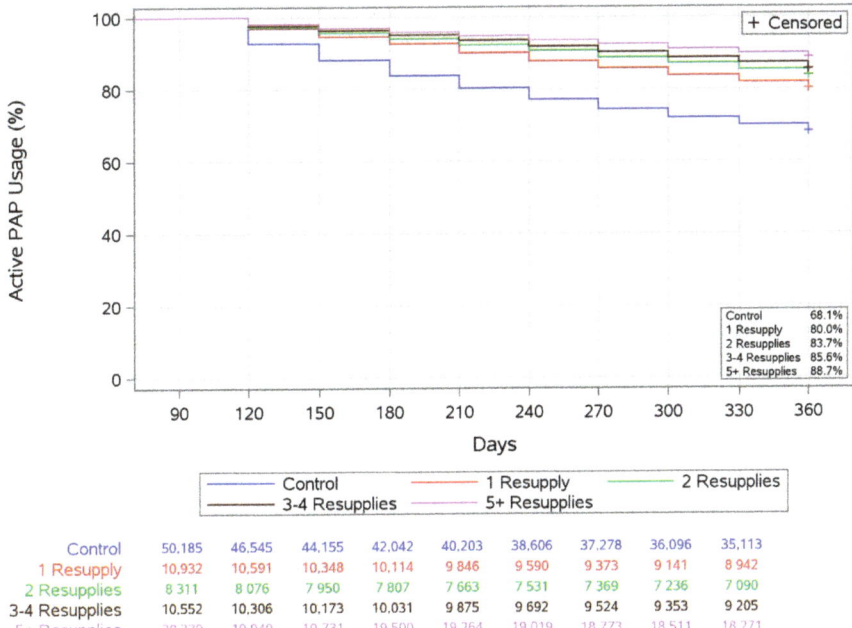

Figure 3. Probability of continuing with the positive airway pressure (PAP) therapy ("survival" of therapy) from days 91–360 in the control and resupply groups broken down by the number of resupplies shipped (primary analysis population). +Censored, patients whose therapy continued after 360 days were censored at the 360 day time point.

3.4. Respiratory Parameters

The mean AHI and median 95th percentile leak were slightly but statistically significantly lower in the resupply group compared with the control group (both $p < 0.0001$) (Table 2).

3.5. Sensitivity Analysis

The results were almost identical when subjects were matched using a linear score window of 0.2 instead of the propensity score window of 5%. Furthermore, Rubin's three conditions for the reliability of regression adjustment methods [20] were all met: (1) the mean linear score (log-odds of the propensity score) was 0.98785 in the resupply group and 0.98787 in the control group, (2) the standard deviation of the linear score was 0.2667 in the resupply group and 0.2666 in the control group, (3) the ratios of the residual variances of the covariates adjusted for the propensity score in the resupply to the control group ranged from 0.991 to 1.003. Therefore, all three of Rubin's conditions were met in the matched pairs analysis population.

3.6. Longitudinal Analysis

On average, patients' usage decreased by 0.27 min per day before resupply and decreased by 0.13 min per day after resupply, which is an improvement that was statistically significant ($p < 0.0001$). The average total difference in usage over 30 days after resupply (the difference between the two estimated linear regression before and after resupply summed over the 30 days after resupply) showed an increase of 211 min with a 95% confidence interval of 112 to 311 min.

4. Discussion

This study showed that regular mask resupply was associated with better usage of the PAP therapy from 3 months to 1 year after treatment initiation. These findings are unique because, to the best of our knowledge, they represent the first major effort to evaluate adherence to PAP therapy as a function of mask resupply.

The average 1.1 h increase in PAP usage in the resupply group versus the control group is likely to represent a clinically relevant improvement [9,11,22]. Although the database used in this study did not allow for the determination of objective hard outcomes, published data suggest that this degree of improvement in device usage is associated with improvements regarding sleepiness, daily functioning, and blood pressure [9,11,22]. Another important finding is that rates of therapy termination, perhaps the worst form of non-adherence, were significantly lower in the resupply group compared with the control group. Maintaining patients on PAP therapy is an important clinical goal because retention increases the likelihood of achieving PAP-therapy-related benefits. The observation that therapy termination rates decreased as resupply volume increased was also of note. Our novel findings suggest that adequate levels of mask resupply might have a beneficial influence on long-term PAP therapy adherence.

To assess the possibility of reverse causation, we performed a longitudinal analysis using a random sample of 1000 patients before and after the first resupply occurring after the 90 initial days of usage. The possibility existed that ongoing PAP usage drove mask resupply rather than mask resupply yielding improved PAP adherence. A mixed effect piecewise linear regression model was used to define daily usage in the 30 days prior to and 30 days after the resupply event. By using a narrow time window, we alleviated some concern regarding the possibility that ongoing PAP usage drove an ongoing need for masks. Moreover, the improvements observed with resupply in this longitudinal analysis provide reassurance that we have identified important clinical findings that are likely to benefit patients rather than a statistical artifact of an observational study.

A number of interventions have been suggested to improve PAP adherence, although there are inconsistencies in the results between studies, leading to ongoing discussions [23]. Intensive support and education has been linked to good PAP adherence in some, but not all, studies [24]. Furthermore, patient engagement using new technology or other approaches may be beneficial [13]. Financial incentives and group PAP therapy have also been advocated for [25–27], although data in this area are limited. Variable success has been reported in clinical trials investigating the use of pressure relief, humidifiers, and various pressure modes on the adherence to PAP therapy [28–30]. In clinical practice, many patients express a preference for one device/mode over another [31], emphasizing the need for an individualized or personalized approach to PAP delivery. As part of this approach, our findings suggest that telemedicine-based patient support, including regular mask resupply, could contribute to improved adherence to PAP therapy.

There are small amounts of published data available to inform the optimal frequency of mask changes during the regular use of PAP. We are aware of efforts to assess the biofilm that can develop on masks and to perform quantitative cultures on the masks, which have suggested increased colony-forming units after 6 months of consistent use [32]. However, recent data suggest that the use of PAP delivered via a nasal mask or full face mask does not increase the risk of respiratory infection compared to controls with OSA who did not receive PAP [33]. Furthermore, even bacterial colonization of the CPAP humidifier reservoir was not associated with higher rates of chronic rhinosinusitis in regular PAP users [34].

In addition to theories about bacterial loads, another consideration might be the development of mask leaks, which tend to happen as masks get older. Clinical experience and some published data have shown that leaks can develop with ongoing PAP usage as masks age and that leaks are predictive of poor PAP adherence [35]. Thus, in theory, mask resupply may be beneficial for a number of reasons, although potential mechanisms are not yet clear based on the literature and the data available from our study.

Current CMS criteria allow for reimbursement of a new mask system every 3 months and two replacement mask cushions every month [16]. Based on these allowances, patients in our study could have accessed three new mask systems and 18 new cushions (i.e., 21 items in total) for the 9-month study period. Our findings documented an average number of 2.1 resupply shipments per patient with a mean of 2.4 items per shipment, meaning that the total resupply over the study period was about 5 items on average. This frequency is substantially below reimbursement limits and indicates that overall mask resupply is generally not being overutilized. In addition, it is possible that better use of mask resupply allowances could contribute to even better longer-term adherence to PAP therapy. Nevertheless, further work is needed to define the optimal frequency of mask changes during long-term PAP therapy. The optimal strategy may differ between patients based on individual preferences, local temperature and humidity, hours of usage, and other factors, such as the patient microbiome.

Several limitations need to be taken into account when interpreting the findings of this study. First, this was not a randomized clinical trial and therefore definitive conclusions about the causal effects of resupply cannot be drawn. However, propensity matching was used, where this approach helped to limit the contribution of confounding factors to the study results. Furthermore, our longitudinal analysis supported the hypothesis that resupply increased usage. The fact that our findings were independent of traditional predictors of PAP adherence suggests that resupply per se may be quite helpful. Second, we did not have any information about how patients managed their resupply or whether they were part of a formal resupply program. We only have data on supply items coded for reimbursement purposes and could not determine factors that led to the resupply behavior. Thus, we cannot exclude the possibility that patients in the resupply group differed from those in the control group in other important ways, including motivation or socioeconomic status, or some other unrecognized confounder [36]. While we acknowledge the potential impact of the "healthy user effect," the same issue might also arise with randomized controlled trials in which PAP adherence may be a marker of a good prognosis. Finally, by design, our study included patients who had met CMS adherence criteria in the first 90 days of therapy, with the aim toward looking at longer-term adherence. As a result, those with poor early adherence who failed to reach CMS criteria were excluded but perhaps unlikely to benefit from a resupply program. Similarly, patients who did not have access to health care or refused PAP therapy would not have been included. Therefore, the effect of a resupply program on adherence in these patient groups is unknown, and our findings are only applicable to patients who have characteristics that are similar to the study population.

In conclusion, this big data analysis including a large group of well-matched patients treated with PAP therapy in routine clinical practice showed that reasonable resupply of mask interfaces was associated with statistically and clinically significant increases in average daily PAP device usage and lower rates of therapy termination compared with no resupply (control). These improvements in PAP therapy adherence and usage could positively impact clinical outcomes if confirmed in future randomized trials.

Author Contributions: A.V.B., L.M.O., and A.M. conceived and designed the study. L.A.W. and C.K. analyzed the data. The first draft of the manuscript was prepared by A.M., who had unrestricted access to the data. The manuscript was reviewed and edited by A.V.B., L.M.O., L.A.W., C.K., C.M.N. and A.M. All authors made the decision to submit the manuscript for publication and assume responsibility for the accuracy and completeness of the analyses and for the fidelity of this report to the trial protocol. A.M. takes responsibility for the content of the manuscript, including data and analysis. All authors have read and agreed to the published version of the manuscript.

Funding: This work was funded by ResMed. Researchers from ResMed participated in the study, including the design, data collation, data analysis, and critical review of the paper.

Institutional Review Board Statement: The study protocol was reviewed by the Chesapeake institutional review board (IRB) and was deemed exempt from IRB oversight per the Department of Health and Human Services regulations 45 CFR 46.101(b) (4).

Informed Consent Statement: All patients had registered to use AirView™ and provided consent for their data to be used in future analyses.

Data Availability Statement: The data are not publicly available due to privacy and patient consent limitations.

Acknowledgments: Editorial assistance with the manuscript preparation was provided by Nicola Ryan, an independent medical writer funded by ResMed after Atul Malhotra wrote the first draft of the manuscript.

Conflicts of Interest: Adam Benjafield, Liesl Oldstone, and Carlos Nunez are employees of ResMed. Leslee Willes and Colleen Kelly are independent statisticians, funded by ResMed. Atul Malhotra is a principal investigator on National Institutes of Health (NIH) RO1 HL085188, K24 HL132105, and T32 HL134632 and co-investigator on R21 HL121794, RO1 HL 119201, and RO1 HL081823. Atul Malhotra received income from Livanova and Merck for medical education. ResMed, Inc. provided a philanthropic donation to UC San Diego in support of a sleep center. Atul Malhotra has not had personal income from medXcloud or ResMed, Inc. The content is solely the responsibility of the authors and does not necessarily represent the official views of the NIH.

References

1. Mesarwi, O.A.; Loomba, R.; Malhotra, A. Obstructive sleep apnea, hypoxia, and nonalcoholic fatty liver disease. *Am. J. Respir. Crit. Care Med.* **2019**, *199*, 830–841. [CrossRef] [PubMed]
2. Benjafield, A.V.; Ayas, N.T.; Eastwood, P.R.; Heinzer, R.; Ip, M.S.M.; Morrell, M.J.; Nunez, C.M.; Patel, S.R.; Penzel, T.; Pepin, J.D.; et al. Estimation of the global prevalence and burden of obstructive sleep apnoea: A literature-based analysis. *Lancet Respir. Med.* **2019**. [CrossRef]
3. Phillips, C.L.; Grunstein, R.R.; Darendeliler, M.A.; Mihailidou, A.S.; Srinivasan, V.K.; Yee, B.J.; Marks, G.B.; Cistulli, P.A. Health outcomes of continuous positive airway pressure versus oral appliance treatment for obstructive sleep apnea: A randomized controlled trial. *Am. J. Respir. Crit. Care Med.* **2013**, *187*, 879–887. [CrossRef] [PubMed]
4. Kezirian, E.J.; Malhotra, A.; Goldberg, A.N.; White, D.P. Changes in obstructive sleep apnea severity, biomarkers, and quality of life after multilevel surgery. *Laryngoscope* **2010**, *120*, 1481–1488. [CrossRef] [PubMed]
5. Weaver, E.M.; Maynard, C.; Yueh, B. Survival of veterans with sleep apnea: Continuous positive airway pressure versus surgery. *Otolaryngol. Head Neck Surg.* **2004**, *130*, 659–665. [CrossRef] [PubMed]
6. Strollo, P.J., Jr.; Soose, R.J.; Maurer, J.T.; de Vries, N.; Cornelius, J.; Froymovich, O.; Hanson, R.D.; Padhya, T.A.; Steward, D.L.; Gillespie, M.B.; et al. Upper-airway stimulation for obstructive sleep apnea. *N. Engl. J. Med.* **2014**, *370*, 139–149. [CrossRef]
7. Pepperell, J.; Ramdassingh-Dow, S.; Crosthwaite, N.; Mullins, R.; Jenkinson, C.; Stradling, J.; Davies, R. Ambulatory blood pressure after therapeutic and subtherapeutic nasal continuous positive airway pressure for obstructive sleep apnoea: A randomised parallel trial. *Lancet* **2002**, *359*, 204–210. [CrossRef]
8. Jenkinson, C.; Davies, R.J.; Mullins, R.; Stradling, J.R. Comparison of therapeutic and subtherapeutic nasal continuous positive airway pressure for obstructive sleep apnoea: A randomised prospective parallel trial. *Lancet* **1999**, *353*, 2100–2105. [CrossRef]
9. Weaver, T.E.; Mancini, C.; Maislin, G.; Cater, J.; Staley, B.; Landis, J.R.; Ferguson, K.A.; George, C.F.; Schulman, D.A.; Greenberg, H.; et al. CPAP treatment of sleepy patients with milder OSA: Results of the CATNAP randomized clinical trial. *Am. J. Respir. Crit. Care Med.* **2012**. [CrossRef]
10. Wimms, A.J.; Kelly, J.L.; Turnbull, C.D.; McMillan, A.; Craig, S.E.; O'Reilly, J.F.; Nickol, A.H.; Hedley, E.L.; Decker, M.D.; Willes, L.A.; et al. Continuous positive airway pressure versus standard care for the treatment of people with mild obstructive sleep apnoea (MERGE): A multicentre, randomised controlled trial. *Lancet Respir. Med.* **2019**, 349–358. [CrossRef]
11. Weaver, T.E.; Maislin, G.; Dinges, D.F.; Bloxham, T.; George, C.F.; Greenberg, H.; Kader, G.; Mahowald, M.; Younger, J.; Pack, A.I. Relationship between hours of CPAP use and achieving normal levels of sleepiness and daily functioning. *Sleep* **2007**, *30*, 711–719. [CrossRef]
12. Redline, S.; Adams, N.; Strauss, M.E.; Roebuck, T.; Winters, M.; Rosenberg, C. Improvement of mild sleep-disordered breathing with CPAP compared with conservative therapy. *Am. J. Respir. Crit. Care Med.* **1998**, *157*, 858–865. [CrossRef] [PubMed]
13. Malhotra, A.; Crocker, M.E.; Willes, L.; Kelly, C.; Lynch, S.; Benjafield, A.V. Patient engagement using new technology to improve adherence to positive airway pressure therapy: A retrospective analysis. *Chest* **2018**, *153*, 843–850. [CrossRef]
14. Deacon, N.L.; Jen, R.; Li, Y.; Malhotra, A. Treatment of obstructive sleep apnea. Prospects for personalized combined modality therapy. *Ann. Am. Thorac. Soc.* **2016**, *13*, 101–108. [CrossRef] [PubMed]
15. Kline, L.; Carlson, P. Humidification improves NCPAP acceptance and use. *Am. J. Respir. Crit. Care Med.* **1999**, *159*, A427.

16. Centers for Medicare & Medicaid Services. Local Coverage Determination: Positive Airway Pressure (PAP) Devices for the Treatment of Obstructive Sleep Apnea (L33178). Available online: https://www.cms.gov/medicare-coverage-database/details/lcd-details.aspx?LCDId=33718&ver=16&CoverageSelection=Local&ArticleType=All&PolicyType=Final&s=All&CptHcpcsCode=e0601&bc=gAAAACAAAAAA& (accessed on 27 August 2019).
17. Patel, N.; Sam, A.; Valentin, A.; Quan, S.; Parthasarathy, S. Refill rates of accessories for positive airway pressure therapy as a surrogate measure of long-term adherence. *J. Clin. Sleep Med.* **2012**, *8*, 169–175. [CrossRef] [PubMed]
18. Liu, D.; Armitstead, J.; Benjafield, A.; Shao, S.; Malhotra, A.; Cistulli, P.A.; Pepin, J.L.; Woehrle, H. Trajectories of emergent central sleep apnea during CPAP therapy. *Chest* **2017**, *152*, 751–760. [CrossRef] [PubMed]
19. Woehrle, H.; Arzt, M.; Graml, A.; Fietze, I.; Young, P.; Teschler, H.; Ficker, J.H. Predictors of positive airway pressure therapy termination in the first year: Analysis of big data from a German homecare provider. *BMC Pulm. Med.* **2018**, *18*, 186. [CrossRef]
20. Woehrle, H.; Ficker, J.H.; Graml, A.; Fietze, I.; Young, P.; Teschler, H.; Arzt, M. Telemedicine-based proactive patient management during positive airway pressure therapy: Impact on therapy termination rate. *Somnologie (Berl.)* **2017**, *21*, 121–127. [CrossRef]
21. Rubin, D.B. Using propensity scores to help design observational studies: Application to the tobacco litigation. *Health Serv. Outcomes Res. Methodol.* **2001**, *2*, 169–188. [CrossRef]
22. Bakker, J.P.; Edwards, B.A.; Gautam, S.P.; Montesi, S.B.; Duran-Cantolla, J.; Aizpuru, F.; Barbe, F.; Sanchez-de-la-Torre, M.; Malhotra, A. Blood pressure improvement with continuous positive airway pressure is independent of obstructive sleep apnea severity. *J. Clin. Sleep Med.* **2014**, *10*, 365–369. [CrossRef] [PubMed]
23. Cistulli, P.A.; Armitstead, J.; Pepin, J.L.; Woehrle, H.; Nunez, C.M.; Benjafield, A.; Malhotra, A. Short-term CPAP adherence in obstructive sleep apnea: A big data analysis using real world data. *Sleep Med.* **2019**, *59*, 114–116. [CrossRef] [PubMed]
24. Hoy, C.J.; Vennelle, M.; Kingshott, R.N.; Engleman, H.M.; Douglas, N.J. Can intensive support improve continuous positive airway pressure use in patients with the sleep apnea/hypopnea syndrome? *Am. J. Respir. Crit. Care Med.* **1999**, *159*, 1096–1100. [CrossRef]
25. Kuna, S.T.; Shuttleworth, D.; Chi, L.; Schutte-Rodin, S.; Friedman, E.; Guo, H.; Dhand, S.; Yang, L.; Zhu, J.; Bellamy, S.L.; et al. Web-based access to positive airway pressure usage with or without an initial financial incentive improves treatment use in patients with obstructive sleep apnea. *Sleep* **2015**, *38*, 1229–1236. [CrossRef]
26. Tarasiuk, A.; Reznor, G.; Greenberg-Dotan, S.; Reuveni, H. Financial incentive increases CPAP acceptance in patients from low socioeconomic background. *PLoS ONE* **2012**, *7*, e33178. [CrossRef]
27. Ye, L.; Antonelli, M.T.; Willis, D.G.; Kayser, K.; Malhotra, A.; Patel, S.R. Couples' experiences with continuous positive airway pressure treatment: A dyadic perspective. *Sleep Health* **2017**, *3*, 362–367. [CrossRef]
28. Aloia, M.S.; Stanchina, M.; Arnedt, J.T.; Malhotra, A.; Millman, R.P. Treatment adherence and outcomes in flexible vs standard continuous positive airway pressure therapy. *Chest* **2005**, *127*, 2085–2093. [CrossRef]
29. Nilius, G.; Happel, A.; Domanski, U.; Ruhle, K.H. Pressure-relief continuous positive airway pressure vs constant continuous positive airway pressure: A comparison of efficacy and compliance. *Chest* **2006**, *130*, 1018–1024. [CrossRef]
30. Ballard, R.D.; Gay, P.C.; Strollo, P.J. Interventions to improve compliance in sleep apnea patients previously non-compliant with continuous positive airway pressure. *J. Clin. Sleep Med.* **2007**, *3*, 706–712. [CrossRef] [PubMed]
31. Benjafield, A.V.; Pepin, J.D.; Valentine, K.; Cistulli, P.A.; Woehrle, H.; Nunez, C.M.; Armitstead, J.; Malhotra, A. Compliance after switching from CPAP to bilevel for patients with non-compliant OSA: Big data analysis. *BMJ Open Respir. Res.* **2019**, *6*, e000380. [CrossRef]
32. Horowitz, A.; Horowitz, S.; Chun, C. CPAP masks are sources of microbial contamination [abstract]. In Proceedings of the 23rd Annual Meeting of the Associated Professional Sleep Societies 2009, Boston, MA, USA, 6–11 June 2009.
33. Mercieca, L.; Pullicino, R.; Camilleri, K.; Abela, R.; Mangion, S.A.; Cassar, J.; Zammit, M.; Gatt, C.; Deguara, C.; Barbara, C.; et al. Continuous positive airway pressure: Is it a route for infection in those with obstructive sleep apnoea? *Sleep Sci.* **2017**, *10*, 28–34. [CrossRef] [PubMed]
34. Chin, C.J.; George, C.; Lannigan, R.; Rotenberg, B.W. Association of CPAP bacterial colonization with chronic rhinosinusitis. *J. Clin. Sleep Med.* **2013**, *9*, 747–750. [CrossRef] [PubMed]
35. Montesi, S.B.; Bakker, J.P.; Macdonald, M.; Hueser, L.; Pittman, S.; White, D.P.; Malhotra, A. Air leak during CPAP titration as a risk factor for central apnea. *J. Clin. Sleep Med.* **2013**, *9*, 1187–1191. [CrossRef]
36. Platt, A.B.; Kuna, S.T.; Field, S.H.; Chen, Z.; Gupta, R.; Roche, D.F.; Christie, J.D.; Asch, D.A. Adherence to sleep apnea therapy and use of lipid-lowering drugs: A study of the healthy-user effect. *Chest* **2010**, *137*, 102–108. [CrossRef] [PubMed]

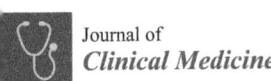

Review

Epidemiology, Physiology and Clinical Approach to Sleepiness at the Wheel in OSA Patients: A Narrative Review

Maria R. Bonsignore [1,2,3,*], Carolina Lombardi [4,5], Simone Lombardo [2] and Francesco Fanfulla [6]

1. PROMISE Department, University of Palermo, 90127 Palermo, Italy
2. Sleep Clinic, Division of Respiratory Medicine, Ospedali Riuniti Villa Sofia-Cervello, 90146 Palermo, Italy; ing.s.lombardo@gmail.com
3. Institute for Biomedical Research and Innovation (IRIB), National Research Council (CNR), 90146 Palermo, Italy
4. Sleep Disorders Center, Department of Cardiology, San Luca Hospital, Istituto Auxologico Italiano, IRCCS, 20145 Milan, Italy; c.lombardi@auxologico.it
5. Department of Medicine and Surgery, University of Milano-Bicocca, 20126 Milan, Italy
6. Respiratory Function and Sleep Unit, Maugeri Clinical and Scientific Institute of Pavia and Montescano, 27100 Pavia, Italy; francesco.fanfulla@icsmaugeri.it
* Correspondence: mariarosaria.bonsignore@unipa.it

Abstract: Sleepiness at the wheel (SW) is recognized as an important factor contributing to road traffic accidents, since up to 30 percent of fatal accidents have been attributed to SW. Sleepiness-related motor vehicle accidents may occur both from falling asleep while driving and from behavior impairment attributable to sleepiness. SW can be caused by various sleep disorders but also by behavioral factors such as sleep deprivation, shift work and non-restorative sleep, as well as chronic disease or the treatment with drugs that negatively affect the level of vigilance. An association between obstructive sleep apnea (OSA) and motor vehicle accidents has been found, with an increasing risk in OSA patients up to sevenfold in comparison to the general population. Regular treatment with continuous positive airway pressure (CPAP) relieves excessive daytime sleepiness and reduces the crash risk. Open questions still remain about the physiological and clinical determinants of SW in OSA patients: the severity of OSA in terms of the frequency of respiratory events (apnea hypopnea index, AHI) or hypoxic load, the severity of daytime sleepiness, concomitant chronic sleep deprivation, comorbidities, the presence of depressive symptoms or chronic fatigue. Herein, we provide a review addressing the epidemiological, physiological and clinical aspects of SW, with a particular focus on the methods to recognize those patients at risk of SW.

Keywords: maintenance of wakefulness test; Epworth Sleepiness Scale; motor vehicle accidents; commercial drivers; driving license

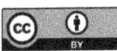

1. Introduction

Obstructive sleep apnea (OSA) is a highly prevalent disease characterized by upper airway occlusion during sleep, intermittent hypoxemia, and sleep fragmentation [1]. Patients with OSA are at an increased risk for cardiometabolic disease and car accidents. The most widely used treatment for OSA is the application of continuous positive airway pressure (CPAP) during sleep, which re-establishes airway patency and prevents the occurrence of upper airway collapse and its functional consequences [1]. However, CPAP is not always accepted or tolerated by many patients, and the compliance with treatment is highly variable. The use of CPAP for at least 4 h on 70% of the nights is considered the threshold for good compliance, but regular and extended CPAP use beyond this threshold is associated with a larger improvement in OSA symptoms, including excessive daytime sleepiness [2].

The role of OSA in increasing sleepiness at the wheel (SW) and the associated risk of driving and occupational accidents has been recognized since the early clinical research studies, as confirmed by several meta-analyses [3–5]. OSA doubles the risk of driving accidents and near-miss accidents, but effective CPAP treatment with good compliance was found to normalize the risk [6–8].

Since the literature on the topic of driving risk in OSA is extensive, the reader is referred to some reviews for a summary of the previous literature [9–11]. A recent systematic review has examined the issue of driving risk in OSA in great detail [10]. The current narrative review aims at providing an overview with a focus on recent updates regarding the epidemiology, the pathophysiology and practical suggestions to evaluate SW in OSA patients.

2. Epidemiology of Driving Accidents in the General Population and in OSA Patients

Excessive daytime sleepiness (EDS) is a non-specific symptom potentially caused by several factors which may be associated with an increased risk of traffic accidents. Most commonly, EDS is the consequence of insufficient sleep, and a recent study comparing the amount of sleep reported by French drivers between 1996 and 2011 found that the sleep time of drivers decreased over 15 years, and this finding was associated with an increased prevalence of SW [12]. Fatigue or sleep-related accidents have been known for a long time to be frequent causes of traffic accidents in the general population [13–15], even though accidents attributable to sleepiness show an estimated rate between 10 and 30% [13,16–18]. Moreover, car crashes related to falling asleep often cause death and severe injury [14]. The death of the driver occurred in 11.4% of sleepiness-related accidents, in contrast with 5.6% of accidents unrelated to sleep [17]. Sleepiness-related motor vehicle accidents (MVA) may result from falling asleep while driving and behavior impairment attributable to sleepiness [18].

Besides OSA, other known causes of EDS are: (1) neurological diseases, such as narcolepsy, idiopathic hypersomnia or Parkinson disease [19,20]; (2) psychiatric disease, especially depression [21]; (3) old age [22]; (4) the use of hypnotics [23]; and (5) diabetes [24]. Sleepiness at the wheel should be specifically investigated, since the risk for car accidents is high in subjects reporting episodes of severe SW [25] and in patients with OSA [26]. Although elderly subjects often report sleepiness, the risk for a poor driving performance associated with sleepiness is lower in old adults compared to young adults, possibly because the former tend to avoid what they perceive as dangerous situations—for example, driving at night [27]. Conversely, risky driving behavior was associated with an increased risk for accidents [28].

The overall picture shows several areas of uncertainty with regard to the factors possibly predictive of SW and sleepiness-related accidents. Nevertheless, the majority of research studies worldwide reported an increased driving risk among those with untreated OSA [10], and meta-analyses further confirmed this finding [2,4,5]. Untreated OSA increases the risk of motor vehicle accidents by 1.5 to 2.5 times compared to the general population, and the risk might be especially high in the excessively sleepy OSA clinical phenotype [29]. The role of OSA in driving accidents is further confirmed by the decreased/normalized accident rate after the initiation of CPAP treatment, evaluated as actual accidents, near-miss accidents or driving simulator performance [7,8].

More recently, in a nationwide cohort study performed in Denmark, Udholm et al., found a prevalence of motor vehicle accidents (MVA) in OSA patients that was 1.4%, higher than the prevalence in the reference population (0.98%) after the adjustment for age, sex, socioeconomic status and co-morbidities. The hazard ratio for MVA in patients with OSA was 1.29 (IC 1.18–1.39), while the incidence rate ratio was 1.3 (1.2–1.42). Interestingly, CPAP therapy determined a statistically significant risk reduction for MVA in comparison to OSA patients that were not treated, with a hazard ratio of 0.82 (0.67–1.02) and an incidence rate ratio of 0.75 (0.6–0.91) [30]. Another recent study was performed in older subjects to assess the effect of sleep apnea on driving behavior. OSA severity, measured by AHI, increased the likelihood of an adverse driving event, with a 1.25 times increase in the odds of an event for each eight-point increase in the AHI [31]. This is the first study that reported a "dose-effect" association between OSA severity and the risk of MVA.

Several studies have tried to identify the predictors of car accidents in OSA patients [10]. The apnea-hypopnea index (AHI), as a marker of OSA severity, was reported to be associated with the occurrence of driving accidents by some studies [32,33], while sleepiness was the principal factor in other studies [26,34–37]. Besides the occurrence of SW, near-miss car accidents in OSA patients could also provide interesting information. SW was reported by 41.3% of OSA patients, but in some cases, it was not associated with excessive daytime sleepiness, as evaluated by the ESS score [37]. SW was predicted by the ESS score, depression and the level of exposure, i.e., the mileage per year. Near-miss accidents were reported by 22% of patients reporting SW and were associated with ESS, depression, habitual sleep duration and the oxygen desaturation index (ODI) [37]. Compared to AHI, the severity of nocturnal hypoxia seems to be a better marker of daytime sleepiness [37–39] or poor performance at psychomotor vigilance tests [40]. The lack of a relationship between AHI and the risk for car accidents could at least partly be explained by the finding that OSA is not always associated with daytime sleepiness, as shown by recent studies on clinical OSA phenotypes [29,41–43]. Excessive sleepiness is common in obesity, independent of coexisting OSA [10].

Some metabolic biomarkers may be related with the occurrence of sleepiness in OSA patients. Among them, increased interleukin-6 (IL-6) has been found during sleep restriction in normal subjects [44] and in OSA patients with objectively documented sleepiness, i.e., a short sleep latency at multiple sleep latency tests, whereas no correlation was shown between IL-6 and subjective sleepiness, as assessed by the Epworth or Stanford Sleepiness scale [45]. In untreated OSA patients, subjective sleepiness was associated with a poor performance for the Psychomotor Vigilance Task (PVT) test but not with IL-6 levels [46]. In women with OSA, increased IL-6 was independently associated with ESS, low physical activity and depression [47], but it was unaffected by CPAP treatment for 12 weeks [48]. Similar findings were reported in a randomized clinical trial in patients with coronary artery disease and non-sleepy OSA after long-term CPAP treatment [49].

C-reactive protein (CRP) is an inflammatory biomarker associated with untreated OSA [50] which decreased shortly after the initiation of CPAP treatment [51]. CRP has recently been assessed as a risk factor for OSA in four prospective studies in population cohorts. Although increased CRP levels at baseline increased the risk for incident OSA, the association was attenuated after the adjustment for BMI, indicating a major role of obesity. The effect of CRP on OSA risk was larger in younger and nonobese subjects [52]. There is currently little evidence for an association of CRP levels with sleepiness [48]. Overall, these results confirm the complexity of the interactions between IL-6, inflammatory markers, OSA, obesity and sleepiness and suggest a limited usefulness of inflammatory biomarkers in predicting EDS in OSA.

Finally, as already discussed, insufficient sleep is a major cause of car accidents in the general population [12], and comorbidities might also contribute, as is the case in depression [21] and diabetes [24].

The results of epidemiological studies on driving risk in OSA should be critically evaluated due to several sources of variability. Firstly, the methods used to assess sleepiness varied, with the majority of studies using the Epworth Sleepiness Scale (ESS) which measures subjective sleepiness in eight situations [53]. The repeatability of the results of ESS has been questioned [54,55], and a low ESS score may be falsely reported despite the occurrence of SW [56]. Secondly, the occurrence of OSA in drivers has been determined as OSA risk by using questionnaires or by the objective documentation of sleep disordered breathing by polysomnography or cardiorespiratory polygraphy [10]. Thirdly, the population under study is a major source of variability, since differences in the results exist between studies in the general population, patients with suspected or diagnosed OSA and non-commercial versus commercial drivers [10]. Fourthly, some studies reported only car accidents that were objectively documented, while other studies derived the risk of car accidents from tests assessing sleepiness, such as the multiple sleep latency test (MSLT) or the maintenance of wakefulness test (MWT) [10]. The use of driving simulators might seem best suited to specifically address driving risk, but the current evidence suggests a limited prediction of sleepiness-related driving risk [57].

Long-haul truck drivers represent a high-risk population due to their high driving distance/year, i.e., increased exposure, frequent sleep debt, and a high prevalence of OSA [11,58,59]. The study by Burks and coworkers in truck drivers in the United States showed that drivers with OSA who were nonadherent to CPAP treatment had a fivefold risk of serious preventable crashes, whereas those adherent to CPAP treatment showed a crash rate similar to the controls [60]. The economic implications are that the motor vehicle-accident-related costs associated with the lack of effective treatment are very high—much higher than those of effective CPAP treatment [60,61]. Legislation on commercial drivers is a very delicate issue, with the interest for public safety on one side and privacy regulations and economic issues on the other side [62,63]. The European Union Directive 2014/85/EU specifically considered the problem of OSA for issuing or renewing a driving license and took into account different safety profiles for commercial and non-commercial drivers [64], but EU Member States have adopted individual measures, and the problem of driving safety in OSA patients is currently heterogeneously addressed throughout Europe.

3. Pathophysiology of Sleepiness at the Wheel in OSA Patients

The identification of risk factors also depends on the methods used to assess sleepiness. Since ESS scores are subjective and show many limitations, the maintenance of wakefulness test (MWT) is currently considered to be the most effective tool to study sleep propensity with regard to SW, especially if the 40 min protocol is used rather than the usual 20 min protocol [65–68]. However, in addition to sleep latency, which is the main result of the MWT, very short episodes of sleep during MWT could be more sensitive markers of the risk to experience car accidents by reflecting drowsiness, i.e., the intermediate state between wakefulness and established sleep. Drowsiness preceding sleep is associated with a lack of control and may be a crucial determinant of car accidents [69–72]. The automatic identification of microsleep episodes may be the first step to develop a new clinical test to identify risky drivers [73]. Age is another important risk factor for car accidents, particularly in patients with OSA. Very recently, Doherty et al., found that higher sleep apnea severity was associated with a higher incidence of adverse driving behavior, such as hard acceleration, braking and speeding. These findings were also observed in cognitively unimpaired old individuals [31].

Another physiological aspect that should be considered is the reduced performance of OSA patients in multi-tasking tests. Driving can be considered a complex and dynamic task that requires the simultaneous performance of intrinsic sub-tasks, such as vehicle control and traffic management, as well as other activities such as radio listening, navigator control, smartphone use, etc. Huang et al., reported that OSA patients showed a reduced performance for divided attention driving simulator trials in comparison to normal age-matched controls [74]. Mazza et al., evaluated the driving performance in a road safety platform, a more natural driving performance test, in a group of OSA patients before and after CPAP treatment [75]. The driving task consisted of avoiding an aquatic obstacle during three real driving conditions: (1) simple condition; (2) distraction condition; (3) anticipation condition. During the simple driving conditions, the patients showed increasing reaction times and a lengthening of the vehicle stopping distance in comparison with the control group. The distraction condition caused a lengthening in reaction times, particularly in OSA patients. Of interest, CPAP therapy determined a statistically significant reduction in the reaction times in OSA patients in comparison to the baseline, as well as a reduction in stopping distance in the distraction and anticipation driving conditions [75]. On the other hand, the ability to perform a multi-tasking trial can be impaired by sleep restriction, including a chronic partial sleep restriction [76]. In this way, OSA per se and partial sleep restriction may have an additive effect on the reduction in driving performance.

Furthermore, Vakulin et al., demonstrated that patients with OSA are more vulnerable than healthy individuals to the effects of alcohol consumption or sleep restriction on driving performance [77].

4. Evaluation of Sleepiness at the Wheel in OSA Patients

Although our knowledge on the determinants of SW has greatly increased, the evaluation of the risk for car accidents in OSA patients remains problematic when considering the number of subjects to be tested for driving license issuing or renewal and the lack of simple and fast tests to be used clinically on a large scale [78]. OSA is recognized as a relevant cause of car accidents worldwide, but the identification of subjects at risk is far from being satisfactory. Figures 1 and 2 schematically depict a possible flow chart for the clinical assessment in subjects with a history of previous car accidents and in subjects with suspected or known OSA, respectively [10].

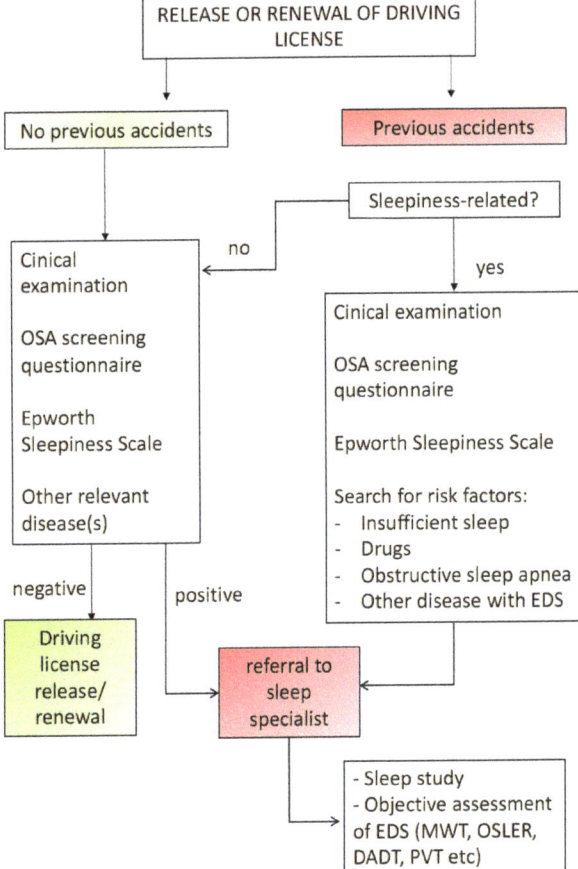

Figure 1. Proposed flowchart to be used for driving license release or renewal. Occurrence of previous sleepiness-related car accidents should be thoroughly investigated. Abbreviations: OSA: Obstructive Sleep Apnea; EDS: Excessive Daytime Sleepiness; MWT: Maintenance of Wakefulness Test; Test; DADT: Divided Attention Driving Task; PVT: Psychomotor Vigilance Test. From [10] with permission.

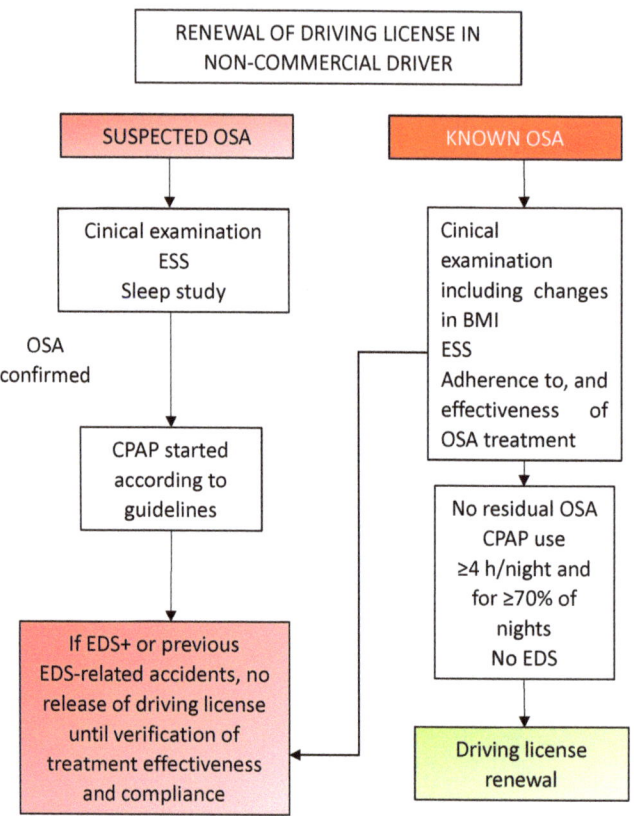

Figure 2. Proposed flowchart to be used for driving license release or renewal. Patients with suspected obstructive sleep apnea (OSA) should be studied and treated whenever the diagnosis of OSA is confirmed. In both newly diagnosed or already known OSA patients, driving licenses should be released or renewed only after the objective documentation of satisfactory compliance with treatment. Abbreviations: ESS: Epworth Sleepiness Scale; BMI: Body Mass Index; CPAP: Continuous Positive Airway Pressure; EDS: Excessive Daytime Sleepiness. Modified from [10] with permission.

Different EEG-derived parameters have been proposed to discriminate patients at risk of poor daytime cognitive performance. Parek et al., demonstrated, in a group of OSA patients, that a sustained run of inspiratory flow limitation determined a significant increment of K-complexes density, with a reduced slow-wave activity associated with delta frequencies. The reduced delta activity (ΔSWAK) was associated with next-day lapses in vigilance during a 20 min psychomotor vigilance test (PVT) [79]. In another study, the same research group demonstrated that the improvement in PVT lapses during CPAP therapy was associated with an increase in ΔSWAK [80]. Mullins et al., observed that sleep EEG microstructure measures recorded during routine PSG were associated with impaired vigilance in OSA patients after sleep deprivation [81]. Eight OSA patients underwent baseline PSG followed by wakefulness for 40 h with repeated PVT tests and driving sessions on a driving simulator. The authors found that a greater EEG slowing during REM sleep was associated with slower PVT reaction times, more PVT lapses and more crashes during driving simulator trials. Furthermore, the decreased spindle density during NREM sleep was also associated with slower PVT reaction times [81]. The study involved a very small number of subjects, highlighting the complexity of such protocols and their obvious limitation for use in large samples.

There is growing evidence that OSA is associated with regional changes in sleep electroencephalography (EEG) pattern, reduced fMRI-measured brain connectivity or reduced functional interhemispheric connectivity [82,83]. Azabarzin et al., recently explored the functional implications of the reduced interhemispheric sleep depth coherence for motor vehicle crash risk in middle-aged and older individuals with OSA [84]. The OSA patients with the highest degree of sleep depth coherence were those with a lower risk of being in an accident [84].

A high level of clinical skills and responsibility is demanded for clinicians who should evaluate the patient's fitness to drive. Specific training would also be useful, since a recent survey reported a high degree of variability in physicians' responses to cases of fitness to drive evaluations [85]. The diagnosis of excessive daytime sleepiness is still based on subjective rather than objective data, and besides the easiest clinical situations—e.g., patients with no previous accidents and no referred daytime sleepiness, patients on CPAP treatment classified as low risk for accidents and patients with clinically evident excessive daytime sleepiness classified as high or very high risk based on ESS—there remains a large and challenging grey area that needs better definition. In this context, a sleep study and MWT remain the best tools to objectively document sleep propensity, evaluated as sleep or microsleep latency at MWT. Psychomotor vigilance tests are promising but far from being standardized for clinical use [10].

5. The New Wake-Promoting Agents

Solriamfetol and pitolisant are new drugs that counteract daytime sleepiness. They are available on the market and are mainly used in neurological disorders such as narcolepsy or idiopathic hypersomnia. Both have been successfully tested in CPAP-treated patients with residual sleepiness and in OSA patients refusing CPAP [86–88]. Little information on the prevention of car accidents with these drugs is available, but solriamfetol improved driving performance [89]. The practical use of solriamfetol or pitolisant in OSA patients is still uncertain, since the clinical features of OSA patients who would benefit most from their use are unclear, and the treatment for sleepiness without concomitant treatment might have detrimental effects on other consequences of OSA, such as cardiometabolic diseases.

6. Conclusions

The role of OSA in increasing the risk for driving accidents is established, and effective CPAP treatment decreases the risk. However, OSA is not the only cause of sleepiness at the wheel, and there are no simple methods to identify the patients at high risk for accidents. From a public health point of view, the risk for driving accidents associated with untreated OSA has been recognized by the EU Commission Directive [64]. Research is exploring new markers of sleepiness, such as the occurrence of microsleep episodes during MWT and polysomnographic indicators of heightened sleep propensity, in order to improve the identification of patients at a high risk. Although new wake-promoting drugs active on daytime sleepiness are available, their clinical indications in OSA patients are still poorly defined.

Author Contributions: Conceptualization, M.R.B., C.L. and F.F.; methodology, M.R.B. and S.L.; writing—original draft preparation, M.R.B. and S.L.; writing—review and editing, C.L. and F.F. All authors have read and agreed to the published version of the manuscript.

Funding: This research received no external funding.

Institutional Review Board Statement: Not applicable.

Informed Consent Statement: Not applicable.

Data Availability Statement: Not applicable.

Conflicts of Interest: The authors declare no conflict of interest.

References

1. Lévy, P.; Kohler, M.; McNicholas, W.T.; Barbé, F.; McEvoy, R.D.; Somers, V.K.; Lavie, L.; Pépin, J.L. Obstructive sleep apnoea syndrome. *Nat. Rev. Dis. Primers* **2015**, *1*, 15015. [CrossRef] [PubMed]
2. Tregear, S.; Reston, J.; Schoelles, K.; Phillips, B. Obstructive sleep apnea and risk of motor vehicle crash: Systematic review and meta-analysis. *J. Clin. Sleep Med.* **2009**, *5*, 573–581. [CrossRef] [PubMed]
3. Weaver, T.E.; Maislin, G.; Dinges, D.F.; Bloxham, T.; George, C.F.; Greenberg, H.; Kader, G.; Mahowald, M.; Younger, J.; Pack, A.I. Relationship Between Hours of CPAP Use and Achieving Normal Levels of Sleepiness and Daily Functioning. *Sleep* **2007**, *30*, 711–719. [CrossRef] [PubMed]
4. Garbarino, S.; Guglielmi, O.; Sanna, A.; Mancardi, G.L.; Magnavita, N. Risk of Occupational Accidents in Workers with Obstructive Sleep Apnea: Systematic Review and Meta-analysis. *Sleep* **2016**, *39*, 1211–1218. [CrossRef]
5. Chou, K.; Tsai, Y.; Yeh, W.; Chen, Y.; Huang, N.; Cheng, H. Risk of work-related injury in workers with obstructive sleep apnea: A systematic review and meta-analysis. *J. Sleep Res.* **2021**, *31*, e13446. [CrossRef]
6. Tregear, S.; Reston, J.; Schoelles, K.; Phillips, B. Continuous Positive Airway Pressure Reduces Risk of Motor Vehicle Crash among Drivers with Obstructive Sleep Apnea: Systematic Review and Meta-analysis. *Sleep* **2010**, *33*, 1373–1380. [CrossRef]
7. Antonopoulos, C.N.; Sergentanis, T.N.; Daskalopoulou, S.S.; Petridou, E.T. Nasal continuous positive airway pressure (nCPAP) treatment for obstructive sleep apnea, road traffic accidents and driving simulator performance: A meta-analysis. *Sleep Med. Rev.* **2011**, *15*, 301–310. [CrossRef]
8. Patil, S.P.; Ayappa, I.A.; Caples, S.M.; Kimoff, R.J.; Patel, S.; Harrod, C.G. Treatment of Adult Obstructive Sleep Apnea with Positive Airway Pressure: An American Academy of Sleep Medicine Systematic Review, Meta-Analysis, and GRADE Assessment. *J. Clin. Sleep Med.* **2019**, *15*, 301–334. [CrossRef]
9. McNicholas, W.T.; Rodenstein, D. Sleep apnoea and driving risk: The need for regulation. *Eur. Respir. Rev.* **2015**, *24*, 602–606. [CrossRef]
10. Bonsignore, M.R.; Randerath, W.; Schiza, S.; Verbraecken, J.; Elliott, M.W.; Riha, R.; Barbe, F.; Bouloukaki, I.; Castrogiovanni, A.; Deleanu, O.; et al. European Respiratory Society statement on sleep apnoea, sleepiness and driving risk. *Eur. Respir. J.* **2020**, *57*, 2001272. [CrossRef]
11. Gurubhagavatula, I.; Tan, M.; Jobanputra, A.M. OSA in Professional Transport Operations. *Chest* **2020**, *158*, 2172–2183. [CrossRef]
12. Quera-Salva, M.A.; Hartley, S.; Sauvagnac-Quera, R.; Sagaspe, P.; Taillard, J.; Contrand, B.; Micoulaud, J.A.; Lagarde, E.; Barbot, F.; Philip, P. Association between reported sleep need and sleepiness at the wheel: Comparative study on French highways between 1996 and 2011. *BMJ Open* **2016**, *6*, e012382. [CrossRef]
13. Connor, J.; Norton, R.; Ameratunga, S.; Robinson, E.; Civil, I.; Dunn, R.; Bailey, J.; Jackson, R. Driver sleepiness and risk of serious injury to car occupants: Population based case control study. *BMJ* **2002**, *324*, 1125. [CrossRef]
14. Horne, J.A.; Reyner, L.A. Driver sleepiness. *J. Sleep Res.* **1995**, *4*, 23–29. [CrossRef]
15. Philip, P.; Vervialle, F.; Le Breton, P.; Taillard, J.; Horne, J.A. Fatigue, alcohol, and serious road crashes in France: Factorial study of national data. *BMJ* **2001**, *322*, 829–830. [CrossRef]
16. Horne, J.; Reyner, L. Vehicle accidents related to sleep: A review. *Occup. Environ. Med.* **1999**, *56*, 289–294. [CrossRef]
17. Garbarino, S.; Nobili, L.; Beelke, M.; De Carli, F.; Ferrillo, F. The contributing role of sleepiness in highway vehicle accidents. *Sleep* **2001**, *24*, 203–206. [CrossRef]
18. Dinges, D.F. An overview of sleepiness and accidents. *J. Sleep Res.* **1995**, *4*, 4–14. [CrossRef]
19. Lammers, G.J.; Bassetti, C.L.; Dolenc-Groselj, L.; Jennum, P.J.; Kallweit, U.; Khatami, R.; Lecendreux, M.; Manconi, M.; Mayer, G.; Partinen, M.; et al. Diagnosis of central disorders of hypersomnolence: A reappraisal by European experts. *Sleep Med. Rev.* **2020**, *52*, 101306. [CrossRef]
20. Lajoie, A.C.; Lafontaine, A.-L.; Kaminska, M. The Spectrum of Sleep Disorders in Parkinson Disease: A review. *Chest* **2021**, *159*, 818–827. [CrossRef]
21. Castro, L.; Castro, J.; Hoexter, M.Q.; Quarantini, L.C.; Kauati, A.; Mello, L.E.; Santos-Silva, R.; Tufik, S.; Bittencourt, L. Depressive symptoms and sleep: A population-based polysomnographic study. *Psychiatry Res.* **2013**, *210*, 906–912. [CrossRef]
22. Choudhury, M.; Miyanishi, K.; Takeda, H.; Tanaka, J. Microglia and the Aging Brain: Are Geriatric Microglia Linked to Poor Sleep Quality? *Int. J. Mol. Sci.* **2021**, *22*, 7824. [CrossRef]
23. Morin, C.M.; Altena, E.; Ivers, H.; Mérette, C.; Leblanc, M.; Savard, J.; Philip, P. Insomnia, hypnotic use, and road collisions: A population-based, 5-year cohort study. *Sleep* **2020**, *43*, zsaa032. [CrossRef]
24. Yusuf, F.L.; Tang, T.S.; Karim, M.E. The association between diabetes and excessive daytime sleepiness among American adults aged 20–79 years: Findings from the 2015–2018 National Health and Nutrition Examination Surveys. *Ann. Epidemiol.* **2022**, *68*, 54–63. [CrossRef]
25. Bioulac, S.; Micoulaud-Franchi, J.-A.; Arnaud, M.M.; Sagaspe, P.; Moore, N.; Salvo, F.; Philip, P. Risk of Motor Vehicle Accidents Related to Sleepiness at the Wheel: A Systematic Review and Meta-Analysis. *Sleep* **2017**, *40*, zsx134, Erratum in *Sleep* **2018**, *41*, zsy075. [CrossRef]
26. Philip, P.; Bailly, S.; Benmerad, M.; Micoulaud-Franchi, J.A.; Grillet, Y.; Sapène, M.; Jullian-Desayes, I.; Joyeux-Faure, M.; Tamisier, R.; Pépin, J.L. Self-reported sleepiness and not the apnoea hypopnoea index is the best predictor of sleepiness-related accidents in obstructive sleep apnoea. *Sci. Rep.* **2020**, *10*, 16267. [CrossRef]

27. Scarpelli, S.; Alfonsi, V.; Gorgoni, M.; Camaioni, M.; Giannini, A.M.; De Gennaro, L. Age-Related Effect of Sleepiness on Driving Performance: A Systematic-Review. *Brain Sci.* **2021**, *11*, 1090. [CrossRef]
28. Pizza, F.; Contardi, S.; Mondini, S.; Cirignotta, F. Simulated driving performance coupled with driver behaviour can predict the risk of sleepiness-related car accidents. *Thorax* **2011**, *66*, 725–726. [CrossRef]
29. Ye, L.; Pien, G.W.; Ratcliffe, S.; Björnsdottir, E.; Arnardottir, E.S.; Pack, A.; Benediktsdottir, B.; Gislason, T. The different clinical faces of obstructive sleep apnoea: A cluster analysis. *Eur. Respir. J.* **2014**, *44*, 1600–1607. [CrossRef]
30. Udholm, N.; Rex, C.E.; Fuglsang, M.; Lundbye-Christensen, S.; Bille, J.; Udholm, S. Obstructive sleep apnea and road traffic accidents: A Danish nationwide cohort study. *Sleep Med.* **2022**, *96*, 64–69. [CrossRef]
31. Doherty, J.M.; Roe, C.M.; Murphy, S.A.; Johnson, A.M.; Fleischer, E.; Toedebusch, C.D.; Redrick, T.; Freund, D.; Morris, J.C.; Schindler, S.E.; et al. Adverse driving behaviors are associated with sleep apnea severity and age in cognitively normal older adults at risk for Alzheimer's disease. *Sleep* **2022**, *45*, zsac070. [CrossRef] [PubMed]
32. Terán-Santos, J.; Jimenez-Gomez, A.; Cordero-Guevara, J. The Association between Sleep Apnea and the Risk of Traffic Accidents. Cooperative Group Burgos-Santander. *N. Engl. J. Med.* **1999**, *340*, 847–851. [CrossRef] [PubMed]
33. Mulgrew, A.T.; Nasvadi, G.; Butt, A.; Cheema, R.; Fox, N.; Fleetham, J.A.; Ryan, C.F.; Cooper, P.; Ayas, N.T. Risk and severity of motor vehicle crashes in patients with obstructive sleep apnoea/hypopnoea. *Thorax* **2008**, *63*, 536–541. [CrossRef] [PubMed]
34. Karimi, M.; Hedner, J.; Lombardi, C.; Mcnicholas, W.T.; Penzel, T.; Riha, R.L.; Rodenstein, D.; Grote, L.; the Esada Study Group. Driving habits and risk factors for traffic accidents among sleep apnea patients—A European multi-centre cohort study. *J. Sleep Res.* **2014**, *23*, 689–699. [CrossRef]
35. Karimi, M.; Hedner, J.; Häbel, H.; Nerman, O.; Grote, L. Sleep Apnea Related Risk of Motor Vehicle Accidents is Reduced by Continuous Positive Airway Pressure: Swedish Traffic Accident Registry Data. *Sleep* **2015**, *38*, 341–349. [CrossRef]
36. Arita, A.; Sasanabe, R.; Hasegawa, R.; Nomura, A.; Hori, R.; Mano, M.; Konishi, N.; Shiomi, T. Risk factors for automobile accidents caused by falling asleep while driving in obstructive sleep apnea syndrome. *Sleep Breath.* **2015**, *19*, 1229–1234. [CrossRef]
37. Fanfulla, F.; Pinna, G.D.; Marrone, O.; Lupo, N.D.; Arcovio, S.; Bonsignore, M.R.; Morrone, E. Determinants of Sleepiness at Wheel and Missing Accidents in Patients with Obstructive Sleep Apnea. *Front. Neurosci.* **2021**, *15*, 656203. [CrossRef]
38. Sabil, A.; Bignard, R.; Gervès-Pinquié, C.; Philip, P.; Le Vaillant, M.; Trzepizur, W.; Meslier, N.; Gagnadoux, F. Risk Factors for Sleepiness at the Wheel and Sleep-Related Car Accidents Among Patients with Obstructive Sleep Apnea: Data from the French Pays de la Loire Sleep Cohort. *Nat. Sci. Sleep* **2021**, *13*, 1737–1746. [CrossRef]
39. Sun, Y.; Ning, Y.; Huang, L.; Lei, F.; Li, Z.; Zhou, G.; Tang, X. Polysomnographic characteristics of daytime sleepiness in obstructive sleep apnea syndrome. *Sleep Breath.* **2012**, *16*, 375–381. [CrossRef]
40. Kainulainen, S.; Duce, B.; Korkalainen, H.; Oksenberg, A.; Leino, A.; Arnardottir, E.S.; Kulkas, A.; Myllymaa, S.; Töyräs, J.; Leppänen, T. Severe desaturations increase psychomotor vigilance task-based median reaction time and number of lapses in obstructive sleep apnoea patients. *Eur. Respir. J.* **2020**, *55*, 1901849. [CrossRef]
41. Saaresranta, T.; Hedner, J.; Bonsignore, M.R.; Riha, R.L.; McNicholas, W.T.; Penzel, T.; Anttalainen, U.; Kvamme, J.A.; Pretl, M.; Sliwinski, P.; et al. Clinical Phenotypes and Comorbidity in European Sleep Apnoea Patients. *PLoS ONE* **2016**, *11*, e0163439. [CrossRef]
42. Mazzotti, D.R.; Keenan, B.T.; Lim, D.C.; Gottlieb, D.J.; Kim, J.; Pack, A.I. Symptom Subtypes of Obstructive Sleep Apnea Predict Incidence of Cardiovascular Outcomes. *Am. J. Respir. Crit. Care Med.* **2019**, *200*, 493–506. [CrossRef]
43. Bailly, S.; Grote, L.; Hedner, J.; Schiza, S.; McNicholas, W.T.; Basoglu, O.K.; Lombardi, C.; Dogas, Z.; Roisman, G.; Pataka, A.; et al. Clusters of sleep apnoea phenotypes: A large pan-European study from the European Sleep Apnoea Database (ESADA). *Respirology* **2021**, *26*, 378–387. [CrossRef]
44. Pejovic, S.; Basta, M.; Vgontzas, A.N.; Kritikou, I.; Shaffer, M.L.; Tsaoussoglou, M.; Stiffler, D.; Stefanakis, Z.; Bixler, E.O.; Chrousos, G.P. Effects of recovery sleep after one work week of mild sleep restriction on interleukin-6 and cortisol secretion and daytime sleepiness and performance. *Am. J. Physiol. Endocrinol. Metab.* **2013**, *305*, E890–E896. [CrossRef]
45. Li, Y.; Vgontzas, A.N.; Fernandez-Mendoza, J.; Kritikou, I.; Basta, M.; Pejovic, S.; Gaines, J.; Bixler, E.O. Objective, but Not Subjective, Sleepiness is Associated with Inflammation in Sleep Apnea. *Sleep* **2017**, *40*, zsw033. [CrossRef]
46. Li, Y.; Vgontzas, A.; Kritikou, I.; Fernandez-Mendoza, J.; Basta, M.; Pejovic, S.; Gaines, J.; Bixler, E.O. Psychomotor Vigilance Test and Its Association with Daytime Sleepiness and Inflammation in Sleep Apnea: Clinical Implications. *J. Clin. Sleep Med.* **2017**, *13*, 1049–1056. [CrossRef]
47. Campos-Rodriguez, F.; Cordero-Guevara, J.; Asensio-Cruz, M.I.; Sanchez-Armengol, A.; Sanchez-Lopez, V.; Arellano-Orden, E.; Gozal, D.; Martinez-Garcia, M.A. Interleukin 6 as a marker of depression in women with sleep apnea. *J. Sleep Res.* **2020**, *30*, e13035. [CrossRef]
48. Campos-Rodriguez, F.; Asensio-Cruz, M.I.; Cordero-Guevara, J.; Jurado-Gamez, B.; Carmona-Bernal, C.; Gonzalez-Martinez, M.; Troncoso, M.F.; Sanchez-Lopez, V.; Arellano-Orden, E.; Garcia-Sanchez, M.I.; et al. Effect of continuous positive airway pressure on inflammatory, antioxidant, and depression biomarkers in women with obstructive sleep apnea: A randomized controlled trial. *Sleep* **2019**, *42*, zsz145. [CrossRef]
49. Thunström, E.; Glantz, H.; Yucel-Lindberg, T.; Lindberg, K.; Saygin, M.; Peker, Y. CPAP Does Not Reduce Inflammatory Biomarkers in Patients with Coronary Artery Disease and Nonsleepy Obstructive Sleep Apnea: A Randomized Controlled Trial. *Sleep* **2017**, *40*, zsx157. [CrossRef]

50. Imani, M.; Sadeghi, M.; Farokhzadeh, F.; Khazaie, H.; Brand, S.; Dürsteler, K.; Brühl, A.; Sadeghi-Bahmani, D. Evaluation of Blood Levels of C-Reactive Protein Marker in Obstructive Sleep Apnea: A Systematic Review, Meta-Analysis and Meta-Regression. *Life* **2021**, *11*, 362. [CrossRef]
51. Wang, Y.; Ni Lin, Y.; Zhang, L.Y.; Li, C.X.; Li, S.Q.; Li, H.P.; Zhang, L.; Li, N.; Yan, Y.R.; Li, Q.Y. Changes of circulating biomarkers of inflammation and glycolipid metabolism by CPAP in OSA patients: A meta-analysis of time-dependent profiles. *Ther. Adv. Chronic Dis.* **2022**, *13*, 20406223211070919. [CrossRef]
52. Huang, T.; Goodman, M.; Li, X.; Sands, S.A.; Li, J.; Stampfer, M.J.; Saxena, R.; Tworoger, S.S.; Redline, S. C-reactive Protein and Risk of OSA in Four US Cohorts. *Chest* **2021**, *159*, 2439–2448. [CrossRef]
53. Johns, M.W. A New Method for Measuring Daytime Sleepiness: The Epworth Sleepiness Scale. *Sleep* **1991**, *14*, 540–545. [CrossRef]
54. Rozgonyi, R.; Dombi, I.; Janszky, J.; Kovács, N.; Faludi, B. Low test–retest reliability of the Epworth Sleepiness Scale within a substantial short time frame. *J. Sleep Res.* **2021**, *30*, e13277. [CrossRef]
55. Lee, J.L.; Chung, Y.; Waters, E.; Vedam, H. The Epworth sleepiness scale: Reliably unreliable in a sleep clinic population. *J. Sleep Res.* **2020**, *29*, e13019. [CrossRef]
56. Baiardi, S.; La Morgia, C.; Sciamanna, L.; Gerosa, A.; Cirignotta, F.; Mondini, S. Is the Epworth Sleepiness Scale a useful tool for screening excessive daytime sleepiness in commercial drivers? *Accid. Anal. Prev.* **2018**, *110*, 187–189. [CrossRef]
57. Schreier, D.R.; Banks, C.; Mathis, J. Driving simulators in the clinical assessment of fitness to drive in sleepy individuals: A systematic review. *Sleep Med. Rev.* **2017**, *38*, 86–100. [CrossRef] [PubMed]
58. Garbarino, S.; Durando, P.; Guglielmi, O.; Dini, G.; Bersi, F.; Fornarino, S.; Toletone, A.; Chiorri, C.; Magnavita, N. Sleep Apnea, Sleep Debt and Daytime Sleepiness Are Independently Associated with Road Accidents. A Cross-Sectional Study on Truck Drivers. *PLoS ONE* **2016**, *11*, e0166262. [CrossRef]
59. Sunwoo, J.-S.; Shin, D.-S.; Hwangbo, Y.; Kim, W.-J.; Chu, M.K.; Yun, C.-H.; Jang, T.; Yang, K.I. High risk of obstructive sleep apnea, insomnia, and daytime sleepiness among commercial motor vehicle drivers. *Sleep Breath.* **2019**, *23*, 979–985. [CrossRef]
60. Burks, S.V.; Anderson, J.E.; Bombyk, M.; Haider, R.; Ganzhorn, D.; Jiao, X.; Lewis, C.; Lexvold, A.; Liu, H.; Ning, J.; et al. Nonadherence with employer-mandated sleep apnea treatment and increased risk of serious truck crashes. *Sleep* **2016**, *39*, 967–975. [CrossRef]
61. Burks, S.V.; Anderson, J.E.; Panda, B.; Haider, R.; Ginader, T.; Sandback, N.; Pokutnaya, D.; Toso, D.; Hughes, N.; Haider, H.S.; et al. Employer-mandated obstructive sleep apnea treatment and healthcare cost savings among truckers. *Sleep* **2020**, *43*, zsz262. [CrossRef] [PubMed]
62. Das, A.M.; Chang, J.L.; Berneking, M.; Hartenbaum, N.P.; Rosekind, M.; Ramar, K.; Malhotra, R.K.; Carden, K.A.; Martin, J.L.; Abbasi-Feinberg, F.; et al. Enhancing public health and safety by diagnosing and treating obstructive sleep apnea in the transportation industry: An American Academy of Sleep Medicine position statement. *J. Clin. Sleep Med.* **2021**, jcsm-9670. [CrossRef]
63. Donovan, L.M.; Kapur, V.K. Screening commercial drivers for sleep apnea: Are profits and public safety aligned? *Sleep* **2020**, *43*, zsaa043. [CrossRef] [PubMed]
64. Commission Directive 2014/85/EU of 1 July 2014, amending Directive 2006/126/EC of the European Parliament and of the Council on Driving Licences. 2014. Available online: https://www.cieca.eu/sites/default/files/legislation/OJ-JOL_2014_194_R_0003-EN-TXT.pdf (accessed on 9 May 2022).
65. Sagaspe, P.; Taillard, J.; Chaumet, G.; Guilleminault, C.; Coste, O.; Moore, N.; Bioulac, B.; Philip, P. Maintenance of wakefulness test as a predictor of driving performance in patients with untreated obstructive sleep apnea. *Sleep* **2007**, *30*, 327–330. [CrossRef]
66. Pizza, F.; Contardi, S.; Mondini, S.; Trentin, L.; Cirignotta, F. Daytime sleepiness and driving performance in patients with obstructive sleep apnea: Comparison of the MSLT, the MWT, and a simulated driving task. *Sleep* **2009**, *32*, 382–391. [CrossRef]
67. Philip, P.; Chaufton, C.; Taillard, J.; Sagaspe, P.; Léger, D.; Raimondi, M.; Vakulin, A.; Capelli, A. Maintenance of Wakefulness Test scores and driving performance in sleep disorder patients and controls. *Int. J. Psychophysiol.* **2013**, *89*, 195–202. [CrossRef]
68. Philip, P.; Guichard, K.; Strauss, M.; Léger, D.; Pepin, E.; Arnulf, I.; Sagaspe, P.; Barateau, L.; Lopez, R.; Taillard, J.; et al. Maintenance of wakefulness test: How does it predict accident risk in patients with sleep disorders? *Sleep Med.* **2020**, *77*, 249–255. [CrossRef]
69. Morrone, E.; Lupo, N.D.; Trentin, R.; Pizza, F.; Risi, I.; Arcovio, S.; Fanfulla, F. Microsleep as a marker of sleepiness in obstructive sleep apnea patients. *J. Sleep Res.* **2020**, *29*, e12882. [CrossRef]
70. Putilov, A.A.; Donskaya, O.G.; Verevkin, E.G. Can we feel like being neither alert nor sleepy? The electroencephalographic signature of this subjective sub-state of wake state yields an accurate measure of objective sleepiness level. *Int. J. Psychophysiol.* **2019**, *135*, 33–43. [CrossRef]
71. Anniss, A.M.; Young, A.; O'Driscoll, D.M. Microsleep assessment enhances interpretation of the Maintenance of Wakefulness Test. *J. Clin. Sleep Med.* **2021**, *17*, 1571–1578. [CrossRef]
72. Hertig-Godeschalk, A.; Skorucak, J.; Malafeev, A.; Achermann, P.; Mathis, J.; Schreier, D.R. Microsleep episodes in the borderland between wakefulness and sleep. *Sleep* **2020**, *43*, zsz163. [CrossRef]
73. Skorucak, J.; Hertig-Godeschalk, A.; Achermann, P.; Mathis, J.; Schreier, D.R. Automatically Detected Microsleep Episodes in the Fitness-to-Drive Assessment. *Front. Neurosci.* **2020**, *14*, 8. [CrossRef]
74. Huang, Y.; Hennig, S.; Fietze, I.; Penzel, T.; Veauthier, C. The Psychomotor Vigilance Test Compared to a Divided Attention Steering Simulation in Patients with Moderate or Severe Obstructive Sleep Apnea. *Nat. Sci. Sleep* **2020**, *12*, 509–524. [CrossRef]

75. Mazza, S.; Pépin, J.L.; Naëgelé, B.; Rauch, E.; Deschaux, C.; Ficheux, P.; Levy, P. Driving ability in sleep apnoea patients before and after CPAP treatment: Evaluation on a road safety platform. *Eur. Respir. J.* **2006**, *28*, 1020–1028. [CrossRef]
76. Haavisto, M.-L.; Porkka-Heiskanen, T.; Hublin, C.; Härmä, M.; Mutanen, P.; Müller, K.; Virkkala, J.; Sallinen, M. Sleep restriction for the duration of a work week impairs multitasking performance. *J. Sleep Res.* **2010**, *19*, 444–454. [CrossRef]
77. Vakulin, A.; Baulk, S.D.; Catcheside, P.G.; Antic, N.A.; Heuvel, C.J.V.D.; Dorrian, J.; McEvoy, R.D. Effects of alcohol and sleep restriction on simulated driving performance in untreated patients with obstructive sleep apnea. *Ann. Intern. Med.* **2009**, *151*, 447–455. [CrossRef]
78. Garbarino, S. Excessive daytime sleepiness in obstructive sleep apnea: Implications for driving licenses. *Sleep Breath.* **2020**, *24*, 37–47. [CrossRef]
79. Parekh, A.; Kam, K.; Mullins, A.E.; Castillo, B.; Berkalieva, A.; Mazumdar, M.; Varga, A.W.; Eckert, D.J.; Rapoport, D.M.; Ayappa, I. Altered K-complex morphology during sustained inspiratory airflow limitation is associated with next-day lapses in vigilance in obstructive sleep apnea. *Sleep* **2021**, *44*, zsab010. [CrossRef]
80. Parekh, A.; Mullins, A.E.; Kam, K.; Varga, A.W.; Rapoport, D.M.; Ayappa, I. Slow-wave activity surrounding stage N2 K-complexes and daytime function measured by psychomotor vigilance test in obstructive sleep apnea. *Sleep* **2019**, *42*, zsy256. [CrossRef]
81. Mullins, A.E.; Kim, J.W.; Wong, K.K.H.; Bartlett, D.J.; Vakulin, A.; Dijk, D.-J.; Marshall, N.S.; Grunstein, R.R.; D'Rozario, A.L. Sleep EEG microstructure is associated with neurobehavioural impairment after extended wakefulness in obstructive sleep apnea. *Sleep Breath.* **2021**, *25*, 347–354. [CrossRef]
82. Canessa, N.; Castronovo, V.; Cappa, S.; Marelli, S.; Iadanza, A.; Falini, A.; Ferini-Strambi, L. Sleep apnea: Altered brain connectivity underlying a working-memory challenge. *NeuroImage Clin.* **2018**, *19*, 56–65. [CrossRef] [PubMed]
83. Rial, R.V.; Gonzalez, J.; Gené, L.; Akaarir, M.; Esteban, S.; Gamundí, A.; Barceló, P.; Nicolau, C. Asymmetric sleep in apneic human patients. *Am. J. Physiol. Integr. Regul. Comp. Physiol.* **2013**, *304*, R232–R237. [CrossRef] [PubMed]
84. Azarbarzin, A.; Younes, M.; Sands, S.A.; Wellman, A.; Redline, S.; Czeisler, C.A.; Gottlieb, D.J. Interhemispheric sleep depth coherence predicts driving safety in sleep apnea. *J. Sleep Res.* **2021**, *20*, e13092. [CrossRef] [PubMed]
85. Dwarakanath, A.; Twiddy, M.; Ghosh, D.; Jamson, S.L.; Baxter, P.D.; Elliott, M.W.; British Thoracic Society. Variability in clinicians' opinions regarding fitness to drive in patients with obstructive sleep apnoea syndrome (OSAS). *Thorax* **2014**, *70*, 495–497. [CrossRef]
86. Lal, C.; Weaver, T.E.; Bae, C.J.; Strohl, K.P. Excessive Daytime Sleepiness in Obstructive Sleep Apnea. Mechanisms and Clinical Management. *Ann. Am. Thorac. Soc.* **2021**, *18*, 757–768. [CrossRef]
87. Craig, S.; Pépin, J.-L.; Randerath, W.; Caussé, C.; Verbraecken, J.; Asin, J.; Barbé, F.; Bonsignore, M.R. Investigation and management of residual sleepiness in CPAP-treated patients with obstructive sleep apnoea: The European view. *Eur. Respir. Rev.* **2022**, *31*, 210230. [CrossRef]
88. Ronnebaum, S.; Bron, M.; Patel, D.; Menno, D.; Bujanover, S.; Kratochvil, B.D.; Lucas, B.E.; Stepnowsky, C. Indirect treatment comparison of solriamfetol, modafinil, and armodafinil for excessive daytime sleepiness in obstructive sleep apnea. *J. Clin. Sleep Med.* **2021**, *17*, 2543–2555. [CrossRef]
89. Vinckenbosch, F.; Asin, J.; Vries, N.; Vonk, P.E.; Donjacour, C.E.H.M.; Lammers, G.J.; Overeem, S.; Janssen, H.; Wang, G.; Chen, D.; et al. Effects of solriamfetol on on-the-road driving performance in participants with excessive daytime sleepiness associated with obstructive sleep apnoea. *Hum. Psychopharmacol. Clin. Exp.* **2022**, e2845. [CrossRef]

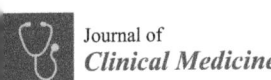

Review

Obstructive Sleep Apnea in Heart Failure: Current Knowledge and Future Directions

Shahrokh Javaheri [1,2,3] and Sogol Javaheri [4,*]

1. Division of Pulmonary and Sleep Medicine, Bethesda North Hospital, Cincinnati, OH 45242, USA; shahrokhjavaheri@icloud.com
2. Division of Cardiology, The Ohio State University, Columbus, OH 43210, USA
3. Division of Pulmonary and Sleep Medicine, University of Cincinnati, Cincinnati, OH 45242, USA
4. Division of Sleep and Circadian Disorders, Brigham and Women's Hospital, Harvard Medical School, Boston, MA 02130, USA
* Correspondence: sjavaheri@bwh.harvard.edu

Abstract: Obstructive sleep apnea (OSA) is highly prevalent among patients with asymptomatic left ventricular systolic and diastolic dysfunction and congestive heart failure, and if untreated may contribute to the clinical progression of heart failure (HF). Given the health and economic burden of HF, identifying potential modifiable risk factors such as OSA and whether appropriate treatment improves outcomes is of critical importance. Identifying the subgroups of patients with OSA and HF who would benefit most from OSA treatment is another important point. This focused review surveys current knowledge of OSA and HF in order to provide: (1) a better understanding of the pathophysiologic mechanisms that may increase morbidity among individuals with HF and comorbid OSA, (2) a summary of current observational data and small randomized trials, (3) an understanding of the limitations of current larger randomized controlled trials, and (4) future needs to more accurately determine the efficacy of OSA treatment among individuals with HF.

Keywords: obstructive sleep apnea; heart failure; continuous positive airway pressure

1. Introduction

According to the American Heart Association 2022 Statistics [1], over 8 million people 18 years or older will have heart failure (HF) in 2030. Despite treatment advances, the prevalence, burden, and costs of HF continue to increase. The healthcare costs associated with HF exceed 30 billion dollars annually and over 50% of these costs are associated with hospitalizations [1]. Obstructive sleep apnea (OSA) is highly prevalent in, and may contribute to the progression of, both HF with reduced ejection fraction (HFrEF) and HF with preserved ejection fraction (HFpEF), potentially reflecting an important modifiable risk factor. The prevalence of OSA ranges from 20% to up to 60% among the HF population, with rates of OSA typically running higher among those with HFpEF as compared with HFrEF [2–6]. Observational data has shown that OSA is independently associated with poor quality of life, excess rehospitalization, and premature mortality among patients with HF [5]. Notably, multiple observational studies have demonstrated that effective treatment of OSA may decrease hospital readmission rates and improve survival [7–9]. To date, there are no randomized controlled trials assessing continuous positive airway pressure (CPAP) therapy in an HF with comorbid OSA population. Prior RCTs using CPAP to treat OSA have shown no benefit on secondary prevention of cardiovascular diseases but have shown improvement in quality-of-life measures. The purpose of this review is to review pathophysiologic mechanisms underlying the association between OSA and HF, to summarize current observational and randomized data, and to characterize the need for trials that can address important questions in real world patients and in specific subgroups of HF patients who may be more likely to benefit from OSA treatment.

2. OSA and HF Pathophysiology

OSA is characterized by repetitive upper airway closure due to soft tissue collapse and genioglossus muscle relaxation in the upper airway resulting in apneas (cessation of breathing for 10 s or longer) and hypopneas (reductions in breathing coupled with desaturation and/or arousal). Obesity and rostral fluid shifts both contribute to upper airway narrowing and collapse. Like the general population, obese individuals with HF are also more prone to upper airway closure related to fat deposition in the upper body, including visceral fat and tongue and throat fat [10]. At the same time, fluid retention and edema, particularly during HF decompensation, can contribute to upper airway closure in the supine position. Translocation of fluid from the lower extremities to the neck may cause vascular congestion and edema of the pharyngeal area [11]. Regardless of the contributing factors, the downstream effects include intermittent hypoxia and hyper-hypocapnia, repetitive arousals, and large negative intrathoracic pressure swings. Hypoxia, hypercapnia, and arousals lead to autonomic dysregulation with heightened sympathetic activity and reduce parasympathetic tone as well as hypothalamic pituitary axis dysregulation. Intermittent hypoxia reoxygenation leads to production of oxygen free radicals, oxidative stress, and upregulation of inflammatory cascades such as NF kb and TNF-alpha. Finally, negative intrathoracic pressure swings may result in increased atrial stretch (facilitating atrial fibrillation), left ventricular transmural pressure and afterload, and myocardial oxygen demand [5,11].

3. Epidemiology

Multiple observational studies suggest that OSA is independently associated with excess hospital readmission [9,10] and that treatment may lower the rate of readmissions [7–9]. Specifically, severe OSA has been independently associated with 1.5 times higher readmission of HF patients when compared with those without OSA [9]. Observational studies also suggest OSA is independently associated with premature mortality in individuals with comorbid HF [7–9,12,13] and that treatment of OSA attenuates this risk [7,9,12,13]. In the largest study, among 30,000 Medicare beneficiaries newly diagnosed with HF, the treatment of SDB was associated with decreased readmission, health care cost, and mortality [7]. Two other studies have shown that effective treatment of OSA with CPAP improves survival in patients with comorbid HF, particularly in those who are compliant with CPAP [9,12]. Long-term randomized control trials (RCTs) in this population are not available, but there is a critical need to assess how effective treatment of OSA affects the clinical course of HF and hard outcomes.

4. Acute Decompensated Heart Failure

Multiple observational studies have shown a high prevalence of SDB, particularly OSA in patients admitted to the hospital for HF decompensation. In a multi-center study from Brazil, consecutive patients with confirmed acute cardiogenic pulmonary edema (ACPE) underwent polygraphy following clinical stabilization [14]. Approximately 100 patients were included in the final analysis, of whom 79 had HFpEF with LVEF greater than or equal to 50%. A total of 61% of the patients had OSA defined as an apnea-hypopnea index (AHI) greater than or equal to 15 events/h based on polygraphy. The mean follow-up was 1 year and the primary outcome was ACPE recurrence. Higher incident rates of ACPE recurrence (25 vs. 6 episodes; $p = 0.01$) and myocardial infarction (15 vs. 0 episodes; $p = 0.0004$) were observed in patients with OSA compared with those without OSA. All 17 deaths occurred in the OSA group ($p = 0.0001$). In a Cox proportional hazards regression analysis, OSA was independently associated with ACPE recurrence (hazard ratio (HR), 3.3 [95% CI, 1.2–8.8], $p = 0.01$), incidence of myocardial infarction (HR, 2.3 [95% CI, 1.1–9.5]; $p = 0.02$), cardiovascular death (HR, 5.4 [95% CI, 1.4–48.4]; $p = 0.004$), and total death (HR, 6.5 [95% CI, 1.2–64.0]; $p = 0.005$). Among the patients with OSA who presented with ACPE recurrence or who died, AHI and hypoxemic burden and rates of sleep-onset ACPE were significantly higher [14].

Given the high prevalence of OSA in HFpEF and HFrEF and supportive observational data, OSA may represent a modifiable risk factor. This is particularly important as HFpEF remains highly prevalent and thus far pharmacological trials have not shown a drug therapy that could improve survival as the primary outcome, though a recent sodium–glucose co-transporter 2 (SGLT-2) inhibitor trial has demonstrated improved survival in the composite endpoint of hospital admission and mortality [15].

One RCT in acute decompensated HF randomized 150 patients with HFrEF who were diagnosed with OSA during hospitalization to a CPAP therapy arm ($n = 75$) or control arm ($n = 75$). All participants received guideline-directed therapy for HF decompensation. Exploratory analysis revealed that 6 months after discharge, there was over a 60% decrease in readmissions for patients who used PAP > 3 h/night compared with those who used PAP < 3 h/night ($p < 0.02$) and compared with controls ($p < 0.04$) [13].

5. Limitations of Randomized Control Trials for OSA Treatment in HF

There have been multiple RCTs, primarily in participants without HF, assessing composite cardiovascular endpoints. Notably, all the trials enrolled individuals with established CVD and/or cerebrovascular disease. The largest OSA RCT to date, the SAVE trial, randomized 2717 patients with established cardiovascular disease (a minority with HF), at least moderate or severe OSA to CPAP, plus usual care versus usual care alone for almost four years. CPAP use did not reduce the composite cardiovascular endpoint, though in secondary analyses there was a lower risk of cerebrovascular events among patients using CPAP for at least 4 h per night [16]. Limitations to this trial (as well as other OSA RCTs) include low adherence to CPAP, minimally symptomatic population selection (largely excluding patients with very severe OSA and/or hypoxia), and reduced generalizability. Regarding adherence, various studies have suggested a linear relationship between hours of CPAP use and change in blood pressure. A metanalysis estimated a 1.39 mm Hg decrease in 24-h mean blood pressure for each 1-h increase in effective nightly use of CPAP [17]. It is feasible that below a certain threshold, too few hours of CPAP use may not confer cardiovascular and metabolic benefit. Additionally, there is data suggesting that sleepier patients [18] and those with more severe hypoxemic burden [19,20] have higher incident cardiovascular risk and therefore might benefit the most with CPAP therapy. However, in most trials, patients with more severe apnea and hypoxemic burden and those with excessive sleepiness are excluded, including the SAVE trial. In the SAVE trial, patients with ESS >15 were excluded and the average ESS was approximately 7 (under 10 is considered within normal limits), suggesting that most patients were not sleepy [16]. Since less symptomatic patients are less likely to benefit from CPAP therapy, this could also contribute to lower CPAP adherence. Overall, participants enrolled had established CVD, did not have severe hypoxic burden, and were generally non-sleepy; the cardinal symptom of OSA for which many patients seek treatment. Yet, observational studies, including the Wisconsin Sleep Cohort Study [21], the Busselton Health Study [22], and the Sleep Heart Health Study [23], revealed that only severe OSA was associated with premature mortality. Similarly, recent studies have suggested that hypoxemic burden is an important predictor of mortality and adverse cardiovascular sequelae [19,20]. Therefore, the patient populations studied in the SAVE trial (as with other RCTs to date) do not reflect the population of patients treated clinically.

6. OSA Phenotyping for Targeting Personalized Therapy

OSA is a heterogeneous disease with distinct endo/phenotypes. Individuals have different symptoms, clinical presentations, and risk factors and may respond differently to the same therapy. Determining which subgroup of patients (whether using symptoms such as sleepiness, PSG measures such as hypoxic burden, or other subtypes such as the insomnia and OSA or COMISA subtype) may have higher CVD risk and respond best to treatment may be a critical point [20,24]. In the Icelandic study, three phenotypes were identified: (1) the disturbed sleep group who were the OSA patients most likely to suffer from insomnia symptoms (and mean ESS < 10), (2) minimally symptomatic OSA patients (most normal ESS scores), and (3) excess daytime sleepiness (mean ESS 15.7 ± 0.6) patients. Differences among the three groups were not explained by obesity, age, sex, or AHI severity [25]. Prior studies have shown that the excessively sleepy subtype may be more strongly associated with a prevalence of HF and may also have a higher degree of CVD risk [26], potentially representing a symptomatic biomarker for CVD risk. Unfortunately, however, these are the very patients who are excluded from RCTs for lack of feasibility and ethical concerns. These patients may be at increased risk of motor vehicle collisions due to drowsy driving and may refuse to participate in a study where they will be in a control arm without effective long-term treatment. In order to effectively study cardiovascular outcomes and mortality, long-term follow up is required, which is ethically complex.

7. Pitfall of the AHI and Alternate Metrics

It is not yet clear what the best metric for measuring OSA disease burden is in HF patients. The AHI does not capture the depth or duration of upper airway obstruction, hypoxic burden, or REM versus NREM preponderance of respiratory events. There may be other metrics to quantify the severity of sleep apnea in the HF population, including measures of hypoxia (i.e., time spent < 90% oxygen saturation, hypoxic burden, measured as the area under the desaturation curve from respiratory event and pre-event baseline). Arousal burden (number and intensity of arousals), REM versus NREM AHI, duration of respiratory events (in addition to frequency), changes in heart rate in response to arousals, or other biomarkers may also present potential metrics of interest. Studies are needed to investigate metrics that may allow for better phenotyping and patient selection first in the general population and then in the HF population. The hypoxic burden and pulse rate response to respiratory events or arousal are currently under investigation [27], however more data on reliability and ease of measurement are needed before clinical application.

8. Other Therapeutic Options

It is widely known that CPAP can be difficult to tolerate, particularly in the HF population. Alternate treatments include oral appliances, hypoglossal nerve stimulation, and positional therapy in patients with supine-dominant OSA. In CPAP-intolerant individuals, custom-made oral appliances and hypoglossal nerve stimulation are recommended, though limited studies are available in HF. Studying the efficacy of alternate therapeutic options, including oral appliance therapy and hypoglossal nerve stimulation, will also be important in the HF population.

9. Summary and Remaining Issues

OSA is highly prevalent in all types of HF. It is biologically plausible that OSA leads to adverse cardiovascular sequelae, and long term pathobiologic consequences of sleep apnea may include sustained increases in sympathetic activity, endothelial dysfunction, oxidate stress, and up-regulation of inflammatory cytokines, ultimately leading to a variety of cerebrocardiovascular complications. Observational studies have demonstrated associations between OSA with excess rehospitalization and mortality among HF patients, and multiple observational studies have demonstrated that effective treatment of OSA decreases hospital readmission and improves survival [10,12,28]. Small prospective [29] and randomized trials [13,30] also show improvement in intermediate outcomes with use of PAP therapy, including reductions in blood pressure and ejection fraction with effective treatment of OSA. However, larger RCTs on composite outcomes have been negative or inconclusive, though they do consistently demonstrate improved quality of life and mood with use of PAP. To date, there are no randomized controlled trials assessing continuous positive airway pressure (CPAP) therapy in an HF with comorbid OSA population, and future studies with improved design and implementation and using alternative therapeutic options, not only PAP devices, are needed to determine whether OSA treatment improves morbidity and mortality in HF patients beyond quality-of-life measures. Additionally, studies are needed to better characterize phenotypes of OSA and objective measures to help determine who may respond best to CPAP (i.e., sleepy versus non-sleepy patients). Use of other metrics beyond the AHI and inclusion of specific OSA phenotypes may allow for more targeted patient selection in future trials. Until then, treatment options should start with evidence-based therapy for HF, and treatment for OSA in HF should be targeted to improve AHI and alleviate patient symptoms with the goal of improving mood, quality of life, and blood pressure. More targeted and thoughtful selection of study populations, larger populations, and higher adherence to PAP are all challenges that must be overcome in OSA RCTs in order to adequately address the pressing questions of whether OSA is indeed a modifiable risk factor for HF and whether CPAP can improve survival and other cardiovascular endpoints.

Author Contributions: Both S.J. (Sogol Javaheri) and S.J. (Shahrokh Javaheri) contributed to the original draft preparation and review and editing of this paper. All authors have read and agreed to the published version of the manuscript.

Funding: This research received no external funding.

Institutional Review Board Statement: Not applicable.

Informed Consent Statement: Not applicable.

Data Availability Statement: Not applicable.

Conflicts of Interest: Sogol Javaheri is a consultant for Jazz Pharmaceuticals and receives grant funding from Zoll Medical. Shahrokh Javaheri has advised Jazz Pharmaceuticals, Fisher Pykel and Harmony Biosciences. He is a consultant for Zoll Medical.

References

1. Bozkurt, B.; Hershberger, R.E.; Butler, J.; Grady, K.L.; Heidenreich, P.A.; Isler, M.L.; Kirklin, J.K.; Weintraub, W.S. 2021 ACC/AHA Key Data Elements and Definitions for Heart Failure: A Report of the American College of Cardiology/American Heart Association Task Force on Clinical Data Standards (Writing Committee to Develop Clinical Data Standards for Heart Failure). *Circ. Cardiovasc. Qual. Outcomes* **2021**, *14*, e000102. [CrossRef] [PubMed]
2. Javaheri, S.; Brown, L.K.; Abraham, W.T.; Khayat, R. Apneas of Heart Failure and Phenotype-Guided Treatments: Part One: OSA. *Chest* **2020**, *157*, 394–402. [CrossRef] [PubMed]
3. Kishan, S.; Rao, M.S.; Ramachandran, P.; Devasia, T.; Samanth, J. Prevalence and Patterns of Sleep-Disordered Breathing in Indian Heart Failure Population. *Pulm. Med.* **2021**, *2021*, 9978906. [CrossRef] [PubMed]
4. Bitter, T.; Faber, L.; Hering, D.; Langer, C.; Horstkotte, D.; Oldenburg, O. Sleep-disordered breathing in heart failure with normal left ventricular ejection fraction. *Eur. J. Heart Fail.* **2009**, *11*, 602–608. [CrossRef]
5. Javaheri, S.; Barbe, F.; Campos-Rodriguez, F.; Dempsey, J.A.; Khayat, R.; Javaheri, S.; Malhotra, A.; Martinez-Garcia, M.A.; Mehra, R.; Pack, A.I.; et al. Sleep Apnea: Types, Mechanism, and Clinical Cardiovascular Consequences. *J. Am. Coll. Cardiol.* **2017**, *69*, 841–858. [CrossRef]
6. Herrscher, T.E.; Akre, H.; Øverland, B.; Sandvik, L.; Westheim, A.S. High prevalence of sleep apnea in heart failure outpatients: Even in patients with preserved systolic function. *J. Card. Fail.* **2011**, *17*, 420–425. [CrossRef]
7. Javaheri, S.; Caref, E.B.; Chen, E.; Tong, K.B.; Abraham, W.T. Sleep apnea testing and outcomes in a large cohort of Medicare beneficiaries with newly diagnosed heart failure. *Am. J. Respir. Crit. Care Med.* **2011**, *183*, 539–546. [CrossRef]
8. Wang, H.; Parker, J.D.; Newton, G.E.; Floras, J.S.; Mak, S.; Chiu, K.; Ruttanaumpawan, P.; Tomlinson, G.; Bradley, T.D. Influence of obstructive sleep apnea on mortality in patients with heart failure. *J. Am. Coll. Cardiol.* **2007**, *49*, 1625–1631. [CrossRef]
9. Khayat, R.N.; Jarjoura, D.; Porter, K.; Sow, A.; Wannemacher, J.; Dohar, R.; Pleister, A.; Abraham, W.T. Sleep disordered breathing and post-discharge mortality in patients with acute heart failure. *Eur. Heart J.* **2015**, *36*, 1463–1469. [CrossRef]
10. Wang, S.H.; Keenan, B.T.; Wiemken, A.; Zang, Y.; Staley, B.; Sarwer, D.B.; Torigian, D.A.; Williams, N.; Pack, A.I.; Schwab, R.J. Effect of Weight Loss on Upper Airway Anatomy and the Apnea-Hypopnea Index: The Importance of Tongue Fat. *Am. J. Respir. Crit. Care Med.* **2020**, *201*, 718–727. [CrossRef]
11. Mehra, R. Sleep apnea and the heart. *Clevel. Clin. J. Med.* **2019**, *86*, 10–18. [CrossRef] [PubMed]
12. Kasai, T.; Narui, K.; Dohi, T.; Yanagisawa, N.; Ishiwata, S.; Ohno, M.; Yamaguchi, T.; Momomura, S. Prognosis of patients with heart failure and obstructive sleep apnea treated with continuous positive airway pressure. *Chest* **2008**, *133*, 690–696. [CrossRef] [PubMed]
13. Khayat, R.N.; Javaheri, S.; Porter, K.; Sow, A.; Holt, R.; Randerath, W.; Abraham, W.T.; Jarjoura, D. In-Hospital Management of Sleep Apnea During Heart Failure Hospitalization: A Randomized Controlled Trial. *J. Card. Fail.* **2020**, *26*, 705–712. [CrossRef] [PubMed]

14. Uchoa, C.H.G.; Pedrosa, R.P.; Javaheri, S.; Geovanini, G.R.; Carvalho, M.M.B.; Torquatro, A.C.S.; Leite, A.P.D.L.; Gonzaga, C.C.; Bertolami, A.; Amodeo, C.; et al. OSA and Prognosis After Acute Cardiogenic Pulmonary Edema: The OSA-CARE Study. *Chest* **2017**, *152*, 1230–1238. [CrossRef] [PubMed]
15. Anker, S.D.; Butler, J.; Filippatos, G.; Ferreira, J.P.; Bocchi, E.; Böhm, M.; Rocca, H.B.; Choi, D.; Chopra, V.; Chuquiure-Valenzuela, E.; et al. Empagliflozin in heart failure with preserved ejection fraction. *N. Engl. J. Med.* **2021**, *385*, 1451–1461. [CrossRef]
16. McEvoy, R.D.; Antic, N.A.; Heeley, E.; Luo, Y.; Ou, Q.; Zhang, X.; Mediano, O.; Chen, R.; Drager, L.F.; Liu, Z.; et al. CPAP for Prevention of Cardiovascular Events in Obstructive Sleep Apnea. *N. Engl. J. Med.* **2016**, *375*, 919–931. [CrossRef]
17. Haentjens, P.; Van Meerhaeghe, A.; Moscariello, A.; De Weerdt, S.; Poppe, K.; Dupont, A.; Velkeniers, B. The impact of continuous positive airway pressure on blood pressure in patients with obstructive sleep apnea syndrome: Evidence from a meta-analysis of placebo-controlled randomized trials. *Arch. Intern. Med.* **2007**, *167*, 757–764. [CrossRef]
18. Robinson, G.V.; Langford, B.A.; Smith, D.M.; Stradling, J.R. Predictors of blood pressure fall with continuous positive airway pressure (CPAP) treatment of obstructive sleep apnoea (OSA). *Thorax* **2008**, *63*, 855–859. [CrossRef]
19. Azarbarzin, A.; Sands, S.A.; White, D.P.; Redline, S.; Wellman, A. The hypoxic burden: A novel sleep apnoea severity metric and a predictor of cardiovascular mortality-Reply to 'The hypoxic burden: Also known as the desaturation severity parameter'. *Eur. Heart J.* **2019**, *40*, 2994–2995. [CrossRef]
20. Azarbarzin, A.; Sands, S.A.; Taranto-Montemurro, L.; Vena, D.; Sofer, T.; Kim, S.W.; Stone, K.L.; White, D.P.; Wellman, A.; Redline, S. The Sleep Apnea-Specific Hypoxic Burden Predicts Incident Heart Failure. *Chest* **2020**, *158*, 739–750. [CrossRef]
21. Young, T.; Finn, L.; Peppard, P.E.; Szklo-Coxe, M.; Austin, D.; Nieto, F.J.; Stubbs, R.; Hla, K.M. Sleep disordered breathing and mortality: Eighteen-year follow-up of the Wisconsin Sleep Cohort. *Sleep* **2008**, *31*, 1071–1078.
22. Marshall, N.S.; Wong, K.K.; Liu, P.Y.; Cullen, S.R.; Knuiman, M.W.; Grunstein, R.R. Sleep apnea as an independent risk factor for all-cause mortality: The Busselton Health Study. *Sleep* **2008**, *31*, 1079–1085. [PubMed]
23. Punjabi, N.M.; Caffo, B.S.; Goodwin, J.L. Sleep-disordered breathing and mortality: A prospective cohort study. *PLoS Med.* **2009**, *6*, e1000132. [CrossRef] [PubMed]
24. Zinchuk, A.; Yaggi, H. Phenotypic Subtypes of OSA: A Challenge and Opportunity for Precision Medicine. *Chest* **2020**, *157*, 403–420. [CrossRef] [PubMed]
25. Ye, L.; Pien, G.W.; Ratcliffe, S.J.; Björnsdottir, E.; Arnardottir, E.S.; Pack, A.I.; Benediktsdottir, B.; Gislason, T. The different clinical faces of obstructive sleep apnoea: A cluster analysis. *Eur. Respir. J.* **2014**, *44*, 1600–1607. [CrossRef]
26. Mazzotti, D.R.; Keenan, B.T.; Lim, D.C.; Gottlieb, D.J.; Kim, J.; Pack, A.I. Symptom Subtypes of Obstructive Sleep Apnea Predict Incidence of Cardiovascular Outcomes. *Am. J. Respir. Crit. Care Med.* **2019**, *200*, 493–506. [CrossRef]
27. Azarbarzin, A.; Sands, S.A.; Taranto-Montemurro, L.; Redline, S.; Wellman, A. Hypoxic burden captures sleep apnoea-specific nocturnal hypoxaemia. *Eur. Heart J.* **2019**, *40*, 2989–2990. [CrossRef]
28. Sommerfeld, A.; Althouse, A.D.; Prince, J.; Atwood, C.W.; Mulukutla, S.R.; Hickey, G.W. Obstructive sleep apnea is associated with increased readmission in heart failure patients. *Clin. Cardiol.* **2017**, *40*, 873–878. [CrossRef]
29. Kourouklis, S.P.; Vagiakis, E.; Paraskevaidis, I.A.; Farmakis, D.; Kostikas, K.; Parissis, J.T.; Katsivas, A.; Kremastinos, D.T.; Anastasiou-Nana, M.; Filippatos, G. Effective sleep apnoea treatment improves cardiac function in patients with chronic heart failure. *Int. J. Cardiol.* **2013**, *168*, 157–162. [CrossRef]
30. Egea, C.J.; Aizpuru, F.; Pinto, J.A.; Ayuela, J.M.; Ballester, E.; Zamarrón, C.; Sojo, A.; Montserrat, J.M.; Barbe, F.; The Spanish Group of Sleep Breathing Disorders; et al. Cardiac function after CPAP therapy in patients with chronic heart failure and sleep apnea: A multicenter study. *Sleep Med.* **2008**, *9*, 660–666. [CrossRef]

Review

A Narrative Review of the Association between Post-Traumatic Stress Disorder and Obstructive Sleep Apnea

Catherine A. McCall [1,2,*] and Nathaniel F. Watson [3,4]

1. Department of Pulmonary, Critical Care and Sleep Medicine, VA Puget Sound Health Care System, Seattle, WA 98108, USA
2. Department of Psychiatry and Behavioral Sciences, University of Washington School of Medicine, Seattle, WA 98195, USA
3. Department of Neurology, University of Washington School of Medicine, Seattle, WA 98195, USA; nwatson@uw.edu
4. University of Washington Medicine Sleep Center, Seattle, WA 98104, USA
* Correspondence: cmccall1@uw.edu

Abstract: Obstructive sleep apnea (OSA) and post-traumatic stress disorder (PTSD) are often co-morbid with implications for disease severity and treatment outcomes. OSA prevalence is higher in PTSD sufferers than in the general population, with a likely bidirectional effect of the two illnesses. There is substantial evidence to support the role that disturbed sleep may play in the pathophysiology of PTSD. Sleep disturbance associated with OSA may interfere with normal rapid eye movement (REM) functioning and thus worsen nightmares and sleep-related movements. Conversely, hyperarousal and hypervigilance symptoms of PTSD may lower the arousal threshold and thus increase the frequency of sleep fragmentation related to obstructive events. Treating OSA not only improves OSA symptoms, but also nightmares and daytime symptoms of PTSD. Evidence suggests that positive airway pressure (PAP) therapy reduces PTSD symptoms in a dose-dependent fashion, but also presents challenges to tolerance in the PTSD population. Alternative OSA treatments may be better tolerated and effective for improving both OSA and PTSD. Further research avenues will be introduced as we seek a better understanding of this complex relationship.

Keywords: post-traumatic stress disorder; obstructive sleep apnea; PTSD; OSA

1. Introduction

Post-traumatic stress disorder (PTSD) is a psychiatric illness occurring after exposure to a traumatic event, in which the individual experiences intrusive memories such as flashbacks, avoidance of trauma reminders, negative changes in mood and cognition, hyperarousal symptoms, and impairment of social, occupational, and interpersonal functioning [1]. Sleep-related symptoms may be particularly prominent and feature nightmares about the event, fear of sleep, night terrors, insomnia, and dream-enactment behavior which often involves thrashing and fighting [2]. Although lifetime trauma exposure estimates worldwide are as high as 70%, PTSD develops in a relatively smaller segment of the population with 8.3% lifetime prevalence [3]. PTSD prevalence also varies considerably with other factors such as the number of trauma exposures and the severity of the trauma [4]. PTSD may resolve in some individuals within a period of weeks to months, whereas in others it becomes a chronic condition [5,6]. One study of rape survivors assessed for PTSD diagnosis every week after their assault found that 94% met criteria for PTSD at the first assessment, 65% met criteria about one month later, and 47% met criteria about three months later. The authors noted a distinct difference between subjects whose PTSD improved over time and those who remained symptomatic [5]. Much attention has been placed in recent years on identifying modifiable factors that may contribute to developing a persistent post-traumatic syndrome resilience protecting against this disorder.

Research over the past decade has uncovered significant evidence for the bidirectionality of sleep problems and PTSD. As many as 70% of PTSD sufferers experience some kind of sleep disturbance [2]. About 41% of individuals with PTSD report trouble initiating sleep versus 13% of those without PTSD, and 47% of PTSD sufferers report difficulty maintaining sleep [7]. Sleep disturbances may also include nightmares as well as dream enactment behaviors that have led to a proposed new sleep disorder, trauma-associated sleep disorder [8–10]. Sleep-related problems were traditionally considered to be symptoms of the disorder rather than separate diagnoses. However, many studies have now suggested that sleep problems preceding a traumatic experience may predict or even predispose to the development of persistent stress and PTSD [11–14].

Compared with patients without sleep complaints, PTSD patients with comorbid sleep disorders experience higher rates of substance abuse, depression, and suicidality [15–17]. Sleep disturbances are predictors of PTSD treatment nonresponse, and may continue even after successful treatment of daytime PTSD symptoms [18–23] This underscores the importance of identifying and managing sleep problems in this population. Treating sleep problems such as nightmares and insomnia is also now understood to improve daytime symptoms of PTSD [24,25] While this may not be surprising given that nightmares and sleep difficulties are core symptoms of PTSD diagnostic criteria, what has been surprising is the more recent evidence showing similar bidirectionality in PTSD and obstructive sleep apnea (OSA) diagnoses and treatment [26–28]. The following sections will highlight research in these domains.

2. The OSA and PTSD Overlap

OSA is a disorder of recurrent partial or complete upper airway collapse during sleep, leading to snoring, reduced ventilation, intermittent and cumulative hypoxemia, frequent arousals from sleep, and alterations in sleep architecture. OSA diagnosis requires a sleep study showing at least five predominantly obstructive events per hour with related symptoms, or 15 events/hour without symptoms [29]. Untreated OSA is associated with a myriad of medical and psychiatric health conditions, including cardiovascular disease [30], metabolic disorders [31], psychiatric disorders [32], motor vehicle accidents [33] and all-cause mortality [34]. The prevalence of OSA is approximately 13% in men and 6% in women aged 30–70 years when using an apnea-hypopnea index (AHI) cutoff of 15 events per hour, whereas 14% of men and 5% of women meet the criteria of AHI > 5 with symptoms of daytime sleepiness [35]. The risk of OSA is higher in individuals with elevated body mass index (BMI), male sex, age > 50 years, neck circumference > 40 cm, and in post-menopausal women [36,37].

A significant co-prevalence has been found between OSA and PTSD. This association has been confirmed in over a dozen studies to date encompassing both military and civilian populations, with a recent meta-analysis of 12 studies showing pooled prevalence rates of 75.7% for AHI $\geq$ 5 and 43.6% for AHI $\geq$ 10 [38], Individuals with OSA and PTSD (OSA + PTSD) may demonstrate fewer "typical" features of OSA such as elevated BMI and older age [16,39]. One study found that age- and sex-matched patients with sleep-disordered breathing and trauma exposure had lower BMI, less snoring, and more insomnia, nightmares, psychotropic medication use, leg jerks, and upper airway resistance findings in PSG than sleep-disordered breathing patients without trauma exposure [39]. Patients with OSA + PTSD have worse symptoms of both disorders than those suffering from either disorder alone, reporting lower quality of life and more somnolence compared to those with OSA only [40], and worse nightmares, sleep quality, anxiety, depression, posttraumatic stress, and quality of life compared to those with PTSD only [16].

There are multiple hypotheses regarding why individuals with PTSD experience significantly higher rates of OSA than the general population. One possibility is that the arousal threshold is lowered in PTSD due to a hyperactive chronic stress response, leading to greater arousal sensitivity to mild obstructive events and thereby increased frequency of hypopneas and respiratory effort-related arousals (RERAs). There is additionally evidence that sleep fragmentation and sleep deprivation may promote airway collapse, which may then further increase arousals [41]. PTSD-triggered sleep fragmentation resulting from hyperarousal processes may also result in lighter sleep, which is associated with respiratory instability [27,42–44]. A low arousal threshold has been found to have high prevalence in veterans with OSA [45] and PTSD [46].

Conversely, upper airway collapse occurring during sleep may have multiple effects that predispose to persistent stress symptomatology. OSA is often worse during rapid eye movement (REM) sleep due normal atonia of accessory respiratory muscles that would otherwise aid in opening the upper airway during collapse. Obstructive events occurring during REM sleep may precipitate increased frequency of arousals that may heighten nightmare awareness and recall. Additionally, awakenings from obstructive events often occur with sympathetic nervous system activation, with associated symptoms of racing heart, shortness of breath, and anxiety, all of which could worsen the experience of a nightmare [47]. OSA has been associated with nightmares even in individuals without PTSD, often with content related to suffocation, choking, drowning, strangulation, burial, and death [48–51]. A study of patients with OSA who slept in a laboratory before and after starting continuous positive airway pressure (CPAP) were awakened after the beginning of every REM period for dream reports. Dream recall was increased after obstructive events, with these dreams being significantly more negative than dreams occurring without obstructive events [52]. Carrasco et al. hypothesized that respiratory events occurring during REM sleep lead to stimulation of the limbic system, which may increase the emotional content of dreams [53].

In the setting of a traumatic stress, OSA-induced REM sleep fragmentation may also interfere with functions of REM sleep itself that are critical for healthy processing of emotional memories. Substantial behavioral and neurophysiological evidence supports the understanding that sleep contributes to emotional memory consolidation, and sleep deprivation negatively impacts it [54–57]. REM sleep in particular appears to play an important role in the acquisition and long-term retention of appropriate fear learning, including the ability to discriminate between threatening and non-threatening stimuli [54,55,58]. REM sleep deficiency is associated with next-day emotional reactivity and amygdala responsivity [54,59,60]. REM sleep is also associated with fear extinction memory performance, as well as fear inhibition [61,62]. Accordingly, disturbed REM sleep is associated with impairments in both conditioned fear and extinction learning [63–65]. Similar impairments in fear learning and emotional dysregulation have also been found with PTSD [66,67], along with evidence of REM sleep abnormalities [59,68,69]. This body of evidence supports hypotheses that REM sleep disturbance may play a role in the development and persistence of PTSD.

The association between PTSD and OSA is additionally supported by studies finding that OSA diagnosis prior to trauma exposure also predicts the development of PTSD [2,28]. Furthermore, individuals with comorbid PTSD and OSA show impairments in fear discrimination, inhibition, and extinction that improve with OSA treatment [70]. OSA occurring during REM sleep could thus be implicated as a potential cause of REM sleep fragmentation and contribute to PTSD pathology. These data in total strongly suggest that there is likely a bidirectional relationship between OSA and PTSD in which each condition mutually reinforces the other [26–28,59]. The cycle of stress-induced arousals and insomnia promotes sleep fragmentation, which worsens PTSD symptoms.

The implications for the role of OSA in PTSD may reach beyond the development of post-traumatic stress symptoms. The most effective treatments for PTSD are recognized to be trauma-focused psychotherapies, including exposure-based therapies such as prolonged exposure (PE) therapy and cognitive processing therapy (CPT) [22,71–73]. These therapies rely on the patient's ability to effectively generalize extinction memory. Sleep-disordered breathing has been found to negatively impact the effectiveness of PE, possibly by disrupting the extinction memory consolidation and generalization that normally occurs during sleep [23]. OSA may thus not only play a role in the development and persistence of PTSD, but also hamper the effectiveness of core therapies to treat it.

Research on treatment strategies for addressing sleep concerns has yielded insight into alternative treatments to improve PTSD severity and outcomes. Successful treatment of nightmares and insomnia is known to have a positive impact on daytime PTSD symptoms [25,74]. As our understanding of the OSA+PTSD connection has developed, a growing body of evidence has suggested that treating OSA may also improve PTSD symptoms. There are several potential advantages to targeting PTSD symptoms using sleep treatments. Despite the evidence base demonstrating effectiveness of PTSD psychotherapies, 13–39% of patients prematurely discontinue exposure therapy for PTSD [71] and 20% of veterans do not experience clinically significant improvement after PE [72]. Possible reasons for this include difficulty tolerating trauma-related memories and emotions, and/or stigma of receiving mental health treatment. Studies in veteran populations have shown that individuals with PTSD report greater willingness to seek sleep medicine treatments over explicitly PTSD-focused care [75,76]. The following sections detail the benefits and challenges of addressing PTSD-related symptoms through treatment of OSA.

3. Impacts of OSA Treatment on PTSD

3.1. PAP Therapy

The cornerstone of OSA treatment is preventing collapse of the upper airway during sleep. As such, the current gold-standard treatment of OSA is PAP therapy [77,78]. CPAP devices deliver pressurized room air through a hose and mask in order to splint the upper airway. This effectively prevents obstruction by the tongue, soft palate and surrounding tissues, enables normal respiratory processes, and minimizes respiratory-related arousals. CPAP has demonstrated clinically significant reduction in disease severity, daytime sleepiness, hypertension, motor vehicle accidents, and quality of life [78]. Meta-analyses of treatment impacts on cardiovascular events, cognitive function and mood have produced mixed results [78–80].

Studies on the effects of CPAP in patients with OSA+PTSD have shown improvement in PTSD-related symptoms in those who were adherent to CPAP. (Table 1) In 1998, a case report was published in which a Veteran with OSA+PTSD experienced dramatic improvement in sleep quality, nightmare frequency, and daytime sleepiness after starting CPAP therapy [81]. A retrospective review in 15 patients in 2000 found that 75% of those using CPAP reported improvement in PTSD symptoms, while those who declined CPAP experienced worsening symptoms [82]. A larger study in 2014 not only found that CPAP improved nightmares, but also noted a dose-dependent relationship, with every 10% improvement in CPAP adherence decreasing the mean number of nightmares by one nightmare/week [83]. El-Solh et al. likewise found that an increased number of hours/night using CPAP was associated with improvement in PTSD symptoms in veterans. Subjects with severe OSA experienced greater improvements in PTSD symptoms than those with mild to moderate OSA over a period of 3 months, but both groups reported reduced nightmare distress and nightmare frequency [84]. Veterans with PTSD and a new diagnosis of OSA reported significant reductions of PTSD symptoms, sleepiness, and depressions, as well as improved sleep quality, daytime functioning, and quality of life over a period of 6 months [85]. A study of Veterans with PTSD and subclinical PTSD found that CPAP therapy reduced PTSD symptoms and nightmare frequency in both groups, though the subclinical PTSD group required higher adherence to achieve symptom improvement. Poor adherence to CPAP resulted in increased PTSD Checklist (PCL) scores in the subclinical PTSD group, and the authors speculated that untreated OSA may predispose to the development of overt PTSD [86].

Despite the well-documented improvements in PTSD-related symptoms with OSA treatment, several notable challenges occur in this population. Adherence to PAP therapy is problematic in the general population, with 29–83% of patients using CPAP under 4 h per night [87]. Adherence is significantly lower in the PTSD population. The meta-analysis of Zhang et al. found three studies showing that patients with PTSD demonstrated significantly lower adherence to PAP therapy, including regular use and average duration of use per night, compared to those with OSA alone [38]. One study showed 40% adherence in PTSD patients after 30-day follow-up, versus 70% adherence in non-PTSD controls. Reasons given for non-adherence included factors that were similar between PTSD and non-PTSD groups, including mask discomfort, air hunger, and high pressure; claustrophobia was reported slightly more frequently in the PTSD group. Nightmares and absence of sleepiness were also predictors of non-adherence [88].

Anecdotally, patients with OSA and PTSD have also reported reluctance to use PAP therapy due to fear of becoming less aware or unable to respond to the potential threats in the environment, which speaks to issues arising from hypervigilance-related symptoms. Other common complaints by patients with OSA + PTSD in the clinical environment have included challenges in feeling tangled or restrained by the hosing, particularly in those with disruptive sleep behaviors. In military populations, reminders of wearing masks during military training and combat are frequent reasons cited for CPAP intolerance. The presence of comorbid anxiety and insomnia have also been speculated to contribute to difficulty sleeping while wearing a mask [88,89]. The presence of insomnia with OSA is often referred to as "comorbid insomnia with OSA" (COMISA) or "complex insomnia" and has been found to reduce PAP adherence and effectiveness due to the sufferer's inability to initiate and maintain sleep while using PAP therapy [90]. Figure 1 shows the complexity of comorbid sleep disorders seen with PTSD, and how they may interact to complicate treatment efforts.

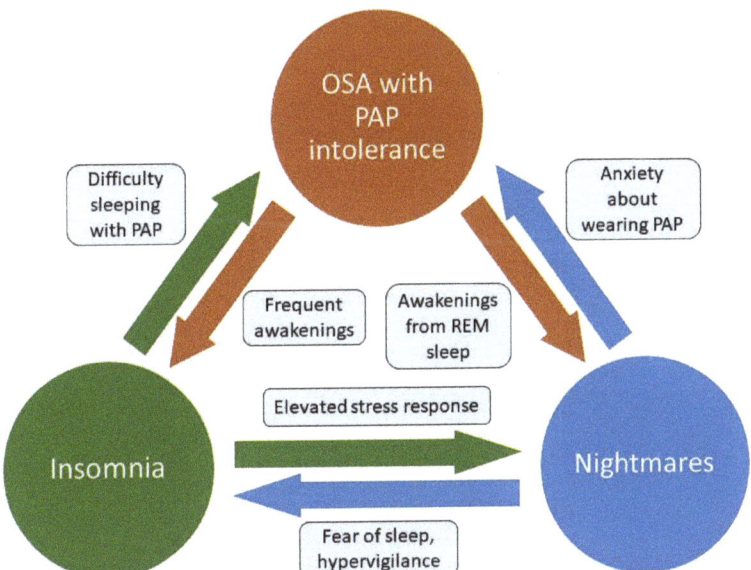

Figure 1. Factors contributing to untreated OSA, insomnia, and nightmares in PTSD sufferers. Untreated sleep apnea may lead to frequent awakenings which precipitate and/or perpetuate insomnia, as well as arousals from REM sleep leading to increased nightmare intensity and recall. Difficulty initiating and maintaining sleep interferes with the ability to tolerate PAP therapy, and hyperarousal related to insomnia may increase nightmares via elevated stress response during REM sleep. The presence of nightmares often leads to fear of sleep, hypervigilance, and poor sleep hygiene (e.g., leaving lights on) that worsen insomnia. Nightmares may also reduce PAP tolerance due to increased anxiety and hypervigilance. OSA, obstructive sleep apnea. PAP, positive airway pressure. REM, rapid eye movement.

Even when patients adhere to treatment, those with PTSD may experience less benefit than those without PTSD. One study found that resolution of sleepiness occurred in 82% of patients without PTSD who were adherent to PAP therapy, but only 62.5% of PAP-adherent patients with PTSD. Quality of life normalization with PAP therapy was also achieved by fewer patients with PTSD (56.3%) than by those without PTSD (72%) [40]. These issues, as well as problems in tolerating PAP therapy in patients with OSA+PTSD, have led to research efforts exploring alternative treatments for OSA in this population.

3.2. Alternative OSA Treatments

Beyond CPAP, alternative treatments for OSA include oral appliances, positional therapy, weight loss, and surgery. Few of these treatments have been studied in the OSA +PTSD population. Oral appliances, sometimes referred to as mandibular repositioning devices (MRD) or mandibular advancement devices (MAD), are a frequently explored treatment option in those patients who cannot tolerate CPAP. MRDs are customized appliances that facilitate protrusion of the mandible, thus preventing collapse of the tongue and soft tissues of the airway. MRDs are considered more beneficial in mild to moderate cases of OSA, and may be less effective with severe OSA [91]. Studies on long-term usage have shown subjective adherence is excellent, with retained effectiveness in treating snoring and sleepiness, but with mild reductions in efficacy over time for nocturia, mouth opening, headache, unrefreshing sleep, and tiredness [92]. Long-term adherence may be affected by adverse dental effects, device features, device wear, and/or progression in severity of OSA [93–96].

El-Solh et al. used a randomized crossover trial to evaluate the effectiveness and adherence of CPAP versus MRD in Veterans with OSA+PTSD. [89] They found that the mean residual number of obstructive events after titration with each treatment was 26.3 events per hour with MRD versus 3.9 events per hour with CPAP. Overall, 71% of CPAP-titrated patients experienced complete resolution of OSA, versus 14% of those with MRDs. However, patients using MRD exhibited longer sleep time and higher sleep efficiency during the titration than those using CPAP. Adherence was improved in the MRD condition, with 58% reporting preference for MRD and 29% preferring CPAP. Despite the differences in OSA treatment effectiveness between CPAP and MRD, the effect size improvements in PTSD symptoms were comparable for both treatments. Likewise, excessive sleepiness and sleep quality also improved with both treatments, though sleep quality was more improved with CPAP. This suggests that some components of treatment effectiveness are not captured solely by reduction in AHI. As this study evaluated only short-term treatment effects, the long-term effects and adherence in this population are not known.

Other alternative OSA treatments that have been studied in PTSD patients include hypoglossal nerve stimulation (HNS). This implanted device causes contraction of the genioglossus muscle with tongue protrusion during inspiration to prevent upper airway collapse during sleep. HNS was approved in 2014 in the US for the treatment of OSA in patients meeting specific criteria for AHI, BMI, airway collapse pattern on drug-induced sleep endoscopy, and history of PAP intolerance. A study of 46 OSA patients (26 with PTSD and 17 without PTSD) who underwent HNS implantation found complete control of OSA (defined as AHI < 5 events/hour), improvement in excessive sleepiness, and mean best adherence were similar for patients with and without PTSD [97]. PTSD patients with COMISA had significantly lower adherence than those without insomnia. The authors noted that PTSD symptom questionnaire scores did not significantly change pre/post-surgery, though 5 of 7 patients showed a slight downward trend in scores.

Surgical options for treating OSA also include modification of the upper airway soft tissue, including the palate, tongue base, and lateral pharyngeal walls [98]. We were unable to find studies evaluating the effects of this treatment specifically in PTSD patients.

Table 1. Studies evaluating OSA treatment effects on PTSD. PAP, positive airway pressure. MRD, mandibular repositioning device. HNS, hypoglossal nerve stimulation. REM, rapid eye movement sleep. NREM, non-rapid eye movement sleep. PCL-M, PTSD checklist-military. PCL-S, PTSD checklist-specific. PCL-5, PTSD checklist for the Diagnostic and Statistical Manual of Mental Disorders, Fifth Edition.

Authors	Year	Study Type	Study Population	Age (Mean Years ± SD)	Sex (% Male)	Treatment Type	Main Findings
Youakim et al. [81]	1998	Case Report	Veteran	42	100	PAP therapy	Nightmare frequency and intensity was improved after 4 months of PAP therapy, as well as daytime PTSD symptoms.
Krakow et al. [82]	2000	Retrospective	Civilians	Treatment: 43.8 ± 14.1 No treatment: 50.8 ± 14.9	Not reported	PAP therapy	PAP users reported a median 75% improvement in PTSD symptoms; subjects without PAP therapy reported worsening symptoms.
Tamanna et al. [83]	2014	Retrospective	Veterans	58 ± 12.05	97	PAP therapy	The mean number of nightmares per week was reduced over 6 months of PAP therapy. Reduced nightmare frequency was best predicted by PAP adherence.
El-Solh et al. [84]	2017a	Prospective cohort	Veterans	52.6 ± 14.2	92.5	PAP therapy	PCL-M scores improved after 3 months of PAP therapy, in a dose-dependent manner. PAP usage was the only significant predictor of overall PTSD symptom improvement.
Orr et al. [85]	2017	Prospective cohort	Veterans	52 (range 43–65)	87.5	PAP therapy	PCL-S scores improved over 6 months of PAP therapy. The percentage of nights in which PAP was used, but not mean hours used per night, predicted improvement.
Ullah et al. [86]	2017	Prospective cohort	Veterans	51.24 ± 14.74	Not reported	PAP therapy	PCL-M scores improved after 6 months of PAP therapy in PTSD patients, whereas non-PTSD patients with low adherence showed worsening of PCL-M scores.

Table 1. Cont.

Authors	Year	Study Type	Study Population	Age (Mean Years ± SD)	Sex (% Male)	Treatment Type	Main Findings
El-Solh et al. [89]	2017b	Randomized crossover trial	Veterans	52.7 ± 11.6	Not reported	MRD compared to PAP therapy	71% of CPAP users and 14% of MRD users had complete OSA resolution during titration studies; however MRD users had longer sleep time, higher sleep efficiency and better adherence to treatment. Both treatments showed similar improvements in PCL-M scores after 3 months.
El-Solh et al. [90]	2018	Prospective	Veterans	PTSD with comorbid OSA and insomnia: 47.2 ± 10.8 PTSD with OSA: 52.7 ± 9.7	PTSD with comorbid OSA and insomnia: 72 PTSD with OSA: 86	PAP therapy	PCL-M scores improved after 3 months of PAP therapy in patients with and without insomnia. The change in PCL-M scores was smaller in those with insomnia. PAP adherence was also lower in the insomnia group.
Patil et al. [97]	2021	Retrospective and prospective case series	Veterans	59.3 ± 10.6	96.2	HNS	Resolution of OSA and adherence were similar for patients with and without PTSD; adherence was lower in PTSD patients with insomnia. PCL-5 scores obtained 6–12 months after surgery did not significantly change from baseline.

There is limited evidence for treatments that target OSA in conjunction with insomnia and/or nightmares. Some small studies have investigated the use of sedative-hypnotics to raise the arousal threshold and improve CPAP adherence, with mixed results [44,99–101]. This approach would necessitate caution with regards to potential risks of using sedating medications if OSA were not fully treated. Many medications, including novel agents, have not been tested as OSA monotherapy in the OSA + PTSD population [102]. Another medication consideration is that antidepressant usage (selective serotonin reuptake inhibitors or SSRIs, and serotonin-norepinephrine reuptake inhibitors or SNRIs) has been associated with higher odds of low arousal threshold, as well as risk of abnormal sleep-related movements and dream enactment behaviors [10,46,103]. This adds a further layer of complexity, given that SSRIs and SNRIs are among the first-line pharmacotherapies for the treatment of PTSD [104,105]. Managing both psychiatric and sleep problems with PTSD thus presents additional challenges. Further research is needed to determine best clinical practice for the treatment of PTSD with comorbid sleep disorders.

4. Conclusions

Recent decades have shown a strong, bidirectional relationship between PTSD and sleep problems, with OSA being an increasingly recognized contributor. Individuals with both OSA and PTSD experience worse symptoms of both disorders than those with only one of these illnesses. The direction of initial causality is not clear, though potential pathology may arise from sleep disturbance around the time of trauma exposure and/or stress-related hyperarousal, sleep fragmentation, and respiratory instability leading to impaired REM sleep function. Evidence-based treatments for PTSD may not address the crucial component of sleep disturbance from OSA. Research on the impact of OSA treatment in the OSA+PTSD has shown substantial clinical benefits for both disorders with PAP therapy, with the limiting factor of significant intolerance in this population. Second-line treatments, including MRD and HNS, have shown benefit with improved adherence, though studies are limited thus far. It is important to note that there is a paucity of randomized controlled trials evaluating OSA treatment effects on PTSD, particularly in women and non-veterans. Further research is needed in this area.

Many patients with PTSD suffer from multiple sleep problems, including OSA, insomnia, nightmares, and dream enactment behaviors, with each disorder presenting challenges in the treatment of the others. Future research will also optimally test combinations of treatments for these complex comorbidities.

Funding: This research received no external funding.

Conflicts of Interest: The authors declare no conflict of interest.

References

1. American Psychiatric Association. *Diagnostic and Statistical Manual of Mental Disorders*, 5th ed.; American Psychiatric Association: Washington, DC, USA, 2013.
2. Babson, K.A.; Feldner, M.T. Temporal relations between sleep problems and both traumatic event exposure and PTSD: A critical review of the empirical literature. *J. Anxiety Disord.* **2010**, *24*, 1–15. [CrossRef]
3. Kilpatrick, D.G.; Resnick, H.S.; Milanak, M.E.; Miller, M.; Keyes, K.M.; Friedman, M.J. National Estimates of Exposure to Traumatic Events and PTSD Prevalence UsingDSM-IVandDSM-5Criteria. *J. Trauma. Stress* **2013**, *26*, 537–547. [CrossRef]
4. Yehuda, R.; Hoge, C.W.; McFarlane, A.C.; Vermetten, E.; Lanius, R.A.; Nievergelt, C.M.; Hobfoll, S.E.; Koenen, K.C.; Neylan, T.C.; Hyman, S.E. Post-traumatic stress disorder. *Nat. Rev. Dis. Prim.* **2015**, *1*, nrdp201557. [CrossRef] [PubMed]
5. Rothbaum, B.O.; Foa, E.B.; Riggs, D.S.; Murdock, T.; Walsh, W. A prospective examination of post-traumatic stress disorder in rape victims. *J. Trauma. Stress* **1992**, *5*, 455–475. [CrossRef]
6. Cahill, S.P.; Pontoski, K. Post-traumatic stress disorder and acute stress disorder I: Their nature and assessment considerations. *Psychiatry* **2005**, *2*, 14–25. [PubMed]
7. Ohayon, M.M.; Shapiro, C.M. Sleep disturbances and psychiatric disorders associated with posttraumatic stress disorder in the general population. *Compr. Psychiatry* **2000**, *41*, 469–478. [CrossRef] [PubMed]
8. El-Solh, A.A.; Riaz, U.; Roberts, J. Sleep Disorders in Patients with Posttraumatic Stress Disorder. *Chest* **2018**, *154*, 427–439. [CrossRef] [PubMed]

9. Mysliwiec, V.; O'Reilly, B.; Polchinski, J.; Kwon, H.P.; Germain, A.; Roth, B.J. Trauma Associated Sleep Disorder: A Proposed Parasomnia Encompassing Disruptive Nocturnal Behaviors, Nightmares, and REM without Atonia in Trauma Survivors. *J. Clin. Sleep Med.* **2014**, *10*, 1143–1148. [CrossRef]
10. Feemster, J.C.; Smith, K.L.; McCarter, S.J.; Louis, E.K.S. Trauma-Associated Sleep Disorder: A Posttraumatic Stress/REM Sleep Behavior Disorder Mash-Up? *J. Clin. Sleep Med.* **2019**, *15*, 345–349. [CrossRef]
11. Breslau, N.; Roth, T.; Rosenthal, L.; Andreski, P. Sleep disturbance and psychiatric disorders: A longitudinal epidemiological study of young Adults. *Biol. Psychiatry* **1996**, *39*, 411–418. Available online: http://www.ncbi.nlm.nih.gov/pubmed/8679786 (accessed on 25 February 2018). [CrossRef]
12. Ford, D.E.; Kamerow, D.B. Epidemiologic study of sleep disturbances and psychiatric disorders. An opportunity for prevention? *JAMA* **1989**, *262*, 1479–1484. [CrossRef] [PubMed]
13. Wright, K.M.; Britt, T.W.; Bliese, P.D.; Adler, A.B.; Picchioni, D.; Moore, D. Insomnia as predictor versus outcome of PTSD and depression among Iraq combat veterans. *J. Clin. Psychol.* **2011**, *67*, 1240–1258. [CrossRef] [PubMed]
14. Bryant, R.A.; Creamer, M.; O'Donnell, M.; Silove, D.; McFarlane, A.C. Sleep Disturbance Immediately Prior to Trauma Predicts Subsequent Psychiatric Disorder. *Sleep* **2010**, *33*, 69–74. Available online: http://www.ncbi.nlm.nih.gov/pubmed/20120622 (accessed on 2 August 2018). [CrossRef] [PubMed]
15. Gupta, M.A.; Jarosz, P. Obstructive Sleep Apnea Severity is Directly Related to Suicidal Ideation in Posttraumatic Stress Disorder. *J. Clin. Sleep Med.* **2018**, *14*, 427–435. [CrossRef]
16. Krakow, B.; Melendrez, D.; Johnston, L.; Warner, T.D.; Clark, J.O.; Pacheco, M.; Pedersen, B.; Koss, M.; Hollifield, M.; Schrader, R. Sleep-disordered breathing, psychiatric distress, and quality of life impairment in sexual assault survivors. *J. Nerv. Ment. Dis.* **2002**, *190*, 442–452. [CrossRef]
17. Krakow, B.; Artar, A.; Warner, T.D.; Melendrez, D.; Johnston, L.; Hollifield, M.; Germain, A.; Koss, M. Sleep Disorder, Depression, and Suicidality in Female Sexual Assault Survivors. *Crisis* **2000**, *21*, 163–170. [CrossRef]
18. Walters, E.M.; Jenkins, M.M.; Nappi, C.M.; Clark, J.; Lies, J.; Norman, S.B.; Drummond, S.P.A. The impact of prolonged exposure on sleep and enhancing treatment outcomes with evidence-based sleep interventions: A pilot study. *Psychol. Trauma Theory Res. Pract. Policy* **2020**, *12*, 175–185. [CrossRef]
19. Zayfert, C.; DeViva, J.C. Residual insomnia following cognitive behavioral therapy for PTSD. *J. Trauma. Stress* **2004**, *17*, 69–73. [CrossRef]
20. Pruiksma, K.E.; Taylor, D.J.; Wachen, J.S.; Mintz, J.; Young-McCaughan, S.; Peterson, A.L.; Yarvis, J.S.; Borah, E.V.; Dondanville, K.A.; Litz, B.; et al. Residual sleep disturbances following PTSD treatment in active duty military personnel. *Psychol. Trauma Theory Res. Pract. Policy* **2016**, *8*, 697–701. [CrossRef]
21. Gutner, C.A.; Casement, M.; Gilbert, K.S.; Resick, P.A. Change in sleep symptoms across Cognitive Processing Therapy and Prolonged Exposure: A longitudinal perspective. *Behav. Res. Ther.* **2013**, *51*, 817–822. [CrossRef]
22. López, C.M.; Lancaster, C.L.; Wilkerson, A.; Gros, D.F.; Ruggiero, K.J.; Acierno, R. Residual Insomnia and Nightmares Postintervention Symptom Reduction Among Veterans Receiving Treatment for Comorbid PTSD and Depressive Symptoms. *Behav. Ther.* **2019**, *50*, 910–923. [CrossRef] [PubMed]
23. Reist, C.; Gory, A.; Hollifield, M. Sleep-Disordered Breathing Impact on Efficacy of Prolonged Exposure Therapy for Posttraumatic Stress Disorder. *J. Trauma. Stress* **2017**, *30*, 186–189. [CrossRef] [PubMed]
24. Harb, G.C.; Cook, J.M.; Phelps, A.J.; Gehrman, P.R.; Forbes, D.; Localio, R.; Harpaz-Rotem, I.; Gur, R.C.; Ross, R.J. Randomized Controlled Trial of Imagery Rehearsal for Posttraumatic Nightmares in Combat Veterans. *J. Clin. Sleep Med.* **2019**, *15*, 757–767. [CrossRef]
25. Yücel, D.E.; van Emmerik, A.A.; Souama, C.; Lancee, J. Comparative efficacy of imagery rehearsal therapy and prazosin in the treatment of trauma-related nightmares in adults: A meta-analysis of randomized controlled trials. *Sleep Med. Rev.* **2020**, *50*, 101248. [CrossRef] [PubMed]
26. Krakow, B.; Melendrez, D.; Pedersen, B.; Johnston, L.; Hollifield, M.; Germain, A.; Koss, M.; Warner, T.D.; Schrader, R. Complex insomnia: Insomnia and sleep-disordered breathing in a consecutive series of crime victims with nightmares and PTSD. *Biol. Psychiatry* **2001**, *49*, 948–953. [CrossRef]
27. Krakow, B.J.; Ulibarri, V.A.; Moore, B.A.; McIver, N.D. Posttraumatic stress disorder and sleep-disordered breathing: A review of comorbidity research. *Sleep Med. Rev.* **2015**, *24*, 37–45. [CrossRef] [PubMed]
28. Jaoude, P.; Vermont, L.N.; Porhomayon, J.; El-Solh, A.A. Sleep-Disordered Breathing in Patients with Post-traumatic Stress Disorder. *Ann. Am. Thorac. Soc.* **2015**, *12*, 259–268. [CrossRef]
29. American Academy of Sleep Medicine. *The International Classification of Sleep Disorders*, 3rd ed.; American Academy of Sleep Medicine: Darien, IL, USA, 2014.
30. Abu Salman, L.; Shulman, R.; Cohen, J.B. Obstructive Sleep Apnea, Hypertension, and Cardiovascular Risk: Epidemiology, Pathophysiology, and Management. *Curr. Cardiol. Rep.* **2020**, *22*, 6. [CrossRef]
31. Jehan, S.; Myers, A.K.; Zizi, F.; Pandi-Perumal, S.R.; Louis, G.J.; McFarlane, S.I. Obesity, obstructive sleep apnea and type 2 diabetes mellitus: Epidemiology and pathophysiologic insights. *Sleep Med. Disord. Int. J.* **2018**, *2*, 52–58. [CrossRef]
32. Gupta, M.A.; Simpson, F. Obstructive Sleep Apnea and Psychiatric Disorders: A Systematic Review. *J. Clin. Sleep Med.* **2015**, *11*, 165–175. [CrossRef]

33. Young, T.; Blustein, J.; Finn, L.; Palta, M. Sleep-disordered breathing and motor vehicle accidents in a population-based sample of employed adults. *Sleep* **1997**, *20*, 608–613. [CrossRef]
34. Punjabi, N.M.; Caffo, B.S.; Goodwin, J.L.; Gottlieb, D.J.; Newman, A.B.; O'Connor, G.; Rapoport, D.; Redline, S.; Resnick, H.E.; Robbins, J.A.; et al. Sleep-Disordered Breathing and Mortality: A Prospective Cohort Study. *PLoS Med.* **2009**, *6*, e1000132. [CrossRef] [PubMed]
35. Peppard, P.E.; Young, T.; Barnet, J.H.; Palta, M.; Hagen, E.W.; Hla, K.M. Increased Prevalence of Sleep-Disordered Breathing in Adults. *Am. J. Epidemiol.* **2013**, *177*, 1006–1014. [CrossRef]
36. Young, T.; Peppard, P.E.; Gottlieb, D.J. Epidemiology of Obstructive Sleep Apnea: A population health perspective. *Am. J. Respir. Crit. Care Med.* **2002**, *165*, 1217–1239. [CrossRef] [PubMed]
37. Young, T.; Finn, L.; Austin, D.; Peterson, A. Menopausal Status and Sleep-disordered Breathing in the Wisconsin Sleep Cohort Study. *Am. J. Respir. Crit. Care Med.* **2003**, *167*, 1181–1185. [CrossRef]
38. Zhang, Y.; Weed, J.G.; Ren, R.; Tang, X.; Zhang, W. Prevalence of obstructive sleep apnea in patients with posttraumatic stress disorder and its impact on adherence to continuous positive airway pressure therapy: A meta-analysis. *Sleep Med.* **2017**, *36*, 125–132. [CrossRef] [PubMed]
39. Krakow, B.; Melendrez, D.; Warner, T.D.; Clark, J.O.; Sisley, B.N.; Dorin, R.; Harper, R.M.; Leahigh, L.K.; Lee, S.A.; Sklar, D.; et al. Signs and Symptoms of Sleep-Disordered Breathing in Trauma Survivors: A matched comparison with classic sleep apnea patients. *J. Nerv. Ment. Dis.* **2006**, *194*, 433–439. [CrossRef]
40. Lettieri, C.; Williams, S.G.; Collen, J.F. OSA Syndrome and Posttraumatic Stress Disorder: Clinical Outcomes and Impact of Positive Airway Pressure Therapy. *Chest* **2016**, *149*, 483–490. [CrossRef]
41. Series, F.; Roy, N.; Marc, I. Effects of sleep deprivation and sleep fragmentation on upper airway collapsibility in normal subjects. *Am. J. Respir. Crit. Care Med.* **1994**, *150*, 481–485. [CrossRef] [PubMed]
42. Trinder, J.; Whitworth, F.; Kay, A.; Wilkin, P. Respiratory instability during sleep onset. *J. Appl. Physiol.* **1992**, *73*, 2462–2469. [CrossRef]
43. Thomson, S.; Morrell, M.J.; Cordingley, J.J.; Semple, S.J. Ventilation is unstable during drowsiness before sleep onset. *J. Appl. Physiol.* **2005**, *99*, 2036–2044. [CrossRef] [PubMed]
44. Eckert, D.J.; Younes, M.K. Arousal from sleep: Implications for obstructive sleep apnea pathogenesis and treatment. *J. Appl. Physiol.* **2014**, *116*, 302–313. [CrossRef]
45. Foster, B.; Kravitz, S.; Collen, J.; Holley, A. 0490 Insomnia Among Military Members with OSA. *Sleep* **2019**, *42*, A196. [CrossRef]
46. A El-Solh, A.; Lawson, Y.; Wilding, G.E. Impact of low arousal threshold on treatment of obstructive sleep apnea in patients with post-traumatic stress disorder. *Sleep Breath.* **2021**, *25*, 597–604. [CrossRef]
47. Narkiewicz, K.; Somers, V.K. Sympathetic nerve activity in obstructive sleep apnoea. *Acta Physiol. Scand.* **2003**, *177*, 385–390. [CrossRef] [PubMed]
48. Schredl, M.; Schmitt, J.; Hein, G.; Schmoll, T.; Eller, S.; Haaf, J. Nightmares and oxygen desaturations: Is sleep apnea related to heightened nightmare frequency? *Sleep Breath.* **2006**, *10*, 203–209. [CrossRef]
49. Bahammam, A.S.; Almeneessier, A.S. Dreams and Nightmares in Patients with Obstructive Sleep Apnea: A Review. *Front. Neurol.* **2019**, *10*, 1127. [CrossRef]
50. Fisher, S.; Lewis, K.; Bartle, I.; Ghosal, R.; Davies, L.; Blagrove, M. Emotional Content of Dreams in Obstructive Sleep Apnea Hypopnea Syndrome Patients and Sleepy Snorers attending a Sleep-Disordered Breathing Clinic. *J. Clin. Sleep Med.* **2011**, *7*, 69–74. [CrossRef] [PubMed]
51. BaHammam, A.S.; Al-Shimemeri, S.A.; Salama, R.I.; Sharif, M.M. Clinical and polysomnographic characteristics and response to continuous positive airway pressure therapy in obstructive sleep apnea patients with nightmares. *Sleep Med.* **2013**, *14*, 149–154. [CrossRef]
52. Gross, M.; Lavie, P. Dreams in sleep apnea patients. *Dreaming* **1994**, *4*, 195–204. [CrossRef]
53. Carrasco, E.; Santamaria, J.; Iranzo, A.; Pintor, L.; De Pablo, J.; Solanas, A.; Kumru, H.; Rodriguez, J.E.M.; Boget, T. Changes in dreaming induced by CPAP in severe obstructive sleep apnea syndrome patients. *J. Sleep Res.* **2006**, *15*, 430–436. [CrossRef]
54. Walker, M.P.; Stickgold, R. Sleep-Dependent Learning and Memory Consolidation. *Neuron* **2004**, *44*, 121–133. [CrossRef]
55. Tempesta, D.; Socci, V.; De Gennaro, L.; Ferrara, M. Sleep and emotional processing. *Sleep Med. Rev.* **2018**, *40*, 183–195. [CrossRef] [PubMed]
56. Goldstein, A.N.; Walker, M.P. The Role of Sleep in Emotional Brain Function. *Annu. Rev. Clin. Psychol.* **2014**, *10*, 679–708. [CrossRef] [PubMed]
57. Wagner, U.; Gais, S.; Born, J. Emotional Memory Formation Is Enhanced across Sleep Intervals with High Amounts of Rapid Eye Movement Sleep. *Learn. Mem.* **2001**, *8*, 112–119. [CrossRef] [PubMed]
58. Menz, M.; Rihm, J.; Salari, N.; Born, J.; Kalisch, R.; Pape, H.; Marshall, L.; Büchel, C. The role of sleep and sleep deprivation in consolidating fear memories. *NeuroImage* **2013**, *75*, 87–96. [CrossRef] [PubMed]
59. Murkar, A.L.; De Koninck, J. Consolidative mechanisms of emotional processing in REM sleep and PTSD. *Sleep Med. Rev.* **2018**, *41*, 173–184. [CrossRef]
60. van der Helm, E.; Yao, J.; Dutt, S.; Rao, V.; Saletin, J.; Walker, M.P. REM Sleep Depotentiates Amygdala Activity to Previous Emotional Experiences. *Curr. Biol.* **2011**, *21*, 2029–2032. [CrossRef]

61. Menz, M.M.; Rihm, J.S.; Büchel, C. REM Sleep Is Causal to Successful Consolidation of Dangerous and Safety Stimuli and Reduces Return of Fear after Extinction. *J. Neurosci.* **2016**, *36*, 2148–2160. [CrossRef] [PubMed]
62. Pace-Schott, E.F.; Milad, M.R.; Orr, S.P.; Rauch, S.L.; Stickgold, R.; Pitman, R.K. Sleep Promotes Generalization of Extinction of Conditioned Fear. *Sleep* **2009**, *32*, 19–26. [CrossRef]
63. Pace-Schott, E.F.; Germain, A.; Milad, M.R. Sleep and REM sleep disturbance in the pathophysiology of PTSD: The role of extinction memory. *Biol. Mood Anxiety Disord.* **2015**, *5*, 3. [CrossRef] [PubMed]
64. Pace-Schott, E.F.; Germain, A.; Milad, M.R. Effects of sleep on memory for conditioned fear and fear extinction. *Psychol. Bull.* **2015**, *141*, 835–857. [CrossRef] [PubMed]
65. Spoormaker, V.; Sturm, A.; Andrade, K.; Schröter, M.; Goya-Maldonado, R.; Holsboer, F.; Wetter, T.; Sämann, P.; Czisch, M. The neural correlates and temporal sequence of the relationship between shock exposure, disturbed sleep and impaired consolidation of fear extinction. *J. Psychiatr. Res.* **2010**, *44*, 1121–1128. [CrossRef]
66. Norrholm, S.D.; Jovanovic, T. Fear Processing, Psychophysiology, and PTSD. *Harv. Rev. Psychiatry* **2018**, *26*, 129–141. [CrossRef] [PubMed]
67. Fitzgerald, J.M.; DiGangi, J.A.; Phan, K.L. Functional Neuroanatomy of Emotion and Its Regulation in PTSD. *Harv. Rev. Psychiatry* **2018**, *26*, 116–128. [CrossRef]
68. Germain, A. Sleep Disturbances as the Hallmark of PTSD: Where Are We Now? *Am. J. Psychiatry* **2013**, *170*, 372–382. [CrossRef]
69. Ross, R.J.; Ball, W.A.; Dinges, D.F.; Kribbs, N.B.; Morrison, A.R.; Silver, S.M.; Mulvaney, F.D. Rapid eye movement sleep disturbance in posttraumatic stress disorder. *Biol. Psychiatry* **1994**, *35*, 195–202. [CrossRef]
70. Reist, C.; Jovanovic, T.; Kantarovich, D.; Weingast, L.; Hollifield, M.; Novin, M.; Khalaghizadeh, S.; Jafari, B.; George, R.; Riser, M.; et al. An analysis of fear inhibition and fear extinction in a sample of veterans with obstructive sleep apnea (OSA): Implications for co-morbidity with post-traumatic stress disorder (PTSD). *Behav. Brain Res.* **2021**, *404*, 113172. [CrossRef]
71. Acierno, R.; Gros, D.F.; Ruggiero, K.J.; Dha, M.A.H.-T.; Knapp, R.G.; Lejuez, C.; Muzzy, W.; Frueh, C.B.; Egede, L.E.; Tuerk, P.W. Behavioral activation and therapeutic exposure for posttraumatic stress disorder: A noninferiority trial of treatment delivered in person versus home-based telehealth. *Depress. Anxiety* **2016**, *33*, 415–423. [CrossRef]
72. Rauch, S.A.M.; Defever, E.; Favorite, T.; Duroe, A.; Garrity, C.; Martis, B.; Liberzon, I. Prolonged exposure for PTSD in a Veterans Health Administration PTSD clinic. *J. Trauma. Stress* **2009**, *22*, 60–64. [CrossRef]
73. Tran, K.; Moulton, K.; Santesso, N.; Rabb, D. *Cognitive Processing Therapy for Post-Traumatic Stress Disorder: A Systematic Review and Meta-Analysis*; Canadian Agency for Drugs and Technologies in Health: Ottawa, ON, Canada, 2016. Available online: https://www.ncbi.nlm.nih.gov/books/NBK362346/ (accessed on 27 November 2021).
74. Ho, F.Y.-Y.; Chan, C.S.; Tang, K.N.-S. Cognitive-behavioral therapy for sleep disturbances in treating posttraumatic stress disorder symptoms: A meta-analysis of randomized controlled trials. *Clin. Psychol. Rev.* **2016**, *43*, 90–102. [CrossRef]
75. Baddeley, J.L.; Gros, D.F. Cognitive Behavioral Therapy for Insomnia as a Preparatory Treatment for Exposure Therapy for Posttraumatic Stress Disorder. *Am. J. Psychother.* **2013**, *67*, 203–214. [CrossRef]
76. Gutner, C.A.; Pedersen, E.R.; Drummond, S. Going direct to the consumer: Examining treatment preferences for veterans with insomnia, PTSD, and depression. *Psychiatry Res.* **2018**, *263*, 108–114. [CrossRef]
77. Kapur, V.K.; Auckley, D.H.; Chowdhuri, S.; Kuhlmann, D.C.; Mehra, R.; Ramar, K.; Harrod, C.G. Clinical Practice Guideline for Diagnostic Testing for Adult Obstructive Sleep Apnea: An American Academy of Sleep Medicine Clinical Practice Guideline. *J. Clin. Sleep Med.* **2017**, *13*, 479–504. [CrossRef] [PubMed]
78. Patil, S.P.; Ayappa, I.A.; Caples, S.M.; Kimoff, R.J.; Patel, S.; Harrod, C.G. Treatment of Adult Obstructive Sleep Apnea with Positive Airway Pressure: An American Academy of Sleep Medicine Clinical Practice Guideline. *J. Clin. Sleep Med.* **2019**, *15*, 335–343. [CrossRef] [PubMed]
79. Pollicina, I.; Maniaci, A.; Lechien, J.R.; Iannella, G.; Vicini, C.; Cammaroto, G.; Cannavicci, A.; Magliulo, G.; Pace, A.; Cocuzza, S.; et al. Neurocognitive Performance Improvement after Obstructive Sleep Apnea Treatment: State of the Art. *Behav. Sci.* **2021**, *11*, 180. [CrossRef]
80. McEvoy, R.D.; Antic, N.A.; Heeley, E.; Luo, Y.; Ou, Q.; Zhang, X.; Mediano, O.; Chen, R.; Drager, L.F.; Liu, Z.; et al. CPAP for Prevention of Cardiovascular Events in Obstructive Sleep Apnea. *N. Engl. J. Med.* **2016**, *375*, 919–931. [CrossRef]
81. Youakim, J.M.; Doghramji, K.; Schutte, S.L. Posttraumatic Stress Disorder and Obstructive Sleep Apnea Syndrome. *J. Psychosom. Res.* **1998**, *39*, 168–171. [CrossRef]
82. Krakow, B.; Lowry, C.; Germain, A.; Gaddy, L.; Hollifield, M.; Koss, M.; Tandberg, D.; Johnston, L.; Melendrez, D. A retrospective study on improvements in nightmares and post-traumatic stress disorder following treatment for co-morbid sleep-disordered breathing. *J. Psychosom. Res.* **2000**, *49*, 291–298. [CrossRef]
83. Tamanna, S.; Parker, J.D.; Lyons, J.; Ullah, M.I. The Effect of Continuous Positive Air Pressure (CPAP) on Nightmares in Patients with Posttraumatic Stress Disorder (PTSD) and Obstructive Sleep Apnea (OSA). *J. Clin. Sleep Med.* **2014**, *10*, 631–636. [CrossRef]
84. El-Solh, A.A.; Vermont, L.; Homish, G.; Kufel, T. The effect of continuous positive airway pressure on post-traumatic stress disorder symptoms in veterans with post-traumatic stress disorder and obstructive sleep apnea: A prospective study. *Sleep Med.* **2017**, *33*, 145–150. [CrossRef] [PubMed]
85. Orr, J.; Smales, C.; Alexander, T.H.; Stepnowsky, C.; Pillar, G.; Malhotra, A.; Sarmiento, K.F. Treatment of OSA with CPAP Is Associated with Improvement in PTSD Symptoms among Veterans. *J. Clin. Sleep Med.* **2017**, *13*, 57–63. [CrossRef] [PubMed]

86. Ullah, M.I.; Campbell, D.G.; Bhagat, R.; Lyons, J.A.; Tamanna, S. Improving PTSD Symptoms and Preventing Progression of Subclinical PTSD to an Overt Disorder by Treating Comorbid OSA with CPAP. *J. Clin. Sleep Med.* **2017**, *13*, 1191–1198. [CrossRef] [PubMed]
87. Weaver, T.E.; Grunstein, R.R. Adherence to Continuous Positive Airway Pressure Therapy: The Challenge to Effective Treatment. *Proc. Am. Thorac. Soc.* **2008**, *5*, 173–178. [CrossRef]
88. El-Solh, A.A.; Ayyar, L.; Akinnusi, M.; Relia, S.; Akinnusi, O. Positive Airway Pressure Adherence in Veterans with Posttraumatic Stress Disorder. *Sleep* **2010**, *33*, 1495–1500. [CrossRef]
89. El-Solh, A.A.; Homish, G.G.; DiTursi, G.; Lazarus, J.; Rao, N.; Adamo, D.; Kufel, T. A Randomized Crossover Trial Evaluating Continuous Positive Airway Pressure Versus Mandibular Advancement Device on Health Outcomes in Veterans With Posttraumatic Stress Disorder. *J. Clin. Sleep Med.* **2017**, *13*, 1327–1335. [CrossRef]
90. El-Solh, A.A.; Adamo, D.; Kufel, T. Comorbid insomnia and sleep apnea in Veterans with post-traumatic stress disorder. *Sleep Breath.* **2018**, *22*, 23–31. [CrossRef] [PubMed]
91. Sharples, L.D.; Clutterbuck-James, A.L.; Glover, M.; Bennett, M.S.; Chadwick, R.; Pittman, M.A.; Quinnell, T.G. Meta-analysis of randomised controlled trials of oral mandibular advancement devices and continuous positive airway pressure for obstructive sleep apnoea-hypopnoea. *Sleep Med. Rev.* **2016**, *27*, 108–124. [CrossRef]
92. Attali, V.; Chaumereuil, C.; Arnulf, I.; Golmard, J.-L.; Tordjman, F.; Morin, L.; Goudot, P.; Similowski, T.; Collet, J.-M. Predictors of long-term effectiveness to mandibular repositioning device treatment in obstructive sleep apnea patients after 1000 days. *Sleep Med.* **2016**, *27–28*, 107–114. [CrossRef] [PubMed]
93. Martínez-Gomis, J.; Willaert, E.; Nogues, L.; Pascual, M.; Somoza, M.; Monasterio, C. Five Years of Sleep Apnea Treatment with a Mandibular Advancement Device: Side effects and technical complications. *Angle Orthod.* **2010**, *80*, 30–36. [CrossRef]
94. Pliska, B.T.; Nam, H.; Chen, H.; Lowe, A.A.; Almeida, F.R. Obstructive Sleep Apnea and Mandibular Advancement Splints: Occlusal Effects and Progression of Changes Associated with a Decade of Treatment. *J. Clin. Sleep Med.* **2014**, *10*, 1285–1291. [CrossRef]
95. Vanderveken, O.M.; Van De Heyning, P.; Braem, M.J. Retention of mandibular advancement devices in the treatment of obstructive sleep apnea: An in vitro pilot study. *Sleep Breath.* **2013**, *18*, 313–318. [CrossRef]
96. Marklund, M.; Franklin, K.A. Treatment of elderly patients with snoring and obstructive sleep apnea using a mandibular advancement device. *Sleep Breath.* **2014**, *19*, 403–405. [CrossRef]
97. Patil, R.D.; Sarber, K.M.; Epperson, M.V.; Tabangin, M.; Altaye, M.; Mesa, F.; Ishman, S.L. Hypoglossal Nerve Stimulation: Outcomes in Veterans with Obstructive Sleep Apnea and Common Comorbid Post-Traumatic Stress Disorder. *Laryngoscope* **2021**, *131*, S1–S11. [CrossRef]
98. Gottlieb, D.J.; Punjabi, N.M. Diagnosis and Management of Obstructive Sleep Apnea: A review. *JAMA* **2020**, *323*, 1389–1400. [CrossRef]
99. Carter, S.G.; Berger, M.S.; Carberry, J.; Bilston, L.E.; Butler, J.; Tong, B.; Martins, R.T.; Fisher, L.P.; McKenzie, D.K.; Grunstein, R.R.; et al. Zopiclone Increases the Arousal Threshold without Impairing Genioglossus Activity in Obstructive Sleep Apnea. *Sleep* **2016**, *39*, 757–766. [CrossRef]
100. Smith, P.R.; Sheikh, K.L.; Costan-Toth, C.; Forsthoefel, D.; Bridges, E.; Andrada, T.F.; Holley, A.B. Eszopiclone and Zolpidem Do Not Affect the Prevalence of the Low Arousal Threshold Phenotype. *J. Clin. Sleep Med.* **2017**, *13*, 115–119. [CrossRef] [PubMed]
101. Schmickl, C.N.; Lettieri, C.J.; Orr, J.E.; Deyoung, P.; Edwards, B.A.; Owens, R.L.; Malhotra, A. The Arousal Threshold as a Drug Target to Improve Continuous Positive Airway Pressure Adherence: Secondary Analysis of a Randomized Trial. *Am. J. Respir. Crit. Care Med.* **2020**, *202*, 1592–1595. [CrossRef] [PubMed]
102. Earl, D.C.; Van Tyle, K.M. New pharmacologic agents for insomnia and hypersomnia. *Curr. Opin. Pulm. Med.* **2020**, *26*, 629–633. [CrossRef] [PubMed]
103. Yang, C.; White, D.P.; Winkelman, J.W. Antidepressants and Periodic Leg Movements of Sleep. *Biol. Psychiatry* **2005**, *58*, 510–514. [CrossRef]
104. Department of Veterans Affairs; Department of Defense. VA/DOD Clinical Practice Guideline for the Management of Posttraumatic Stress Disorder and Acute Stress Disorder. 2017. Available online: www.tricare.mil (accessed on 28 November 2021).
105. American Psychological Association. Clinical Practice Guideline for the Treatment of Posttraumatic Stress Disorder (PTSD) in Adults. 2017. Available online: https://www.apa.org/ptsd-guideline/ptsd.pdf (accessed on 28 November 2021).

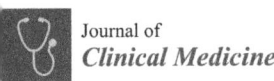

Review

Obstructive Sleep Apnea and Cardiac Arrhythmias: A Contemporary Review

Balint Laczay and Michael D. Faulx *

Department of Cardiovascular Medicine, Heart, Vascular and Thoracic Institute, Cleveland Clinic, Cleveland, OH 44195, USA; laczayb@ccf.org
* Correspondence: faulxm@ccf.org; Tel.: +1-216-445-7212

Abstract: Obstructive sleep apnea (OSA) is a highly prevalent disorder with a growing incidence worldwide that closely mirrors the global obesity epidemic. OSA is associated with enormous healthcare costs in addition to significant morbidity and mortality. Much of the morbidity and mortality related to OSA can be attributed to an increased burden of cardiovascular disease, including cardiac rhythm disorders. Awareness of the relationship between OSA and rhythm disorders is variable among physicians, a fact that can influence patient care, since the presence of OSA can influence the incidence, prevalence, and successful treatment of multiple rhythm disorders. Herein, we provide a review of this topic that is intentionally broad in scope, covering the relationship between OSA and rhythm disorders from epidemiology and pathophysiology to diagnosis and management, with a particular focus on the recognition of undiagnosed OSA in the general clinical population and the intimate relationship between OSA and atrial fibrillation.

Keywords: obstructive sleep apnea (OSA); atrial fibrillation (AF); continuous positive airway pressure (CPAP); ventricular tachycardia (VT); atrioventricular (AV) block

1. Sleep Apnea and Cardiac Rhythm Disorders: An Introduction

Sleep apnea is a highly prevalent disorder among patients with all forms of cardiovascular disease. Decades of data from several large prospective patient registries have revealed that sleep apnea—in particular, obstructive sleep apnea (OSA)—is practically endemic in cardiology clinics and cardiac inpatient wards across the globe [1,2]. OSA has been closely associated with prevalent and incident hypertension [3], ischemic heart disease [4,5], heart failure [6], stroke [7], and all forms of cardiac rhythm disturbance [8]. Additionally, central sleep apnea (CSA) or combined OSA and CSA often affects patients with heart failure and stroke [9]. Sleep apnea and cardiovascular disease are so intertwined with respect to their epidemiology and shared pathophysiology that one can think of them as being two components of a global, multi-system metabolic syndrome driven largely by obesity.

In this review, we will focus on OSA and its relationship to cardiac rhythm disorders. We do this because OSA is the most common form of sleep apnea, and its presence appears to have a greater overall impact on cardiac rhythm disorders than other forms of sleep apnea or sleep-disordered breathing [8]. Additionally, there is a rich and growing body of clinical and basic scientific evidence linking OSA and cardiac rhythm disorders, particularly atrial fibrillation, at multiple levels, which deserves a thorough review [10,11]. Lastly, OSA risk can be readily assessed in the clinical setting by allowing for appropriate testing and subsequent referral for a number of validated treatment options—most commonly, positive airway pressure (PAP) device management. Appropriate treatment can have a positive impact on a patient's morbidity, mortality, and quality of life, irrespective of its impact on rhythm disorders per se.

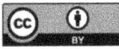

Citation: Laczay, B.; Faulx, M.D. Obstructive Sleep Apnea and Cardiac Arrhythmias: A Contemporary Review. *J. Clin. Med.* **2021**, *10*, 3785. https://doi.org/10.3390/jcm10173785

Academic Editor: Yuksel Peker

Received: 22 July 2021
Accepted: 20 August 2021
Published: 24 August 2021

Publisher's Note: MDPI stays neutral with regard to jurisdictional claims in published maps and institutional affiliations.

Copyright: © 2021 by the authors. Licensee MDPI, Basel, Switzerland. This article is an open access article distributed under the terms and conditions of the Creative Commons Attribution (CC BY) license (https://creativecommons.org/licenses/by/4.0/).

2. Hiding in Plain Sight? The Epidemiology of Obstructive Sleep Apnea

OSA is a global health crisis that parallels the global obesity epidemic. Obesity and OSA are associated to the extent that it is credible to think of OSA as a consequence of obesity in a majority of cases, although there are certainly patients with OSA who are not obese. In the United States, OSA affects 17% of adult women and 34% of adult men, and incident cases are on the rise [12]. Across the world, OSA prevalence rates vary, but share the trend of rising on every continent [2]. OSA is often associated with features of the metabolic syndrome or "Syndrome X", including insulin resistance, dyslipidemia, hypertension, and central adiposity, so often so that some authors have proposed the adoption of a "Syndrome Z" to account for the frequent presence of OSA [13]. This association with the metabolic syndrome and its attendant effects on inflammation, oxidative stress, and endothelial dysfunction likely accounts for a large portion of the association between OSA and cardiovascular disease [14].

OSA is often symptomatic, with its principal symptom being excessive daytime sleepiness or fatigue. Historical features that are strongly suggestive of OSA include loud snoring and witnessed apneas or gasping for air during sleep. This element of the history often requires an interview with the patient's bed partner for confirmation. Other symptomatic manifestations of OSA include difficult concentration, declining work performance, depressed mood, and a heightened risk for motor vehicle accidents. There are a number of valid and simple screening tools that can be easily applied during a patient interview to predict the presence of OSA with fair accuracy. Of these, the STOP-BANG questionnaire (Table 1) appears to have the best sensitivity and specificity for the detection of OSA [15–17]. Although many patients with OSA do not volunteer that they are symptomatic, screening for symptoms can nonetheless be helpful. The Epworth sleepiness scale (ESS), an eight-item questionnaire administered during a clinical encounter (Table 2), can prove useful in establishing whether significant OSA symptoms are present [18]. While it is not solely specific to sleepiness caused by sleep apnea, the ESS scale has been well validated in the OSA population and is a reliable gauge for symptom severity. This matters because the presence of subjective and objective sleepiness correlates with greater expression of pro-inflammatory biomarkers and a greater overall risk for adverse cardiac events than the absence of OSA symptoms [19]. The presence of symptoms also justifies OSA treatment, irrespective of any interest in cardiac risk mitigation.

Table 1. The STOP-BANG questionnaire and its accuracy in detecting moderate or severe sleep apnea (AHI $\geq$15/hour). Score one point for each finding.

Snoring		Typically loud and disruptive		
Tiredness		Tired, fatigued, or sleepy during the day		
Observed apnea		Often observed by bed partner		
Pressure		History of hypertension treatment		
BMI		BMI > 35 kg/m^2		
Age		>50 years		
Neck circumference		>40 cm		
Gender		Male		
STOP BANG Score	**Sensitivity**	**Specificity**	**PPV**	**NPV**
1	100	1	67	100
2	99	10	68	79
3	94	32	73	74
4	81	51	76	58
5	60	72	80	48
6	35	89	86	42
7	14	96	88	37
8	3	100	95	35

AHI, apnea–hypopnea index; BMI, body mass index, PPV, positive predictive value; NPV, negative predictive value. The table was created from data taken from references [17] and [19].

Table 2. The Epworth Sleepiness Scale (ESS) and its relationship to OSAS risk. Each question is scored from 0 to 3. ESS score range is from 0–24.

Activity	Likelihood of Dozing 0 = Never, 1 = Slight, 2 = Moderate, 3 = High
Sitting and reading	
Watching television	
Sitting inactively in a public place	
As a car passenger for one uninterrupted hour	
Lying down in the afternoon when able	
Sitting and talking to someone	
Sitting quietly after lunch with no alcohol	
In a car, while stopped for a few minutes in traffic	

Mean RDI	Mean ESS	ESS Range	Interpretation
8.8 ± 2.3	9.5 ± 3.3	1–9	No or little OSAS risk
21.1 ± 4.0	11.5 ± 4.2	10–15	Moderate OSAS risk
49.5 ± 9.6	16.0 ± 4.4	16–24	High OSAS risk

RDI, respiratory disturbance index; OSAS, obstructive sleep apnea syndrome. The table was adapted from reference [20].

When OSA is strongly suspected after screening, the diagnosis is typically confirmed or excluded with an attended, laboratory-based polysomnogram (PSG) or a home sleep apnea test (HSAT). PSG is considered the gold standard for the diagnosis of sleep disorders owing to its multi-channel data acquisition, which includes brainwave activity and cardiac telemetry to allow for sleep staging, arousal assessment, and assessment of heart rate variability. Major disadvantages of PSG include its limited availability despite rising demand and lack of access in the setting of the ongoing coronavirus disease 2019 (COVID-19) pandemic [20]. In contrast, HSAT offers a simpler dataset that includes continuous oximetry and airflow assessment. The device is worn in the patient's home and is often more readily available than PSG. HSAT is most appropriate for patients with few medical comorbidities in whom there is a high index of suspicion for OSA, rather than central or mixed apnea. There are even algorithms that allow for the assessment of heart rate variability based on data obtained from continuous oximetry, a feature that may prove useful in the prediction of incident rhythm disorders, such as atrial fibrillation [21].

OSA severity may be assessed in several ways. The most commonly reported metric of OSA severity is the apnea hypopnea index (AHI), which measures the number of times that a patient stops breathing (apnea) or experiences a significant reduction in airflow (hypopnea) per hour of sleep time. An apnea is defined as a lack of an air flow for at least 10 s with an associated oxygen desaturation of at least 4%. Hypopnea is defined as a 50% or greater reduction in airflow for at least 10 s with an associated oxygen desaturation of at least 4%. The AHI is easy to reproduce and is, without question, the most widely reported OSA severity metric in clinical trials. However, the AHI may underrepresent OSA severity when viewed in isolation, and there are data to support focusing more on indices of oxygen desaturation as a gauge of OSA severity [22]. Recent studies have suggested that measures of oxygen desaturation, such as the percentage of sleep time spent with an oxygenation saturation below 90% (T90) or 88% (T88) or the lowest saturation achieved during sleep, may better predict adverse cardiac events than the AHI [23].

3. Guilt by Association or Public Enemy Number One? Obstructive Sleep Apnea and Cardiac Arrhythmogenesis

OSA impacts the development of cardiac arrhythmias through direct and indirect mechanisms (Figure 1). The direct effects of OSA on arrhythmia development include the acute physiologic changes that occur as a consequence of airway collapse during sleep, including the development of hypoxemia and hypercapnia [24], changes in sympathetic and parasympathetic tone [25], and fluctuations in thoracic pressure [26]. Indirectly, OSA alters the structure of the heart and is a risk factor for the development of structural heart disease. The indirect effects include the development of cardiovascular disease, including hypertension [3,27], heart failure, and coronary artery disease [28], which form the underlying substrate for arrhythmia development. While atrial fibrillation is the arrhythmia most commonly associated with OSA [29], there is evidence linking OSA to the development of arrhythmias at the level of the sinus node [30], atrial arrhythmias [31], ventricular arrhythmias, and sudden cardiac death [32]. In this section, we will review the pathophysiologic impact of sleep apnea on cardiac arrhythmia and explore the relationship with each disease entity in turn.

The basis of arrhythmogenesis includes changes in myocardial automaticity, triggered activity, and reentrant mechanisms [33]. Abnormal automaticity refers to the formation of cardiac impulses in normally quiescent cardiac cells and is controlled by multiple factors, including sympathetic and parasympathetic tone, acid–base status, and electrolyte disturbances at the membrane and sub-membrane levels [34]. OSA causes repetitive, cyclical changes in sympathetic tone. During apneic events, increased vagal tone causes bradycardia followed by sympathetic discharge as a result of hypoxemia and hypercapnia. Increased vagal tone has been shown to shorten the effective refractory period of the atrium in porcine models of AF and to lead to easier inducibility of AF [35]. The following sympathetic discharge, in turn, promotes increased arrhythmia formation due to beta-adrenergic stimulation [26,36] The repetitive hypoxemia is also thought to increase reactive oxygen species and alter potassium regulation during sleep, which affects the automaticity of cardiac tissue [37]. OSA has also been shown to decrease the atrial effective refractory period (ERP) in canine models, thus leaving the atria more vulnerable to automatic depolarization and ectopy during periods of sleep-disordered breathing [38]. Triggered activity refers to spontaneous depolarizations that are able to cross the membrane potential required to trigger an action potential. These individual extrasystoles can precipitate tachyarrhythmias in both the atrial and ventricular chambers [38]. Well-established causes of triggered activity include hypoxemia, acidemia, and increased sympathetic tone, all of which occur during the repetitive cycles of apnea that characterize OSA. Re-entrant mechanisms are postulated to arise from heterogenous myocardial conduction as a result of abnormal cardiac remodeling in the setting of structural heart disease that accompanies OSA [24].

The mechanistic link between OSA and heart failure is complex and likely bidirectional, with each entity contributing to the other [39]. Obstructive apnea and hypopnea are associated with respiratory efforts against the collapsed upper airway, with associated changes in intrathoracic pressure as high as 60 to 80 mmHg [40] These repetitive, acute swings have a significant impact on cardiac preload and afterload. Simulation of OSA by means of the Mueller maneuver, which involves breathing in against a forced resistance by means of a nose clip and mouthpiece with a 21 G needle, was shown to reproduce changes in intrathoracic pressure in healthy human subjects [38]. This experiment showed that the effect of these intrathoracic pressure swings includes increases in left ventricle (LV) end-systolic volumes, decreased cardiac performance, and abrupt swings in left atrial volumes due to mural stress on the more pliable left atrial wall. Likewise, in patients undergoing cardiac catheterization with measurement of aortic and left ventricular pressures, negative intrathoracic pressures by means of the Mueller maneuver caused increases in LV contraction load as well as an increase in the LV relaxation coefficient (tau) [41,42]. These pathophysiologic changes play a possible role in the observation that severe OSA is associated with ventricular diastolic dysfunction in a dose-dependent fashion [42]. The sum of these interactions is that OSA predisposes one to the development of structural heart disease and heart failure, and the development of these disease states, in turn, predisposes one to and perpetuates the development of OSA.

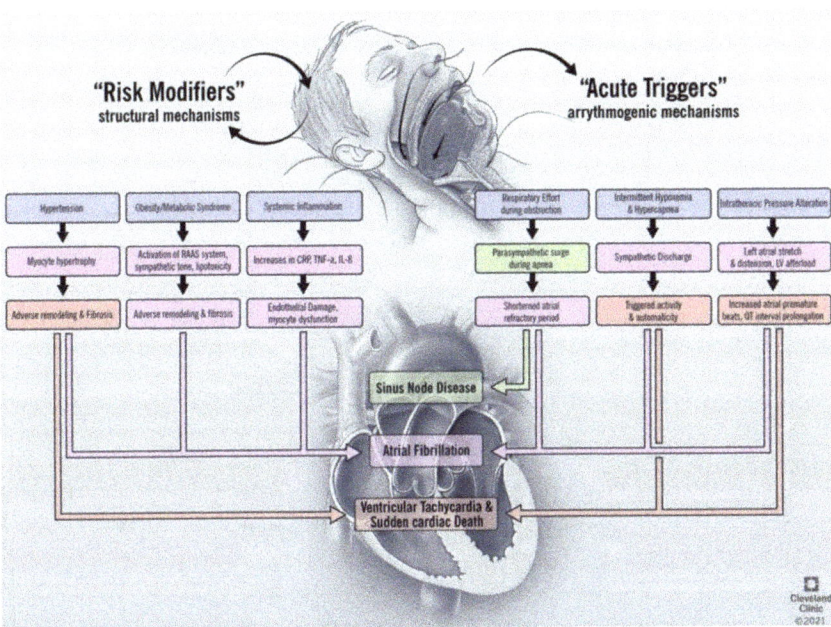

Figure 1. Proposed mechanisms linking obstructive sleep apnea and cardiac arrhythmias. RAAS, renin angiotensin aldosterone system; CRP, c-reactive protein; TNF, tumor necrosis factor; IL, interleukin; LV, left ventricle.

Sick sinus syndromes, including bradycardia with chronotropic incompetence, sinoatrial exit block, and tachycardia–bradycardia syndromes, are recognized to be more common in OSA patients than in the general population [43–45]. One study using Holter monitoring of 239 consecutive patients with a new diagnosis of OSA found that bradyarrhythmias occurred in as many as 20% of the patients and that there was a dose–response effect with respect to oxygen saturation nadir during sleep [46]. Early studies in using tracheostomy as a treatment for OSA in the context of "Pickwickian Syndrome" showed that the treatment of recurrent apneic episodes with tracheostomy normalized both sleep patterns and bradyarrhythmias in this population [47]. These studies were among the first to postulate that hypoxia-induced vagal tone at nighttime could be a significant cause of bradyarrhythmias. A study of patients with excessive daytime sleepiness and sleep-related breathing disorders showed that these patients had increased sympathetic and parasympathetic surges when looking at changes in R-R intervals overnight, showing a link between parasympathetic tone and bradyarrhythmia in this population [48]. A study of six consecutive patients with sleep apnea showed that bradycardia correlated with apneic events and that the duration and severity of bradycardia correlated with the degree of hypoxemia during the apneic events [49] These observations can be explained by the natural diving reflex that is elicited during upper airway obstruction. During upper airway obstruction, there is sympathetic vasoconstriction of arteries to muscles and viscera, with resultant hypertension and vagal tone causing bradycardia [48,50]. This association between OSA and bradycardia is also seen in reverse: Patient cohorts not known to have sleep apnea were shown to have an excessively high prevalence of OSA, regardless of the indication for pacing [51]. Studies of OSA patients referred for pulmonary vein isolation have shown slower sinus node recovery times, suggesting that OSA also impacts the structural integrity of the sinus node [52].

Atrial fibrillation (AF) is the most common arrhythmia in the United States and is estimated to affect more than 3 million individuals [53]. The pathogenesis of atrial fibrillation is complex and incompletely understood, but is accepted to involve both abnormal atrial substrates and triggers of abnormal electrical activity. The initiation of abnormal electrical activity in the pulmonary veins and their subsequent spread and activation of the atrium has been described, and the isolation of said pulmonary veins is the mainstay of catheter-based ablation of atrial fibrillation [54]. In addition to the pulmonary veins, additional areas of abnormal electrical activity have been implicated in AF pathogenesis, including the superior vena cava, the left atrial appendage, the ligament of Marshall, and scarred areas of the left atrium [53]. Additionally, small spiral wave fronts called rotors have been implicated in initiating atrial fibrillation from areas of the atrium outside the traditional pulmonary vein foci [55]. The progression of structural disease, including scarring and fibrosis of the left atrium, has also been implicated in the development and progression of atrial fibrillation [56]. In these patients, the abnormal atrial tissue is considered an additional instigator of atrial fibrillation in addition to the pulmonary veins [57,58]. Parasympathetic tone is also thought to impact the development of atrial fibrillation, with the ganglionated plexi of the left atrium located near the pulmonary vein ostia being an ongoing target of investigation in atrial fibrillation management [59]. The prevalence of OSA is as high as 50–80% in atrial fibrillation patients [59–61], and conversely, the prevalence of atrial fibrillation is higher in OSA patients compared to controls (4.8 vs. 1.9%) [44]. OSA predisposes one to the development of atrial fibrillation both through its acute effects in modulating autonomic tone and by acutely changing intrathoracic pressure dynamics, as well as by modulating chronic changes in the underlying atrial substrate [62].

The impact of OSA on structural changes in the left atrium is well described in an increasing body of literature. Studies using mice models of OSA have shown that the repetitive induction of apneic events has direct effects on connexin protein regulation, atrial fibrous tissue content, and structural changes, including slowed atrial conduction [63]. Similar mimics of OSA in rats were shown to selectively increase the fraction of interstitial collagen in the atria of mice, without any similar findings in murine ventricles [64]. This study further showed that Interleukin 6 and Antiogensin-1 Converting Enzyme were significantly upregulated and correlated with the degree of atrial fibrosis [64]. Relating to these laboratory findings, a study of 40 patients undergoing AF ablation showed that while patients with OSA had no differences in baseline AF risk factors compared to controls, they had slower conduction velocities in atrial tissue and more complex electrograms in the atrium [54]. In a study of patients referred for pulmonary vein isolation, 43 patients with OSA were compared to 43 control patients and were shown to have lower atrial voltage amplitude, slower conduction velocity, and more fractionation of electrograms [65].

In addition to the chronic structural changes attributed to OSA, acute changes in physiology account for an additional risk factor for AF development. A retrospective review of overnight polysomnograms from the Sleep Heart Health Study showed that the odds of an arrhythmia were 18 times higher during a period of respiratory disturbance compared to normal breathing during sleep [66]. One acute factor that has been shown to contribute to AF development is hypercapnia. In a study of a sheep model of hypercapnia, there was an increase in vulnerability to the development of atrial fibrillation during the post-hypercapnic phase of airway obstruction [67]. In this experiment, hypercapnia caused a lengthening of the atrial effective refractory period and an increase in conduction time, which resolved with resolution of hypercapnia. Vulnerability to atrial fibrillation development was assessed by evaluating the response to an early electrical stimulus to the atrium, with more development of atrial fibrillation in response to this stimulus during the return to normal carbon dioxide levels.

4. Why Will This Patient Not Get Better? The Impact of Obstructive Sleep Apnea on Treatment and Outcomes in Cardiac Rhythm Disorders

As previously mentioned, the prevalence of recognized and unrecognized OSA among patients with cardiac arrhythmias in general and atrial fibrillation in particular is quite high. Thus, screening patients with rhythm disorders for OSA would be reasonable for no other reason than to identify subjects with symptomatic OSA who might benefit from treatment. While altruistic, routine screening of patients with rhythm disorders may also provide insight regarding rhythm management as well, particularly among patients with treatment-resistant rhythm disorders. Obesity and OSA are tightly linked to one another, and both conditions have been recognized as contributors to the reoccurrence of atrial fibrillation after both cardioversion and successful catheter-based ablation [68,69]. The presence of OSA has been associated with a greater rotor burden in patients with atrial fibrillation, with a proclivity for right atrial rotors in particular [70]. OSA has been implicated as a contributor to secondary rhythm-related complications of other cardiovascular diagnoses, including myocardial infarction and heart failure [71,72]. Among patients with permanent pacemakers that are largely implanted for sinus or AV nodal diseases, the prevalence of previously unrecognized OSA is quite high, raising the question of whether appropriate OSA treatment might have resulted in fewer device implants [73]. In patients with non-ischemic cardiomyopathies who have implanted cardiac defibrillators for the primary prevention of sudden death, OSA has been associated with an increased rate of inappropriate shocks [74]. Current clinical guidelines recommend screening all patients with treatment-resistant atrial fibrillation for the presence of OSA, and one should strongly consider screening patients with tachy-brady syndrome or ventricular tachycardia and survivors of sudden cardiac death if OSA risk factors are present [53].

5. Do I Really Need to Wear This Mask Every Night? The Impact of Obstructive Sleep Apnea Treatment on Outcomes in Cardiac Rhythm Disorders

Most of the research done to assess the impact of OSA treatment on outcomes in patients with cardiac arrhythmias has focused on PAP devices. To date, there are no published data supporting the use of mandibular advancement device therapy or hypoglossal nerve stimulation for the express purpose of reducing arrhythmic or other cardiovascular events. It has been observed that surgical weight loss can reduce the likelihood for AF recurrence in a dose-dependent fashion, but large-scale randomized clinical trials with rhythm-related endpoints are lacking [75]. While observational cohort data suggest that PAP therapy improves outcomes in rhythm disorders such as atrial fibrillation and lessens the burden of premature ventricular contractions and non-sustained ventricular tachycardia in patients with heart failure [76–79], recent randomized controlled clinical trials involving subjects with OSA treated with PAP or either sham PAP or no PAP have failed to demonstrate any significant benefits in patients with atrial fibrillation or other arrhythmias [80–82]. The reason for this disconnect between observational and randomized trial data is likely multifactorial, but patient adherence to therapy selection probably plays a large role. Current randomized controlled trials involving PAP tend to enroll asymptomatic or minimally sleepy patients due to ethical concerns about not treating sleep patients with PAP. These are also the patients who are less likely to adhere to PAP therapy. Many of these studies also exclude patients with more extreme obesity. There are data linking OSA symptoms to greater OSA morbidity and mortality, so by excluding these patients from clinical trials, we may be testing a lower-risk population than that seen in everyday clinical practice [83,84]. Thus, current randomized clinical trials are likely excluding patients who would be expected to benefit the most from PAP therapy.

6. Where Do We Go from Here? Parting Thoughts and Future Directions

Based on a review of the available data, it seems clear that the presence of OSA increases one's likelihood for developing incident atrial fibrillation, nocturnal pauses, bradycardia, sustained and non-sustained ventricular arrhythmias, and individual ectopic ventricular complexes. The growing body of basic scientific data supporting the causal role of OSA-related events in the genesis of rhythm disorders is quite robust. Observational data also strongly suggest that the presence of unrecognized and untreated OSA interferes with the success of conventional rhythm management, especially in patients with AF. What has yet to be clearly established is whether OSA treatment—and PAP treatment in particular—actually improves rhythm-related outcomes in patients with OSA. It is well known that the presence of objective and subjective sleepiness in OSA is associated with poorer cardiac outcomes for reasons that are not entirely clear, but may be related to a greater degree of oxidative stress and the expression of pro-inflammatory molecules in these sleepy patients [83,84] While randomized clinical trial data looking at the effect of PAP treatment on cardiac outcomes have been admittedly disappointing [80,85], these trials enrolled patients with few or no OSA symptoms for ethical reasons, and many of these trials studied patients who were much less obese than the average "real-world" OSA patient. PAP compliance also remains a limitation in many clinical trials [86]. These facts raise significant doubts about the true efficacy of PAP treatment in such patients, and future trials should look to include sleepy patients with higher BMIs to see if this lack of treatment effects persists. Since recent randomized clinical trials have called into question whether PAP therapy provides any cardiovascular therapy at all, it may be time to revisit the ethics of randomizing sleepy patients in PAP trials or to utilize different study designs to address these questions, such as observational studies using propensity scoring [86]. In addition, the role of a multi-faceted intervention for OSA, such as combining PAP with structured weight loss, exercise, and lifestyle and nutritional counseling, deserves more exploration, as there are data that suggest that these approaches may benefit patients with rhythm disorders more than PAP therapy alone [87].

Author Contributions: B.L. was responsible for the primary literature review pertaining to the mechanistic relationship between sleep apnea and rhythm disorders, for primary authorship of the manuscript sections pertaining to these mechanisms, and for the design of Figure 1. M.D.F. was responsible for the overall conceptualization and methodolgy of the manuscript, the primary literature review pertaining to OSA epidemiology and the impact of OSA treatment on rhythm outcomes, the creation of tables and for authoring these portions of the manuscript. All authors have read and agreed to the published version of the manuscript.

Funding: This research received no external funding.

Conflicts of Interest: The authors declare no conflict of interest.

References

1. Tietjens, J.R.; Claman, D.; Kezirian, E.J.; De Marco, T.; Mirzayan, A.; Sadroonri, B.; Goldberg, A.N.; Long, C.; Gerstenfeld, E.P.; Yeghiazarians, Y. Obstructive Sleep Apnea in Cardiovascular Disease: A Review of the Literature and Proposed Multidisciplinary Clinical Management Strategy. *J. Am. Hear. Assoc.* **2019**, *8*, e010440. [CrossRef]
2. Senaratna, C.V.; Perret, J.L.; Lodge, C.J.; Lowe, A.J.; Campbell, B.E.; Matheson, M.C.; Hamilton, G.S.; Dharmage, S.C. Prevalence of obstructive sleep apnea in the general population: A systematic review. *Sleep Med. Rev.* **2016**, *34*, 70–81. [CrossRef]
3. Guillot, M.; Sforza, E.; Crawford, E.A.; Maudoux, D.; Martin, M.S.; Barthélémy, J.-C.; Roche, F. Association between severe obstructive sleep apnea and incident arterial hypertension in the older people population. *Sleep Med.* **2013**, 838–842. [CrossRef] [PubMed]
4. Cepeda-Valery, B.; Acharjee, S.; Romero-Corral, A.; Pressman, G.S.; Gami, A.S. Obstructive Sleep Apnea and Acute Coronary Syndromes: Etiology, Risk, and Management. *Curr. Cardiol. Rep.* **2014**, *16*, 1–7. [CrossRef] [PubMed]
5. Gottlieb, D.J.; Yenokyan, G.; Newman, A.B.; O'Connor, G.T.; Punjabi, N.M.; Quan, S.F.; Redline, S.; Resnick, H.E.; Tong, E.K.; West, M.D.; et al. Prospective study of obstructive sleep apnea and incident coronary heart disease and heart failure: The sleep heart health study. *Circulation* **2010**, *22*, 52–360. [CrossRef] [PubMed]
6. Hetland, A.; Vistnes, M.; Haugaa, K.H.; Liland, K.H.; Olseng, M.; Edvardsen, T. Obstructive sleep apnea versus central sleep apnea: Prognosis in systolic heart failure. *Cardiovasc. Diagn. Ther.* **2020**, *10*, 396–404. [CrossRef] [PubMed]
7. Mansukhani, M.; Calvin, A.D.; Kolla, B.P.; Brown, R.D.; Lipford, M.C.; Somers, V.K.; Caples, S.M. The association between atrial fibrillation and stroke in patients with obstructive sleep apnea: A population-based case-control study. *Sleep Med.* **2013**, *14*, 243–246. [CrossRef] [PubMed]
8. Acharya, R.; Basnet, S.; Tharu, B.; Koirala, A.; Dhital, R.; Shrestha, P.; Poudel, D.; Ghimire, S.; Kafle, S. Obstructive Sleep Apnea: Risk Factor for Arrhythmias, Conduction Disorders, and Cardiac Arrest. *Cureus* **2020**, *12*, e9992. [CrossRef] [PubMed]

9. Baillieul, S.; Revol, B.; Jullian-Desayes, I.; Joyeux-Faure, M.; Tamisier, R.; Pépin, J.-L. Diagnosis and management of central sleep apnea syndrome. *Expert Rev. Respir. Med.* **2019**, *13*, 545–557. [CrossRef]
10. Yu, L.; Li, X.; Huang, B.; Zhou, X.; Wang, M.; Zhou, L.; Meng, G.; Wang, Y.; Wang, Z.; Deng, J.; et al. Atrial Fibrillation in Acute Obstructive Sleep Apnea: Autonomic Nervous Mechanism and Modulation. *J. Am. Hear. Assoc.* **2017**, *6*. [CrossRef] [PubMed]
11. Chahal, A.A.; Somers, V.K.; Chan, W.; Coutts, S.B.; Hanly, P.; Jiang, N.; Zhou, A.; Prasad, B.; Zhou, L.; Doumit, J.; et al. Ion Channel Remodeling—A Potential Mechanism Linking Sleep Apnea and Sudden Cardiac Death. *J. Am. Hear. Assoc.* **2016**, *5*. [CrossRef] [PubMed]
12. Peppard, P.E.; Young, T.; Barnet, J.H.; Palta, M.; Hagen, E.W.; Hla, K.M. Increased Prevalence of Sleep-Disordered Breathing in Adults. *Am. J. Epidemiology* **2013**, *177*, 1006–1014. [CrossRef]
13. Jehan, S.; Myers, A.K.; Zizi, F.; Perumal, S.R.P.; Louis, G.J.; McFarlane, S.I. Obesity, obstructive sleep apnea and type diabetes mellitus: Epidemiology and pathophysiologic insights. *Sleep Med. Disord. Int. J.* **2018**, *2*, 52–58.
14. Jean-Louis, G.; Zizi, F.; Clark, L.T.; Brown, C.D.; McFarlane, S.I. Obstructive Sleep Apnea and Cardiovascular Disease: Role of the Metabolic Syndrome and Its Components. *J. Clin. Sleep Med.* **2008**, *4*, 261–272. [CrossRef]
15. Chung, F.; Abdullah, H.R.; Liao, P. STOP-Bang Questionnaire: A Practical Approach to Screen for Obstructive Sleep Apnea. *Chest* **2016**, *149*, 631–638. [CrossRef]
16. Chiu, H.-Y.; Chen, P.-Y.; Chuang, L.-P.; Chen, N.-H.; Tu, Y.-K.; Hsieh, Y.-J.; Wang, Y.-C.; Guilleminault, C. Diagnostic accuracy of the Berlin questionnaire, STOP-BANG, STOP, and Epworth sleepiness scale in detecting obstructive sleep apnea: A bivariate meta-analysis. *Sleep Med. Rev.* **2017**, *6*, 57–70. [CrossRef] [PubMed]
17. Nagappa, M.; Liao, P.; Wong, J.; Auckley, D.; Ramachandran, S.K.; Memtsoudis, S.G.; Mokhlesi, B.; Chung, F. Validation of the STOP-Bang Questionnaire as a Screening Tool for Obstructive Sleep Apnea among Different Populations: A Systematic Review and Meta-Analysis. *PLOS ONE* **2015**, *10*, e0143697. [CrossRef]
18. Johns, M.W. Daytime sleepiness, snoring, and obstructive sleep apnea. The Epworth Sleepiness Scale. *Chest* **1993**, *103*, 30–36. [CrossRef]
19. Mehra, R.; Wang, L.; Andrews, N.; Tang, W.W.; Young, J.B.; Javaheri, S.; Foldvary-Schaefer, N. Dissociation of Objective and Subjective Daytime Sleepiness and Biomarkers of Systemic Inflammation in Sleep-Disordered Breathing and Systolic Heart Failure. *J. Clin. Sleep Med.* **2017**, *13*, 1411–1422. [CrossRef]
20. Johnson, K.G.; Sullivan, S.S.; Rastegar, A.N.V.; Gurubhagavatula, I. The impact of the COVID-19 pandemic on sleep medicine practices. *J. Clin. Sleep Med.* **2021**, *7*, 79–87. [CrossRef]
21. Blanchard, M.; Gervès-Pinquié, C.; Feuilloy, M.; Le Vaillant, M.; Trzepizur, W.; Meslier, N.; Paris, A.; Pigeanne, T.; Racineux, J.-L.; Balusson, F.; et al. Association of Nocturnal Hypoxemia and Pulse Rate Variability with Incident Atrial Fibrillation in Patients Investigated for Obstructive Sleep Apnea. *Ann. Am. Thorac. Soc.* **2021**, *18*, 1043–1051. [CrossRef]
22. Kainulainen, S.; Töyräs, J.; Oksenberg, A.; Korkalainen, H.; Sefa, S.; Kulkas, A.; Leppänen, T. Severity of Desaturations Reflects OSA-Related Daytime Sleepiness Better Than AHI. *J. Clin. Sleep Med.* **2019**, *15*, 1135–1142. [CrossRef]
23. Xie, J.; Kuniyoshi, F.H.S.; Covassin, N.; Singh, P.; Gami, A.S.; Wang, S.; Chahal, C.A.A.; Wei, Y.; Somers, V.K. Nocturnal Hypoxemia Due to Obstructive Sleep Apnea Is an Independent Predictor of Poor Prognosis After Myocardial Infarction. *J. Am. Hear. Assoc.* **2016**, *5*. [CrossRef]
24. May, A.M.; van Wagoner, D.R.; Mehra, R. OSA. Cardiac Arrhythmogenesis: Mechanistic Insights. *Chest* **2017**, *51*, 225–241. [CrossRef] [PubMed]
25. Leung, R.S. Sleep-Disordered Breathing: Autonomic Mechanisms and Arrhythmias. *Prog. Cardiovasc. Dis.* **2009**, *51*, 324–338. [CrossRef] [PubMed]
26. Drager, L.F.; Silva, L.D.; Diniz, P.M.; Bortolotto, L.A.; Pedrosa, R.P.; Couto, R.B.; Marcondes, B.; Giorgi, D.M.A.; Filho, G.L.; Krieger, E.M. Obstructive sleep apnea, hypertension, and their interaction on arterial stiffness and heart remodeling. *Chest* **2007**, *31*, 1379–1386. [CrossRef] [PubMed]
27. Marin, J.M.; Agusti, A.; Villar, I.; Forner, M.; Nieto, D.; Carrizo, S.J.; Barbé, F.; Vicente, E.; Wei, Y.; Nieto, F.J.; et al. Association Between Treated and Untreated Obstructive Sleep Apnea and Risk of Hypertension. *JAMA* **2012**, *07*, 2169–2176. [CrossRef]
28. Shahar, E.; Whitney, C.W.; Redline, S.; Lee, E.T.; Newman, A.B.; Nieto, F.J.; O'Connor, G.T.; Boland, L.L.; Schwartz, J.E.; Samet, J.M. Sleep-disordered Breathing and Cardiovascular Disease. *Am. J. Respir. Crit. Care Med.* **2001**, *163*, 19–25. [CrossRef]
29. Chung, M.K.; Eckhardt, L.L.; Chen, L.Y.; Ahmed, H.M.; Gopinathannair, R.; Joglar, J.A.; Noseworthy, P.A.; Pack, Q.R.; Sanders, P.; Trulock, K.M. Lifestyle and Risk Factor Modification for Reduction of Atrial Fibrillation: A Scientific Statement From the American Heart Association. *Circulation* **2020**, *41*, e750–e772.
30. Almor, J.M.; López, J.J.; Casteigt, B.; Conejos, J.; Valles, E.; Farré, N.; Flor, M.F. Prevalence of obstructive sleep apnea syndrome in patients with sick sinus syndrome. *Rev. Esp. Cardiol.* **2006**, *9*, 28–32.
31. Hoffstein, V.; Mateika, S. Cardiac arrhythmias, snoring, and sleep apnea. *Chest* **1994**, *106*, 466–471. [CrossRef]
32. Gami, A.S.; Howard, D.E.; Olson, E.J.; Somers, V.K. Day-night pattern of sudden death in obstructive sleep apnea. *N. Engl. J. Med.* **2005**, *52*, 1206–1214. [CrossRef]
33. Mann, D.; Zipes, D.; Libby, P.; Bonow, R. *Braunwald's Heart Disease: A Textbook of Cardiovascular Medicine*, 11th ed.; Elsevier/Saunders: Philadelphia, PA, USA, 2015.
34. Vetulli, H.M.; Elizari, M.V.; Naccarelli, G.V.; Gonzalez, M.D. Cardiac automaticity: Basic concepts and clinical observations. *J. Interv. Card. Electrophysiol.* **2018**, *52*, 263–270. [CrossRef]

35. Linz, D.; Schotten, U.; Neuberger, H.-R.; Böhm, M.; Wirth, K. Negative tracheal pressure during obstructive respiratory events promotes atrial fibrillation by vagal activation. *Hear. Rhythm.* **2011**, *8*, 1436–1443. [CrossRef]
36. Chadda, K.R.; Fazmin, I.T.; Ahmad, S.; Valli, H.; E Edling, C.; Huang, C.L.-H.; Jeevaratnam, K. Arrhythmogenic mechanisms of obstructive sleep apnea in heart failure patients. *Sleep* **2018**, *41*. [CrossRef]
37. Lu, Z.; Nie, L.; He, B.; Yu, L.; Salim, M.; Huang, B.; Cui, B.; He, W.; Wu, W.; Jiang, H. Increase in vulnerability of atrial fibrillation in an acute intermittent hypoxia model: Importance of autonomic imbalance. *Auton. Neurosci.* **2013**, *177*, 148–153. [CrossRef]
38. Tse, G. Mechanisms of cardiac arrhythmias. *J. Arrhythmia* **2015**, *32*, 75–81. [CrossRef]
39. Selim, B.J.; Ramar, K. Management of Sleep Apnea Syndromes in Heart Failure. *Sleep Med. Clin.* **2017**, *12*, 107–121. [CrossRef] [PubMed]
40. Orban, M.; Bruce, C.J.; Pressman, G.S.; Leinveber, P.; Romero-Corral, A.; Korinek, J.; Konecny, T.; Villarraga, H.R.; Kara, T.; Caples, S.M.; et al. Dynamic Changes of Left Ventricular Performance and Left Atrial Volume Induced by the Mueller Maneuver in Healthy Young Adults and Implications for Obstructive Sleep Apnea, Atrial Fibrillation, and Heart Failure. *Am. J. Cardiol.* **2008**, *102*, 1557–1561. [CrossRef] [PubMed]
41. Fung, J.W.; Li, T.S.; Choy, D.K.; Yip, G.W.; Ko, F.W.; Sanderson, J.E.; Hui, D.S. Severe Obstructive Sleep Apnea Is Associated With Left Ventricular Diastolic Dysfunction. *Chest* **2002**, *121*, 422–429. [CrossRef]
42. Virolainen, J.; Ventila, M.; Turto, H.; Kupari, M. Effect of negative intrathoracic pressure on left ventricular pressure dynamics and relaxation. *J. Appl. Physiol.* **1995**, *79*, 455–460. [CrossRef]
43. Simantirakis, E.N.; Schiza, S.I.; Marketou, M.E.; Chrysostomakis, S.I.; Chlouverakis, G.I.; Klapsinos, N.C.; Siafakas, N.S.; Vardas, P.E. Severe bradyarrhythmias in patients with sleep apnoea: The effect of continuous positive airway pressure treatment: A long-term evaluation using an insertable loop recorder. *Eur. Heart J.* **2004**, *5*, 1070–1076. [CrossRef]
44. Mehra, R.; Benjamin, E.J.; Shahar, E.; Gottlieb, D.J.; Nawabit, R.; Kirchner, H.L.; Sahadevan, J.; Redline, S. Association of nocturnal arrhythmias with sleep-disordered breathing: The Sleep Heart Health Study. *Am. J. Respir. Crit. Care Med.* **2006**, *73*, 910–916. [CrossRef]
45. Guilleminault, C.; Connolly, S.J.; Winkle, R.A. Cardiac arrhythmia and conduction disturbances during sleep in 400 patients with sleep apnea syndrome. *Am. J. Cardiol.* **1983**, *52*, 490–494. [CrossRef]
46. Becker, H.F.; Koehler, U.; Stammnitz, A.; Peter, J.H. Heart block in patients with sleep apnoea. *Thorax* **1998**, *53*, S29–S32. [CrossRef] [PubMed]
47. Tilkian, A.G.; Guilleminault, C.; Schroeder, J.S.; Lehrman, K.L.; Simmons, F.; Dement, W.C. Sleep-induced apnea syndrome: Prevalence of cardiac arrhythmias and their reversal after tracheostomy. *Am. J. Med.* **1977**, *63*, 348–358. [CrossRef]
48. Cortelli, P.; Lombardi, C.; Montagna, P.; Parati, G. Baroreflex modulation during sleep and in obstructive sleep apnea syndrome. *Auton. Neurosci.* **2012**, *169*, 7–11. [CrossRef] [PubMed]
49. Zwillich, C.; Devlin, T.; White, D.; Douglas, N.; Weil, J.; Martin, R. Bradycardia during sleep apnea. Characteristics and mechanism. *J. Clin. Investig.* **1982**, *69*, 1286–1292. [CrossRef]
50. Daly, M.D.B.; Scott, M.J. The effects of stimulation of the carotid body chemoreceptors on heart rate in the dog. *J. Physiol.* **1958**, *144*, 148–166. [CrossRef]
51. Garrigue, S.; Pépin, J.L.; Defaye, P.; Murgatroyd, F.; Poezevara, Y.; Clémenty, J.; Lévy, P. High Prevalence of Sleep Apnea Syndrome in Patients With Long-Term Pacing. *Circulation* **2007**, *115*, 1703–1709. [CrossRef] [PubMed]
52. Dimitri, H.; Ng, M.; Brooks, A.G.; Kuklik, P.; Stiles, M.K.; Lau, D.H.; Antic, N.; Thornton, A.; Saint, D.A.; McEvoy, D.; et al. Atrial remodeling in obstructive sleep apnea: Implications for atrial fibrillation. *Heart Rhythm* **2012**, 321–327. [CrossRef]
53. Chugh, S.S.; Havmoeller, R.; Narayanan, K.; Singh, D.; Rienstra, M.; Benjamin, E.J.; Gillum, R.F.; Kim, Y.-H.; McAnulty, J.H., Jr.; Zheng, Z.-J.; et al. Worldwide epidemiology of atrial fibrillation: A Global Burden of Disease010 Study. *Circulation* **2014**, *29*, 837–847. [CrossRef]
54. Haïssaguerre, M.; Jaïs, P.; Shah, D.C.; Takahashi, A.; Hocini, M.; Quiniou, G.; Garrigue, S.; Le Mouroux, A.; Le Métayer, P.; Clémenty, J. Spontaneous Initiation of Atrial Fibrillation by Ectopic Beats Originating in the Pulmonary Veins. *New Engl. J. Med.* **1998**, *339*, 659–666. [CrossRef] [PubMed]
55. Nattel, S.; Dobrev, D. Controversies about atrial fibrillation mechanisms: Aiming for order in chaos and whether it matters. *Circ. Res.* **2017**, *20*, 1396–1398. [CrossRef]
56. Akoum, N.; Daccarett, M.; McGann, C.; Segerson, N.; Vergara, G.; Kuppahally, S.; Badger, T.; Burgon, N.; Haslam, T.; Kholmovski, E.; et al. Atrial Fibrosis Helps Select the Appropriate Patient and Strategy in Catheter Ablation of Atrial Fibrillation: A DE-MRI Guided Approach. *J. Cardiovasc. Electrophysiol.* **2010**, *22*, 16–22. [CrossRef]
57. Kottkamp, H. Human atrial fibrillation substrate: Towards a specific fibrotic atrial cardiomyopathy. *Eur. Heart J.* **2013**, *4*, 2731–2738. [CrossRef]
58. Buckley, U.; Rajendran, P.S.; Shivkumar, K. Ganglionated plexus ablation for atrial fibrillation: Just because we can, does that mean we should? *Hear. Rhythm.* **2017**, *14*, 133–134. [CrossRef] [PubMed]
59. Gami, A.S.; Pressman, G.; Caples, S.M.; Kanagala, R.; Gard, J.J.; Davison, D.E.; Malouf, J.F.; Ammash, N.M.; Friedman, P.A.; Somers, V.K. Association of Atrial Fibrillation and Obstructive Sleep Apnea. *Circulation* **2004**, *110*, 364–367. [CrossRef] [PubMed]
60. Braga, B.; Poyares, D.; Cintra, F.; Guilleminault, C.; Cirenza, C.; Horbach, S.; Macedo, D.; Silva, R.; Tufik, S.; De Paola, A. Sleep-disordered breathing and chronic atrial fibrillation. *Sleep Med.* **2009**, *10*, 212–216. [CrossRef] [PubMed]

61. Stevenson, I.H.; Teichtahl, H.; Cunnington, D.; Ciavarella, S.; Gordon, I.; Kalman, J.M. Prevalence of sleep disordered breathing in paroxysmal and persistent atrial fibrillation patients with normal left ventricular function. *Eur. Heart J.* **2008**, *9*, 662–1669. [CrossRef] [PubMed]
62. Shantha, G.; Pelosi, F.; Morady, F. Relationship Between Obstructive Sleep Apnoea and AF. *Arrhythmia Electrophysiol. Rev.* **2019**, *8*, 180–183. [CrossRef]
63. Iwasaki, Y.-K.; Kato, T.; Xiong, F.; Shi, Y.-F.; Naud, P.; Maguy, A.; Mizuno, K.; Tardif, J.-C.; Comtois, P.; Nattel, S. Atrial Fibrillation Promotion With Long-Term Repetitive Obstructive Sleep Apnea in a Rat Model. *J. Am. Coll. Cardiol.* **2014**, *64*, 2013–2023. [CrossRef]
64. Ramos, P.; Rubies, C.; Torres, M.; Batlle, M.; Farre, R.; Brugada, J.; Montserrat, J.M.; Almendros, I.; Mont, L. Atrial fibrosis in a chronic murine model of obstructive sleep apnea: Mechanisms and prevention by mesenchymal stem cells. *Respir. Res.* **2014**, *15*, 54. [CrossRef]
65. Anter, E.; Biase, L.D.; Valdes, F.M.C.; Gianni, C.; Mohanty, S.; Tschabrunn, C.M.; Gonzalez, J.F.V.; Leshem, E.; Buxton, A.E.; Kulbak, G.; et al. Atrial Substrate and Triggers of Paroxysmal Atrial Fibrillation in Patients With Obstructive Sleep Apnea. *Circ. Arrhythmia Electrophysiol.* **2017**, *0*, e005407. [CrossRef] [PubMed]
66. Monahan, K.; Storfer-Isser, A.; Mehra, R.; Shahar, E.; Mittleman, M.; Rottman, J.; Punjabi, N.; Sanders, M.; Quan, S.F.; Resnick, H.; et al. Triggering of Nocturnal Arrhythmias by Sleep-Disordered Breathing Events. *J. Am. Coll. Cardiol.* **2009**, *54*, 1797–1804. [CrossRef]
67. Stevenson, I.H.; Roberts-Thomson, K.C.; Kistler, P.; Edwards, G.A.; Spence, S.; Sanders, P.; Kalman, J.M. Atrial electrophysiology is altered by acute hypercapnia but not hypoxemia: Implications for promotion of atrial fibrillation in pulmonary disease and sleep apnea. *Hear. Rhythm.* **2010**, *7*, 1263–1270. [CrossRef] [PubMed]
68. Trines, S.A.; Stabile, G.; Arbelo, E.; Dagres, N.; Brugada, J.; Kautzner, J.; Pokushalov, E.; Maggioni, A.P.; Laroche, C.; Anselmino, M.; et al. Influence of risk factors in the ESC-EHRA EORP atrial fibrillation ablation long-term registry. *Pacing Clin. Electrophysiol.* **2019**, *42*, 1365–1373. [CrossRef]
69. Kanagala, R.; Murali, N.S.; Friedman, P.A.; Ammash, N.M.; Gersh, B.J.; Ballman, K.V.; Shamsuzzaman, A.S.M.; Somers, V.K. Obstructive Sleep Apnea and the Recurrence of Atrial Fibrillation. *Circulation* **2003**, *107*, 2589–2594. [CrossRef] [PubMed]
70. Friedman, D.J.; Liu, P.; Barnett, A.S.; Campbell, K.B.; Jackson, K.P.; Bahnson, T.D.; Daubert, J.P.; Piccini, J.P. Obstructive sleep apnea is associated with increased rotor burden in patients undergoing focal impulse and rotor modification guided atrial fibrillation ablation. *Europace* **2017**, *20*, f337–f342. [CrossRef] [PubMed]
71. Mehra, R.; Redline, S. Arrhythmia Risk Associated with Sleep Disordered Breathing in Chronic Heart Failure. *Curr. Hear. Fail. Rep.* **2013**, *11*, 88–97. [CrossRef] [PubMed]
72. Wang, L.-J.; Pan, L.-N.; Yan, R.-Y.; Quan, W.-W.; Xu, Z.-H. Obstructive sleep apnea increases heart rhythm disorders and worsens subsequent outcomes in elderly patients with subacute myocardial infarction. *J. Geriatr. Cardiol.* **2021**, *8*, 30–38.
73. Engstrom, N.; Dobson, G.P.; Ng, K.; Letson, H.L. Primary Prevention Implantable Cardiac Defibrillators: A Townsville District Perspective. *Front. Cardiovasc. Med.* **2020**, *7*, 577248. [CrossRef]
74. Yeghiazarians, Y.; Jneid, H.; Tietjens, J.R.; Redline, S.; Brown, D.L.; El-Sherif, N.; Mehra, R.; Bozkurt, B.; Ndumele, C.E.; Somers, V.K. Obstructive Sleep Apnea and Cardiovascular Disease: A Scientific Statement From the American Heart Association. *Circulation* **2021**. [CrossRef] [PubMed]
75. Donnellan, E.; Wazni, O.M.; Elshazly, M.; Kanj, M.; Hussein, A.A.; Baranowski, B.; Kochar, A.; Trulock, K.; Aminian, A.; Schauer, P.; et al. Impact of Bariatric Surgery on Atrial Fibrillation Type. *Circ. Arrhythmia Electrophysiol.* **2020**, *13*, e007626. [CrossRef] [PubMed]
76. Holmqvist, F.; Guan, N.; Zhu, Z.; Kowey, P.R.; Allen, L.A.; Fonarow, G.; Hylek, E.M.; Mahaffey, K.W.; Freeman, J.V.; Chang, P.; et al. Impact of obstructive sleep apnea and continuous positive airway pressure therapy on outcomes in patients with atrial fibrillation—Results from the Outcomes Registry for Better Informed Treatment of Atrial Fibrillation (ORBIT-AF). *Am. Hear. J.* **2015**, *169*, 647–654.e2. [CrossRef]
77. Iwaya, S.; Yoshihisa, A.; Nodera, M.; Owada, T.; Yamada, S.; Sato, T.; Suzuki, S.; Yamaki, T.; Sugimoto, K.; Kunii, H.; et al. Suppressive effects of adaptive servo-ventilation on ventricular premature complexes with attenuation of sympathetic nervous activity in heart failure patients with sleep-disordered breathing. *Hear. Vessel.* **2013**, *29*, 470–477. [CrossRef] [PubMed]
78. Deng, F.; Raza, A.; Guo, J. Treating obstructive sleep apnea with continuous positive airway pressure reduces risk of recurrent atrial fibrillation after catheter ablation: A metaanalysis. *Sleep Med.* **2018**, *46*, 5–11. [CrossRef] [PubMed]
79. Piccini, J.P.; Pokorney, S.D.; Anstrom, K.J.; Oldenburg, O.; Punjabi, N.M.; Fiuzat, M.; Tasissa, G.; Whellan, D.J.; Lindenfeld, J.; Benjafield, A.; et al. Adaptive servo-ventilation reduces atrial fibrillation burden in patients with heart failure and sleep apnea. *Hear. Rhythm.* **2019**, *16*, 91–97. [CrossRef] [PubMed]
80. Traaen, G.M.; Aakerøy, L.; Hunt, T.-E.; Øverland, B.; Bendz, C.; Sande, L.; Akhus, S.; Fagerland, M.W.; Steinshamn, S.; Anfinsen, O.-G.; et al. Effect of Continuous Positive Airway Pressure on Arrhythmia in Atrial Fibrillation and Sleep Apnea: A Randomized Controlled Trial. *Am. J. Respir. Crit. Care Med.* **2021**. [CrossRef]
81. Caples, S.M.; Mansukhani, M.; Friedman, P.A.; Somers, V.K. The impact of continuous positive airway pressure treatment on the recurrence of atrial fibrillation post cardioversion: A randomized controlled trial. *Int. J. Cardiol.* **2019**, *278*, 133–136. [CrossRef]
82. McNicholas, W.T. Obstructive sleep apnoea and comorbidity—An overview of the association and impact of continuous positive airway pressure therapy. *Expert Rev. Respir. Med.* **2019**, *13*, 251–261. [CrossRef] [PubMed]

83. Lombardi, C.; Parati, G.; Cortelli, P.; Provini, F.; Vetrugno, R.; Plazzi, G.; Vignatelli, L.; Di Rienzo, M.; Lugaresi, E.; Mancia, G.; et al. Daytime sleepiness and neural cardiac modulation in sleep-related breathing disorders. *J. Sleep Res.* **2008**, *17*, 263–270. [CrossRef] [PubMed]
84. Choi, J.B.; Nelesen, R.; Loredo, J.S.; Mills, P.J.; Israel, S.A.; Ziegler, M.G.; Dimsdale, J.E. Sleepiness in obstructive sleep apnea: A harbinger of impaired cardiac function? *Sleep* **2006**, *29*, 1531–1536. [CrossRef] [PubMed]
85. McEvoy, R.D.; Antic, N.A.; Heeley, E.; Luo, Y.; Ou, Q.; Zhang, X.; Mediano, O.; Chen, R.; Drager, L.F.; Liu, Z.; et al. CPAP for Prevention of Cardiovascular Events in Obstructive Sleep Apnea. *N. Engl. J. Med.* **2016**, *375*, 919–931. [CrossRef] [PubMed]
86. McEvoy, R.D.; Sánchez-De-La-Torre, M.; Peker, Y.; Anderson, C.S.; Redline, S.; Barbe, F. Randomized clinical trials of cardiovascular disease in obstructive sleep apnea: Understanding and overcoming bias. *Sleep* **2021**, *44*. [CrossRef]
87. Donnellan, E.; Wazni, O.M.; Kanj, M.; Elshazly, M.; Hussein, A.A.; Patel, D.R.; Trulock, K.; Wilner, B.; Baranowski, B.; Cantillon, D.J.; et al. Impact of risk-factor modification on arrhythmia recurrence among morbidly obese patients undergoing atrial fibrillation ablation. *J. Cardiovasc. Electrophysiol.* **2020**, *31*, 1979–1986. [CrossRef]

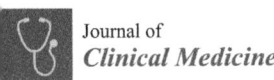

Review

Body Mass Index Reduction and Selected Cardiometabolic Risk Factors in Obstructive Sleep Apnea: Meta-Analysis

Marta Stelmach-Mardas [1,*,†], Beata Brajer-Luftmann [2,†], Marta Kuśnierczak [3], Halina Batura-Gabryel [2], Tomasz Piorunek [2] and Marcin Mardas [3]

1. Department of Treatment of Obesity, Metabolic Disorders and Clinical Dietetics, Poznan University of Medical Sciences, Szamarzewskiego 84 Street, 61-569 Poznan, Poland
2. Department of Pulmonology, Allergology and Pulmonary Oncology, Poznan University of Medical Sciences, Szamarzewskiego 84 Street, 60-569 Poznan, Poland; bbrajer@ump.edu.pl (B.B.-L.); halinagabryel@wp.pl (H.B.-G.); t_piorun@op.pl (T.P.)
3. Department of Oncology, Poznan University of Medical Sciences, Szamarzewskiego 84 Street, 61-569 Poznan, Poland; martakusnierczak@gmail.com (M.K.); marcin.mardas@ump.edu.pl (M.M.)
* Correspondence: stelmach@ump.edu.pl; Tel.: +48-697424245
† Authors equally contributed to the work.

Abstract: Although clinical studies have been carried out on the effects of weight reduction in sleep apnea patients, no direct link has been shown between weight reduction and changes in cardio-metabolic risk factors. We aimed to analyze changes in the apnea–hypopnea index and selected cardio-metabolic parameters (total cholesterol, triglycerides, glucose, insulin, blood pressure) in relation to the reduction in body mass index in obstructive sleep apnea patients. Medline, Web of Science and Cochrane databases were searched to combine results from individual studies in a single meta-analysis. We identified 333 relevant articles, from which 30 papers were assigned for full-text review, and finally 10 (seven randomized controlled trials and three nonrandomized studies) were included for data analysis. One unit of body mass index reduction was found to significantly influence changes in the apnea–hypopnea index (−2.83/h; 95% CI: −4.24, −1.41), total cholesterol (−0.12 mmol/L; 95% CI: −0.22, −0.01), triglycerides (−0.24 mmol/L; 95% CI: −0.46, −0.02), fasting insulin (−7.3 pmol/L; 95% CI: −11.5, −3.1), systolic (−1.86 mmHg; 95% CI: −3.57, −0.15) and diastolic blood pressure (−2.07 mmHg; 95% CI: −3.79, −0.35). Practical application of lifestyle modification resulting in the reduction of one unit of body mass index gives meaningful changes in selected cardio-metabolic risk factors in obstructive sleep apnea patients.

Keywords: biological markers; weight loss; apnea–hypopnea index; blood pressure

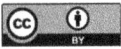

1. Introduction

Obstructive sleep apnea (OSA) is a recognized cardio-metabolic disorder affecting 53% of the middle-to-older age general population, and 36% of OSA subjects having exclusive positional sleep apnea can be treated with positional therapy [1,2]. OSA is characterized by repetitive partial or complete closure of the upper airway during sleep that results in hypoxemia and hypercapnia, is frequently associated with arousals, and leads to an increase in myocardial oxygen demand [3]. The sum of the number of apneas and the number of hypopneas per hour is described by the apnea–hypopnea index (AHI) [4]. The AHI defines four grades of OSA: mild (5.0–14.9), moderate (15.0–29.9) and severe (≥30.0 events per hour) [4].

Currently, continuous positive airway pressure (CPAP) therapy is the 'gold standard' treatment for OSA, with dietary interventions and physical activity promoting weight loss encouraged in obese OSA individuals [5]. An increase of body weight by 10% over time increases the AHI, on average, by 30%, whereas a 10–15% reduction in body weight can reduce the AHI by 50% [6]. It has been shown that the Mediterranean diet improves OSA regardless of CPAP use and weight loss, whereas body-mass reduction itself improves OSA severity and symptoms [7]. Recent results from the Sleep AHEAD Study confirmed that individuals with OSA and type 2 diabetes mellitus receiving intensive lifestyle intervention for weight loss had reduced OSA severity, related to changes in body weight, baseline AHI and intervention independent of weight change at 10 years [8]. Additionally, previously published data have shown that OSA can itself be associated with dyslipidemia, hypertension and impaired glucose (Glc) tolerance independent of obesity [9–11]. OSA increases the risk of heart failure by 140%, the risk of stroke by 60% and the risk of coronary heart disease by 30%, causes significant sleep disturbances, leading to excessive daytime sleepiness and fatigue, depression (21.8%), anxiety (16.7%), posttraumatic stress disorder (11.9%), psychosis (5.1%) and bipolar disorder (3.3%) [12]. Although differentiated lifestyle interventions were applied in OSA individuals [13–17], until now there is no consistent finding that directly translates the effectiveness of lifestyle modification, expressed as body mass index (BMI) reduction, to changes in cardio-metabolic risk factors.

Because of this fact, we aimed this study to analyze changes in the AHI and selected cardio-metabolic parameters (concentration of total cholesterol (TC), triglycerides (TG), Glc, insulin, systolic and diastolic blood pressure (SBP, DBP)) in relation to reductions in the BMI in OSA patients.

2. Materials and Methods

2.1. Search Strategy, Inclusion and Exclusion Criteria

The databases Medline, Cochrane Library and Web of Knowledge were searched for clinical studies carried out between 1958 and November 2020 that reported the effect of lifestyle modification on BMI and selected cardio-metabolic parameters as primary or secondary outcomes in individuals with OSA.

The search strategy was restricted to humans, English language and original articles. The search was based upon the following index terms and titles: #1, sleep or apnea or obstructive sleep apnea or obstructive sleep apnea or sleep-disordered breathing and #2, diet or dietary intervention or diet, fat-restricted or energy intake or energy reduction and #3, weight loss or weight and #4, insulin or insulin resistance or insulin-secreting cells or glucose or lipids or triglycerides or cholesterol, and not animals. The PRISMA Statement was followed [18].

Only studies run with patients suffering from OSA indicating the changes in BMI, AHI and selected blood parameters after lifestyle modification were included. Intervention studies (randomized controlled trial, RCT, and nonrandomized controlled study, NRS) were taken into consideration. The articles that did not meet inclusion criteria were excluded.

2.2. Data Extraction and Analysis

Relevant articles were identified by screening the abstracts, titles and full texts. The study selection process was performed by two independent researchers in parallel for each database, cross-checked by a third reviewer. For each full-text paper, information was extracted including general information (study title, authors, year, journal), study characteristics (study design, country, length of intervention), characteristics of studied population (number, nationality, demographic characteristics of participants), assessment methods (body weight measurement, Glc, insulin, TC, TG and AHI measurements) and type of outcome (BMI changes, changes in selected cardio-metabolic parameters). The relationships between BMI reduction and AHI, TC, TG, Glc and insulin changes respectively were described as mean difference per 1 unit of BMI reduction if the effect of lifestyle modification was linked with reductions or increases in the analyzed parameters.

To assess the study quality, the Cochrane risk of bias for RCTs was used. For NRS, a nine-point scoring system according to the Newcastle–Ottawa scale was applied [19], where a high-quality study was defined by a threshold of ≥ 7 points.

2.3. Statistical Approach

When possible, the recorded Glc, TC and TG concentrations were converted to mmol/L and insulin concentration to pmol/L in order to standardize the results. A meta-analysis was performed to combine the results of the individual studies. Data were analyzed using a random-effects model, which allowed for true effect variation between studies. The effect size of a study was investigated by calculating mean difference per unit of BMI reduction (treated as an objective measurement of body weight change) with a 95% confidence interval.

The heterogeneity of the sum of studies was tested for significance. As a measure for quantifying inconsistencies, I2 was selected [20]. The results of the meta-analysis were visualized using a forest plot, which illustrates the results of the individual studies and the summary effect. The analysis was performed with Review Manager (RevMan) V5.3 (the Nordic Cochrane Centre, the Cochrane Collaboration, Copenhagen, Denmark, 2014).

3. Results

3.1. Search Results, Studies and Population Characteristics

We initially identified 333 potentially relevant publications from which, after title search, 97 articles were included. After duplicate removal, 30 papers were assigned for full-text review and finally 10 articles were included for data extraction and analysis [4,12–17,21–24]. The process outline and workflow is presented in Figure 1.

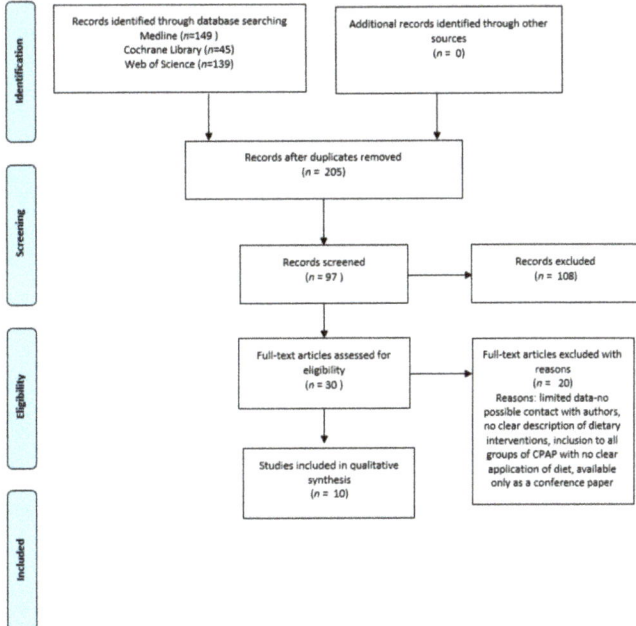

Figure 1. Process of the literature search for dietary intervention and cardio-metabolic risk factors in adults.

The characteristics of clinical studies (randomized and nonrandomized) and populations are presented in Tables 1 and 2, respectively. The population consists of 1069 individuals and was characterized by a mean baseline BMI of >29 kg/m^2, a mean age of 35–70 [13] and a predominance of Caucasian ethnicity. The durations of interventions ranged from 4 week [13] to 24 week [24] (with observations up to 2 year) [16], based on lifestyle modification [4,12–17,21–24].

Table 1. Characteristics of the included studies and changes in BMI and AHI during dietary intervention in the study and control groups.

Study	Study Design	Subjects (n)[§]	Age (Years) Mean ± SD	% of Women	Nationality	Analyzed Groups	Intervention	Time of Intervention	BMI (kg/m²) Mean ± SD		AHI (A + H/h) Mean ± SD	
									Baseline	Intervention	Baseline	Intervention
Barnes et al. 2009 [13]	NRS	12	All: 42.3 ± 10.4	100	Australia	SG	VLED *	16 wk	36.1 ± 4.3	30.1 ± 4.2	24.6 ± 12.0	18.3 ± 11.9
Chakravorty et al. 2002 [21]	RCT	53	All: 49.0 ± 11.0	-	Great Britain	SG CG	CPAP Diet	12 wk	40.0 ± 14.5 32.5 ± 5.5	40.0 ± 12.5 31.7 ± 5.6	55.0 ± 28.7 35.0 ± 19.1	8.0 ± 28.0 34.0 ± 21.0
Chirinos et al. 2014 [24]	RCT	146	48.3 49.8 49.0	41.0 59.7 49.0	American	SG 1 SG 2 CG	Diet CPAP Diet + CPAP	24 wk	38.3 ± 5.5 38.2 ± 7.2 37.7 ± 5.5	-	39.7 ± 20.3 41.2 ± 20.96 47.1 ± 26.86	-
Desplan et al. 2014 [14]	RCT	22	All: 35–70	-	France	SG CG	Diet + EAS * EAS	4 wk	29.9 ± 3.4 31.3 ± 2.5	29.1 ± 3.1 31.3 ± 2.2	40.6 ± 19.2 19,439.8 ± 19.2	28.0 ± 19.3 45.4 ± 22.5
Foster et al. 2009 [4]	RCT	264	All: 61.2 ± 6.5	-	American	SG CG	Diet * Education support	16 wk	−3.8 ± 0.3 −0.2 ± 0.3		−5.4 ± 1.5 4.2 ± 1.4	
Johansson et al. 2011 [22]	NRS	62	All: 48.7 ± 7.3	-	Sweden	SG	VLCD	9 wk	−5.5 ± 2.0		−21 ± 16	
Kuna et al. 2013 [23]	RCT	264	All: 61.3 ± 6.5	59	American	SG CG	Diet * Education support	16 wk	−3.8 ± 0.74 *** −0.2 ± 0.66 ***		−5.7 ± 1.5 4.0 ± 1.4	
Monasterio et al. 2001 [15]	RCT	142	54.0 ± 9.0 53.0 ± 9.0	-	Spain	SG CG	Sleep hyg. + diet Sleep hyg. + diet + CPAP	12 wk	29.5 ± 3.3 29.4 ± 3.7	28.5 ± 3.5 ** 29.5 ± 2.8 **	21.0 ± 6.0 20.0 ± 6.0	17.0 ± 10.0 * 6.0 ± 8.0 *
Nerfeldt et al. 2010 [16]	NRS	33	All: 52(31–68)	27.2	Sweden	SG	VLCD + behavioral support	8-wk (observation: 24mo)	40.0 ± 5.0	35.0 ± 3.0	43.0 ± 24.0	28.0 ± 19.0
Tuomilehto et al. 2009 [17]	RCT	72	51.8 (9.0) 50.9 (8.6)	35	Finland	SG CG	VLCD + lifestyle modification lifestyle modification	12 wk (observation: 12mo)	−3.5 ± 2.1 −0.8 ± 2.0		−4.0 ± 5.6 0.3 ± 8.0	

* physical activity recommended. ** after 6-months,*** calculated, §—the number that completed the study; SD—standard deviation; AHI—the apnea–hypopnea index; BMI—body mass index; CBT—cognitive-behavioral therapy; CG—control group; CPAP—continuous positive airway pressure; EAS—education activity session; NRS—nonrandomized controlled study; RCT—randomized clinical trial; SG—study group; VLCD—very-low-caloric diet, VLED-very low energy density.

Table 2. Mean changes in cardio-metabolic risk factors during dietary intervention in the study and control groups in selected studies.

Study	Analyzed Groups	TC (mmol/L) Mean ± SD		TG (mmol/L) Mean ± SD		Fasting Glc (mmol/L) Mean ± SD		Fasting Insulin (pmol/L) Mean ± SD		SBP/DBP (mmHg) Mean ± SD	
		Baseline	Intervention	Baseline	Intervention	Baseline	Intervention	Baseline	Intervention	Baseline	Intervention
Barnes et al. 2009 [13]	SG	5.3 ± 1.1	4.4 ± 1.0	1.5 ± 0.8	1.0 ± 0.6	6.1 ± 2.2	5.8 ± 1.5	107.6 ± 41.7	74.3 ± 32.6	125.8 ± 14.0/ 77.3 ± 10.6	120.5 ± 9.8/ 73.3 ± 6.3
Chirinos et al. 2014 [24]	SG 1 SG 2 CG	-	-	-0.26 (−0.49 to −0.03) ** −0.08 (−0.27 to 0.11) ** −0.60 (−0.86 to −0.34) **	-	-	-	-	-	−6.8 (−10.8 to −2.7)/ −4.7 (−7.7 to −1.7) ** −3 (−6.5 to 0.5)/ −3.5 (−6.1 to −0.9) ** −14.1 (−18.7 to −9.5)/ −10.6 (−14 to −7.2) **	
Desplan et al. 2014 [14]	SG CG	-	-	1.87 ± 1.01 1.70 ± 0.53	1.20 ± 0.29 1.72 ± 0.81	5.61 (4.94–6.17) * 5.44 (5.17–5.67) *	4.78 (4.5–5.44) * 5.17 (4.89–6.0) *	-	-	141.8 ± 15.8/ 79.0 ± 7.1 128.1 ± 14.4/ 82.5 ± 7.1	145.6 ± 23.2/ 73.0 ± 10.3 128.0 ± 18.2/ 78.8 ± 9.7
Monasterio et al. 2001 [15]	SG CG	-	-	-	-	-	-	-	-	132 ± 17/84 ± 11 126 ± 17 81 ± 12	131 ± 16/84 ± 10 126 ± 15/81 ± 10
Nerfeldt et al. 2010 [16]	SG	5.3 ± 1.1	4.9 ± 1.2	1.8 ± 0.8	1.6 ± 0.7	7.2 ± 2.7	7.0 ± 3.3	147 ± 78	90 ± 52	144 ± 19/89 ± 14	129 ± 10/81 ± 6
Tuomilehto et al. 2009 [17]	SG CG	-	-	−0.48 ± 1.13 −0.006 ± 0.65	-	−0.6 ± 2.3 −0.4 ± 1.4	-	−34.7 ± 48.6 8.33 ± 23.6	-	−1.7 ± 14.7/−1.9 ± 10.6 −1.1 ± 19.6/−0.4 ± 12.6	

* Median, 25%, 75%; ** 95% CI; CG—control group; DBP—diastolic blood pressure; Glc—glucose; SBP—systolic blood pressure; SG—study group; TC-total cholesterol; TG-triglycerides.

The dietary strategies leading to a decrease in energy intake were based on a reduced intake of fat or general caloric restriction [4,12–17,21–24]. After the intervention period, mean BMI values decreased up to 5 units [16,22] and AHI values up to 15 [16] when only diet was used (Table 1).

The quantitative meta-analysis revealed a significant decrease in AHI per 1 unit of BMI change (mean difference: $-2.83/h$; 95% CI: $-4.24, -1.41$; $p < 0.00001$, $I2 = 95\%$) (Figure 2).

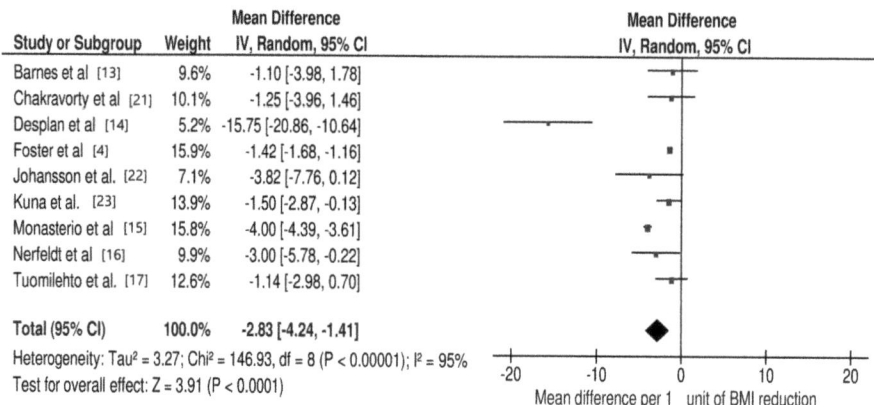

Figure 2. Forest plot for mean apnea–hypopnea index (AHI) change per 1 unit of body mass index (BMI) reduction in selected studies.

For each study, the square represents the point estimate of the effect. Horizontal lines join lower and upper limits of the 95% CI of this effect. The area of shaded squares reflects the relative weight of the study in the meta-analysis. Diamonds represent the subgroup mean difference and pooled mean differences. CI indicates the confidence interval (upper and lower limit) [4,12–17,21–24].

3.2. Changes in Selected Cardio-Metabolic Parameters during Lifestyle Modification in Relation to BMI Reduction

Details about the analyzed biomarkers, at baseline and at the end of the intervention, or mean differences between the concentrations, were reported in only six studies [12–17,24]. The changes in TC concentration were followed by only Barnes et al. [12] and Nerfeld et al. [16]. The changes in TG were analyzed in five studies [12,13,16,17,24], fasting Glc in four studies [12,13,16,17], fasting insulin in three studies [12,16,17] and blood pressure in all six included studies [12–17,24] (Table 2).

Mean decreases ranged from 0.26 mmol/L [24] to 0.67 mmol/L [13] for TG concentrations, from 0.2 mmol/L [16] to 0.83 mmol/L [13] for Glc levels, up to 66.7 pmol/L for insulin levels, with changes in BP being highly differentiated [12–17,24] (Table 2).

The meta-analysis revealed a significant association between changes in the following cardio-metabolic risk factors per 1 unit of BMI change: TC (mean difference: -0.12 mmol/L; 95% CI: $-0.22, -0.01$; $p = 0.03$, $I2 = 0\%$), TG (mean difference: -0.24 mmol/L; 95% CI: $-0.46, -0.02$; $p = 0.03$, $I2 = 92\%$) and fasting insulin (mean difference: -7.3 pmol/L; 95% CI: $-11.5, -3.1$; $p = 0.0007$, $I2 = 0\%$) (Figure 3), as well as in SBP (mean difference: -1.86 mmHg; 95% CI: $-3.57, -0.15$; $p = 0.03$, $I2 = 76\%$) and DBP (mean difference: -2.07 mmHg; 95% CI: $-3.79, -0.35$; $p = 0.02$, $I2 = 90\%$) (Figure 4).

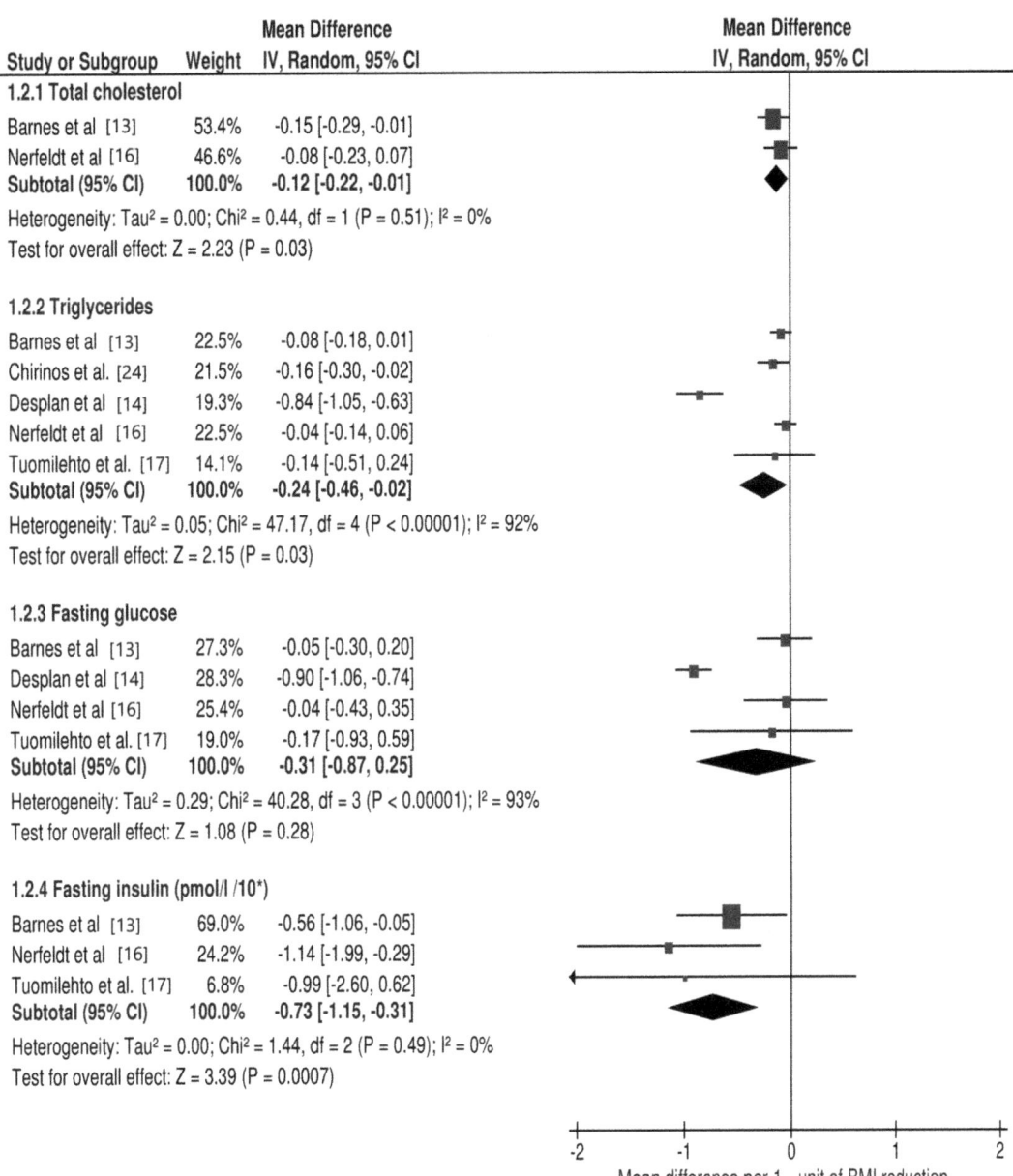

Figure 3. Forest plot for mean cardio-metabolic parameters change in subgroup analysis: total cholesterol, triglycerides, glucose, insulin per 1 unit of body mass index (BMI) reduction in selected studies.

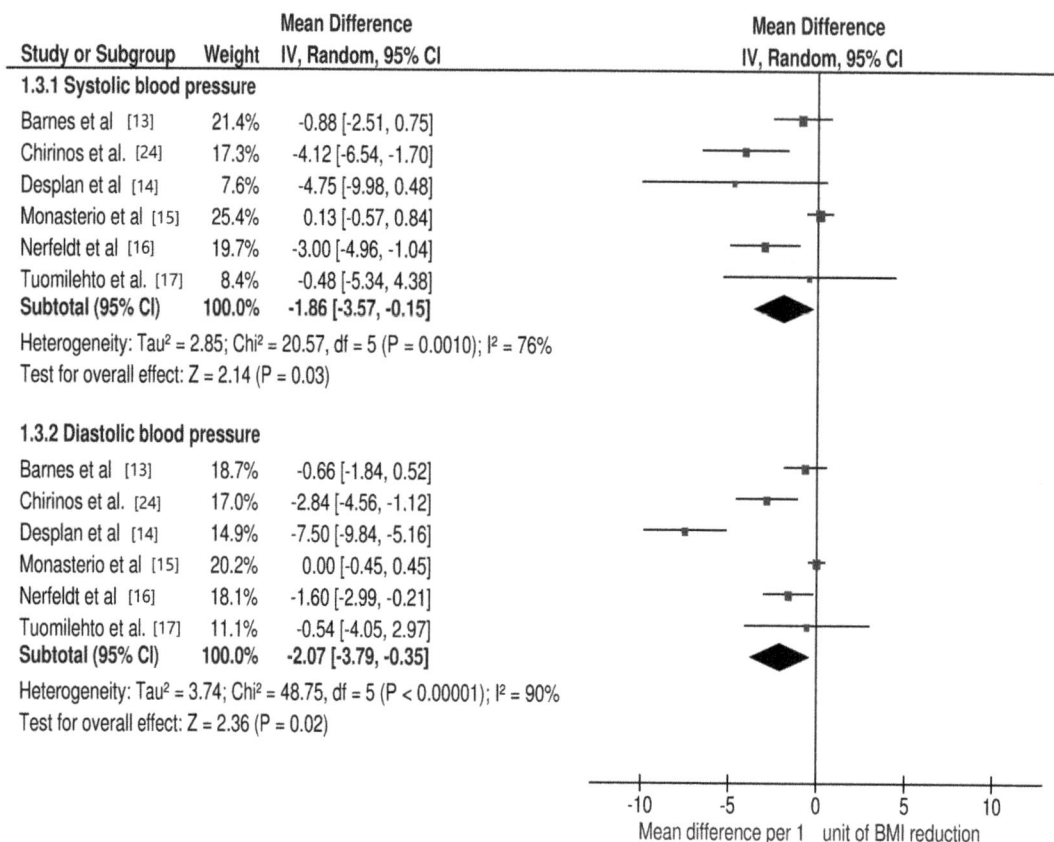

Figure 4. Forest plot for mean cardio-metabolic parameter changes in subgroup analysis: systolic and diastolic blood pressure per 1 unit of body mass index (BMI) reduction in selected studies.

For each study, the square represents the point estimate of the effect. Horizontal lines join lower and upper limits of the 95% CI of this effect. The area of shaded squares reflects the relative weight of the study in the meta-analysis. Diamonds represent the subgroup mean difference and pooled mean differences. CI indicates the confidence interval (upper and lower limit) [12,13,16,17,24].

3.3. Subgroup Analyses

Different subgroup analyses were performed to evaluate the possible influences of BMI reduction on AHI and cardio-metabolic risk-factor changes (study duration, study design and type of lifestyle modification). Nevertheless, none of the subgroup analyses, with regards to AHI changes and cardio-metabolic risk factors, indicated significance ($p > 0.05$)—in some cases, due to the limited number of studies, analysis was not possible (Table 3).

Table 3. Subgroup analyses for possible influences of BMI reduction on AHI and cardio-metabolic risk-factor changes (study duration, study design and type of dietary intervention).

Analyzed Parameter	Duration			Design			Intervention		
	Short-Term	Long-Term	p	RCT	NRS	p	LC Diet	VLCD	p-Value
AHI [A + H/h]	−7.24 (14.15, −0.34)	−1.87 (−3.37, −0.37)	0.14	−2.95 (−4.65, −1.26)	−2.44 (−4.22, −0.65)	0.68	−3.35 (−5.25, −1.46)	−1.81 (−3.09, −0.53)	0.19
TC (mmol/L)	-	-	-	-	-	-	-	-	-
TG (mmol/L)	−0.47 (−1.25, 0.31)	−0.11 (−0.19, −0.03)	0.37	−0.39 (−0.87, 0.10)	−0.08 (−0.18, 0.02)	0.22	−0.50 (−1.16, 0.17)	−0.06 (−0.13, 0.01)	0.21
fasting Glc (mmol/L)	−0.49 (−1.33, 0.35)	−0.06 (−0.30, 0.18)	0.34	−0.63 (−1.32, 0.06)	−0.05 (−0.26, 0.16)	0.11	-	-	-
fasting insulin (pmol/L)	-	-	-	-	-	-	-	-	-
SBP (mmHg)	−3.22 (−5.05, −1.38)	−1.22 (−3.05, 0.62)	0.12	−2.05 (−4.98, 0.89)	−1.87 (−3.94, 0.21)	0.92	−2.49 (−6.11, 1.14)	−1.70 (−3.29, −0.10)	0.70
DBP (mmHg)	−4.47 (−10.25, 1.31)	−0.68 (−1.41, 0.05)	0.20	−2.70 (−6.01, 0.60)	−0.87 (−1.63, −0.10)	0.29	−3.31 (−7.33, 0.71)	−1.02 (−1.89, −0.15)	0.28

AHI—the apnea–hypopnea index; DBP—diastolic blood pressure; Glc—glucose; LC—low caloric; SBP—systolic blood pressure; TC-total cholesterol; TG-triglycerides; NRS—nonrandomized controlled study; p—p-value; RCT—randomized clinical trial; VLCD—very-low-caloric diet.

3.4. Risk of Bias and Publication Bias

The risk of bias for RCTs [4,13,15,17,21,23,24] is summarized in Figure 5 indicating mainly low risk or unclear risk. A high risk of bias was recognized for allocation in one study only [21]. For NRS, the Newcastle–Ottawa scale was applied and the mean score was 7 [12,16,22].

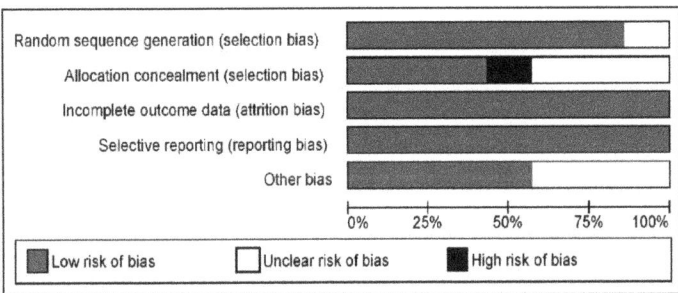

Figure 5. Risk of bias graph: review authors' judgments about each risk of bias item presented as percentages across all included studies.

A funnel plot did not suggest real evidence of a publication bias for changes in AHI per 1 unit of BMI change (Figure 6a). However, funnel plots for other cardio-metabolic risk factors did reveal asymmetry, despite only a few studies being outliers, suggesting evidence of publication bias (Figure 6b,c).

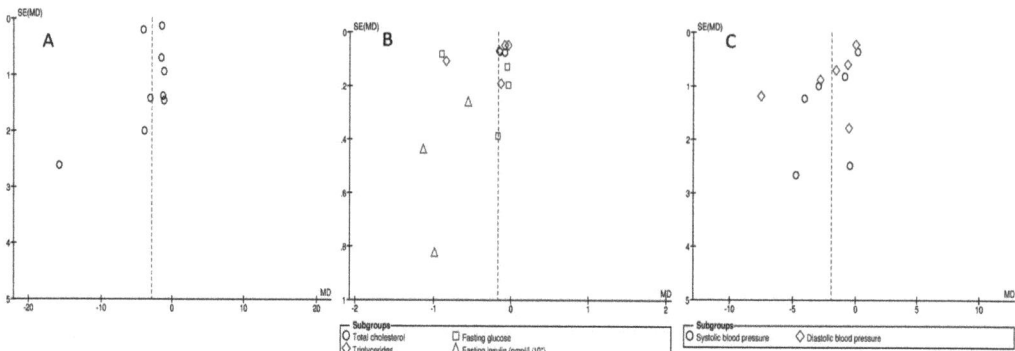

Figure 6. Funnel plot of standard error by standard differences in means of: (**A**) apnea–hypopnea index, (**B**) total cholesterol, triglycerides, glucose and insulin, (**C**) systolic and diastolic blood pressure in selected studies per unit of body mass index reduction.

The summary diamonds at the bottom of the plot represent the summarized effects using fixed and random effects models, where the random effects estimates are considered the primary findings for this study, due to heterogeneity [4,12–17,21–24].

4. Discussion

Here we present the first review summarizing the results from clinical studies performed on OSA with a primary interest in changes of selected cardio-metabolic outcomes as results of BMI reduction after applying lifestyle modification. The findings of the conducted systematic review present the beneficial effects of lifestyle modification on changes in BMI in OSA patients with strong clinical implications for positive changes in cardio-metabolic risk factors (TC, TG, fasting insulin and BP).

It was imperative for the conducted review to show that OSA patients should be recognized as the core group with a prime interest in changing diet being the determinant of "metabolic health". However, only limited data are available with regards to dietary behaviors in OSA. It has to be highlighted that lifestyle change is very unlikely in this group of patients; therefore, the likelihood of the positive effect in OSA patients could be even smaller. It has been shown by Fogelholm et al. [25] that patients with OSA are more likely to suffer from increased excessive daytime sleepiness, sedentary behaviors associated with more time to eat, an increase in appetite and a liking for high-fat food. Therefore, an estimated 60–70% of patients with OSA can be categorized as obese, with a BMI greater than 30 kg/m^2 [26]. Increasing body weight may predict an increase in clinical indicators of OSA severity, such as the AHI, which measures respiratory events during sleep [26,27]. For data consistency, we have expressed the changes in analyzed parameters per unit of BMI reduction. As a result, the differentiated duration of included dietary interventions could not influence the interpretation of obtained results. As previously shown in a prospective cohort study conducted from 1989 to 2000, a 10% weight gain may predict an approximate increase of 32% in the AHI. In contrast, a 10% weight loss may predict a 26% decrease in the AHI [27]. As shown by our meta-analysis, an improvement in AHI of more than 2.8/h per unit of BMI reduction may have practical significance. According to data published by Tuomilehto et al. [28], sustained improvement in body weight reduction and AHI can also be observed in 2 year post-intervention follow-ups. In clinical practice, changes from severe to either moderate or mild OSA may improve quality of life and reduce sleepiness in OSA patients. Specifically, it is worth noting that obesity itself contributes to daytime somnolence independent of OSA [12]. In clinical practice, it is possible without great efforts to have patients consult with dieticians in a way that will result in successful weight loss with long-term body weight maintenance [29,30]. We did not assess the benefits from applied dietary intervention in subgroup analysis with regards to overweight or obese-status analyzed individuals, as individuals in both conditions were included in the study population at baseline. The application of a very-low-caloric diet in routine practice needs replication of intervention studies in large-scale cohort studies and involvement of experienced nutritionists. It seems that the energy density of food is a simple and effective measure to manage weight in obese individuals with the aim of weight reduction [31]. A diet with self-regulation of dietary intake seems to be given a prominent role in the strategy of successful long-term weight loss among the obese [30]. Nevertheless, this measure could be combined with behavior therapy and physical activity and tailored to the individual situation [30]. A previously published study [29], based on individualized dietary counseling for obese subjects, indicated the mean percentage of body weight changes can be as follows: in the 6th week—5.9%, in the 12th week—10.9% and in the 52nd week—9.7% ($p < 0.0001$). These data are similar to those published on the OSA group of patients. For example, de Melo et al. [32] has shown that even a one month application of a low-energy diet resulted in body mass reduction in OSA patients (-3.7 ± 2.0 for the low protein group: 0.8 g of protein/kg/day and -4.0 ± 1.5 for the high protein group: 1.6 g of protein/kg/day; $p < 0.001$). It was also confirmed that a long-term lifestyle modification program could be more effective in reducing BMI (-1.8 kg/m^2, 6.0% of the initial BMI $p < 0.001$) in comparison to the usual care of OSA patients (-0.6 kg/m^2, 2.0% of the initial BMI; $p < 0.001$) [33].

The prevalence of cardiovascular diseases is increased in patients with OSA, possibly related to dyslipidemia in these individuals [34]. The findings from a meta-analysis of Dong et al. [35] support the idea that moderate–severe OSA significantly increased cardiovascular risk, in particular, stroke risk. Although insulin resistance is also very often diagnosed in OSA patients, its contribution to the dyslipidemia of OSA remains unclear. Our analysis indicates statistically significant positive changes in TC, TG and fasting insulin per unit of BMI reduction, which was also confirmed in single studies after applied lifestyle modification [12,16,17,24]. However, the change in TC concentration was analyzed based solely on data from two studies, but with 0% of heterogeneity. Nevertheless, the observed particular change in TG concentration seems to be more valuable as a marker for the assessment of dyslipidemia in the current study. Taking into account the results obtained from a 16 week intervention, based on a low-caloric diet, in a group of obese women sufferers of dyslipidemia, we could expect changes in TG around 13% [36]. Therefore, obtaining a similar result when expressed per unit of BMI reduction is sufficient for OSA to reach a goal of complementary use of diet with medical treatment. Reductions in hepatic TG content are strongly associated with improved hepatic insulin sensitivity and lipoprotein metabolism through different mechanisms, including the effect of inflammatory intermediates on insulin receptor signaling and very-low-density lipoprotein synthesis [37]. In contrast, no effect on peripheral insulin resistance can be observed, which may support the hypothesis that a relatively small pool of intrahepatic lipids may be responsible for dysregulated hepatic Glc metabolism [38,39]. In our analysis, no significant change in Glc concentration was observed, which may suggest long-term dysregulation in Glc metabolism. Although, the overall effect of diet on SBP and DBP expressed per unit of BMI reduction was also significant (between 1.86 and 2.07 mmHg per unit of BMI reduction) in our study, it can be interpret as minor from a clinical point of view. Nevertheless, as reported by Tuomilehto et al. [17], a notable number of patients were able to discontinue drug treatment for hypertension, diabetes and hypercholesterolemia after lifestyle modification. It seems justified to consider the relationship between BMI reduction and changes in cardio-metabolic biomarkers in obese and overweight individuals when evaluating patients found to have OSA. It should be highlighted that, currently, more personalized attention to patients is present, and more focus on different phenotypes of OSA is recognized, such as REM-dependent phenotype or positional phenotype, which in future studies also should be considered when analyzing the effect of diet on cardio-metabolic factors [40,41]. Finally, a recent meta-analysis including 39 RCTs with 6954 subjects has shown that there is a risk of an increase in BMI in patients with OSA following CPAP treatment, especially in those with less than 5 h/night of CPAP use [42]. In this context, the greatest reduction in BP observed in the study by Chirinos et al. (Table 2) was when CPAP was combined with diet therapy [24], which further emphasizes the importance of lifestyle modifications, especially in obese individuals with OSA.

5. Limitations

Despite an increasing number of dietary intervention studies, the body of evidence remains limited by either small sample size (an inclusion-only arm of intervention without use of devices) or inclusion of nonrandomized trials and studies with behavioral support. Only future clinical trials with long-term follow-up periods can address this limitation. Moreover, no information on possible comorbidities of individuals in the analyzed studies was provided, which could also influence obtained data. Furthermore, the present findings are based on limited ethnicity (Caucasian); therefore, results could vary as a function of ethnic background. Although, the duration of the interventions in analyzed studies was relatively long (up to 24 weeks), we could observe long-term follow-up changes of analyzed cardio-metabolic parameters in a few studies. We did not analyze interventions based on physical activity, which is commonly recommended to OSA patients with standard therapy and applied as a pragmatic strategy (hard to accept by patients having stable behavior habits), though alone it does not provide significant clinical benefits [39]. It must be highlighted that only studies that could show the effectiveness of lifestyle modification (either diet alone or diet with physical activity) were included. Some studies published in the grey literature may have been missed by our literature search.

6. Conclusions

In conclusion, we find that lifestyle modification resulting in the reduction of one unit of BMI gives meaningful and positive changes in selected cardio-metabolic risk factors such as TC, TG, fasting insulin and BP in OSA patients. Broader interventional studies are needed to assess different dietary approaches in OSA individuals.

Author Contributions: Conceptualization, M.S.-M., M.M., B.B.-L., methodology, M.S.-M., B.B.-L., and M.M.; software, M.M.; validation, T.P. and H.B.-G.; formal analysis, M.S.-M. and M.M.; investigation, M.K., B.B.-L. and T.P., resources, B.B.-L.,T.P., M.K.; data curation, M.S.-M., B.B.-L., M.M.; writing-original draft preparation, B.B.-L., M.S.-M. and M.M; writing-review and editing, B.B.-L., M.S.-M. T.P., H.B.-G. and M.M; visualization, M.M.; supervision, H.B.-G., T.P. and M.M.; project administration, M.S.-M. and B.B.-L.; funding acquisition—not applicable. All authors have read and agreed to the published version of the manuscript.

Funding: This research received no external funding.

Institutional Review Board Statement: The single studies included in this SLR were conducted according to the guidelines of the Declara-tion of Helsinki, and approved by the single Institutional Review Boards (or Ethics Committees). As the design of this study was systematic literature review it does not require additional review board approval.

Informed Consent Statement: Not applicable.

Data Availability Statement: To get an access to secondary data please contact correspondence author.

Conflicts of Interest: The authors declare no conflict of interest.

References

1. Heinzer, R.; Petitpierre, N.J.; Marti-Soler, H.; Haba-Rubio, J. Prevalence and characteristics of positional sleep apnea in the HypnoLaus population-based cohort. *Sleep Med.* **2018**, *48*, 157–162. [CrossRef]
2. Mirrakhimov, A.E. Obstructive sleep apnea and kidney disease: Is there any direct link? *Sleep Breath.* **2011**, *16*, 1009–1016. [CrossRef] [PubMed]
3. Dorasamy, P. Obstructive sleep apnea and cardiovascular risk. *Ther. Clin. Risk Manag.* **2007**, *3*, 1105–1111.

4. Foster, G.D.; Borradaile, K.E.; Sanders, M.H.; Millman, R.; Zammit, G.; Newman, A.B.; Wadden, T.A.; Kelley, D.; Wing, R.R.; Kuna, S.T.; et al. A randomized study on the effect of weight loss on obstructive sleep apnea among obese patients with type 2 diabetes: The Sleep AHEAD study. *Arch. Intern. Med.* **2009**, *169*, 1619–1626. [CrossRef]
5. Thomasouli, M.-A.; Brady, E.M.; Davies, M.J.; Hall, A.P.; Khunti, K.; Morris, D.H.; Gray, L.J. The impact of diet and lifestyle management strategies for obstructive sleep apnoea in adults: A systematic review and meta-analysis of randomised controlled trials. *Sleep Breath.* **2013**, *17*, 925–935. [CrossRef] [PubMed]
6. Smith, P.L.; Gold, A.R.; Meyers, D.A.; Haponik, E.F.; Bleecker, E.R. Weight Loss in Mildly to Moderately Obese Patients with Obstructive Sleep Apnea. *Ann. Intern. Med.* **1985**, *103*, 850–855. [CrossRef]
7. Georgoulis, M.; Yiannakouris, N.; Kechribari, I.; Lamprou, K.; Perraki, E.; Vagiakis, E.; Kontogianni, M.D. The effectiveness of a weight-loss Mediterranean diet/lifestyle intervention in the management of obstructive sleep apnea: Results of the "MIMOSA" randomized clinical trial. *Clin. Nutr.* **2021**, *40*, 850–859. [CrossRef]
8. Kuna, S.T.; Reboussin, D.M.; Strotmeyer, E.S.; Millman, R.P.; Zammit, G.; Walkup, M.P.; Wadden, T.A.; Wing, R.R.; Pi-Sunyer, F.X.; Spira, A.P.; et al. Effects of Weight Loss on Obstructive Sleep Apnea Severity. Ten-Year Results of the Sleep AHEAD Study. *Am. J. Respir. Crit. Care Med.* **2021**, *15*, 221–229. [CrossRef]
9. Shahar, E.; Whitney, C.W.; Redline, S.; Lee, E.T.; Newman, A.B.; Javier Nieto, F.; Boland, L.L.; Samet, J.M. Sleep-disordered breathing and cardiovascular disease: Cross-sectional results of the Sleep Heart Health Study. *Am. J. Respir. Crit. Care Med.* **2001**, *163*, 19–25. [CrossRef] [PubMed]
10. Tan, K.C.; Chow, W.-S.; Lam, J.C.; Lam, B.; Wong, W.-K.; Tam, S.; Ip, M.S. HDL dysfunction in obstructive sleep apnea. *Atherosclerosis* **2006**, *184*, 377–382. [CrossRef]
11. Al-Delaimy, W.K.; Manson, J.E.; Willett, W.C.; Stampfer, M.J.; Hu, F.B. Snoring as a risk factor for type II diabetes mellitus: A prospective study. *Am. J. Epidemiol.* **2002**, *155*, 387–393. [CrossRef]
12. Jean-Louis, G.; Zizi, F.; Clark, L.T.; Brown, C.D.; McFarlane, S.I. Obstructive Sleep Apnea and Cardiovascular Disease: Role of the Metabolic Syndrome and Its Components. *J. Clin. Sleep Med.* **2008**, *4*, 261–272. [CrossRef]
13. Barnes, M.; Goldsworthy, U.R.; Cary, B.A.; Hill, C.J. A Diet and Exercise Program to Improve Clinical Outcomes in Patients with Obstructive Sleep Apnea—A Feasibility Study. *J. Clin. Sleep Med.* **2009**, *5*, 409–415. [CrossRef]
14. Desplan, M.; Mercier, J.; Sabaté, M.; Ninot, G.; Prefaut, C.; Dauvilliers, Y. A comprehensive rehabilitation program improves disease severity in patients with obstructive sleep apnea syndrome: A pilot randomized controlled study. *Sleep Med.* **2014**, *15*, 906–912. [CrossRef] [PubMed]
15. Monasterio, C.; Vidal, S.; Duran, J.; Ferrer, M.; Carmona, C.; Barbé, F.; Mayos, M.; Gonzalez-Mangado, N.; Juncadella, M.; Navarro, A.; et al. Effectiveness of Continuous Positive Airway Pressure in Mild Sleep Apnea–Hypopnea Syndrome. *Am. J. Respir. Crit. Care Med.* **2001**, *164*, 939–943. [CrossRef] [PubMed]
16. Nerfeldt, P.; Nilsson, B.Y.; Mayor, L.; Uddén, J.; Friberg, D. A Two-Year Weight Reduction Program in Obese Sleep Apnea Patients. *J. Clin. Sleep Med.* **2010**, *6*, 479–486. [CrossRef] [PubMed]
17. Tuomilehto, H.P.; Seppä, J.M.; Partinen, M.M.; Peltonen, M.; Gylling, H.; Tuomilehto, J.O.; Vanninen, E.J.; Randell, J.; Uusitupa, M.; Martikainen, T.; et al. Lifestyle intervention with weight reduction: First-line treatment in mild obstructive sleep apnea. *Am. J. Respir. Crit. Care Med.* **2009**, *179*, 320–327. [CrossRef] [PubMed]
18. Moher, D.; Liberati, A.; Tetzlaff, J.; Altman, D.G.; PRISMA Group. Preferred reporting items for systematic reviews and me-ta-analyses: The PRISMA statement. *PLoS Med.* **2009**, *6*, e1000097. [CrossRef] [PubMed]
19. Wells, G.; Shea, B.; O'Connell, D.; Peterson, J.; Welch, V.; Losos, M.; Tigwell, P. The Newcastle–Ottawa Scale (NOS) for Assessing the Quality of Nonrandomized Studies in Meta-Analyses. Available online: http://www.ohri.ca/programs/clinical_epidemiology/oxford.htm (accessed on 7 August 2015).
20. Borenstein, M.; Hedges, L.V.; Higgins, J.P.T.; Rothstein, H.R. *Introduction to Meta-Analysis*; John Wiley & Sons, Ltd.: Hoboken, NJ, USA, 2009.
21. Chakravorty, I.; Cayton, R.; Szczepura, A. Health utilities in evaluating intervention in the sleep apnoea/hypopnoea syndrome. *Eur. Respir. J.* **2002**, *20*, 1233–1238. [CrossRef] [PubMed]
22. Johansson, K.; Hemmingsson, E.; Harlid, R.; Lagerros, Y.T.; Granath, F.; Rössner, S.; Neovius, M. Longer term effects of very low energy diet on obstructive sleep apnoea in cohort derived from randomised controlled trial: Prospective observational follow-up study. *BMJ* **2011**, *342*, d3017. [CrossRef] [PubMed]
23. Kuna, S.T.; Reboussin, D.M.; Borradaile, K.E.; Sanders, M.H.; Millman, R.P.; Zammit, G.; Newman, A.B.; Wadden, T.A.; Wing, R.R.; Foster, G.D.; et al. Long-term effect of weight loss on obstructive sleep apnea severity in obese patients with type 2 diabetes. *Sleep* **2013**, *36*, 641–649. [CrossRef] [PubMed]
24. Chirinos, J.A.; Gurubhagavatula, I.; Teff, K.; Rader, D.J.; Wadden, T.A.; Townsend, R.; Foster, G.D.; Maislin, G.; Saif, H.; Broderick, P.; et al. CPAP, Weight Loss, or Both for Obstructive Sleep Apnea. *N. Engl. J. Med.* **2014**, *370*, 2265–2275. [CrossRef]
25. Fogelholm, M.; Kronholm, E.; Kukkonen-Harjula, K.; Partonen, T.; Partinen, M.; Härmä, M. Sleep-related disturbances and physical inactivity are independently associated with obesity in adults. *Int. J. Obes.* **2007**, *31*, 1713–1721. [CrossRef]
26. Smith, S.S.; Waight, C.; Doyle, G.; Rossa, K.R.; Sullivan, K.A. Liking for high fat foods in patients with Obstructive Sleep Apneea. *Appetite* **2014**, *78*, 185–192. [CrossRef] [PubMed]
27. Peppard, P.E.; Young, T.; Palta, M.; Dempsey, J.; Skatrud, J. Longitudinal Study of Moderate Weight Change and Sleep-Disordered Breathing. *JAMA* **2000**, *284*, 3015–3021. [CrossRef]

28. Tuomilehto, H.; Gylling, H.; Peltonen, M.; Martikainen, T.; Sahlman, J.; Kokkarinen, J.; Randel, J.; Tukiainen, H.; Vannien, E.; Partinen, M.; et al. Sustained improvement in mild obstructive sleep apnea after a diet- and physical activity-based lifestyle intervention: Postinterventional follow-up. *Am. J. Clin. Nutr.* **2010**, *92*, 688–696. [PubMed]
29. Stelmach-Mardas, M.; Mardas, M.; Warchoł, W.; Jamka, M.; Walkowiak, J. Successful maintenance of body weight reduction after individualized dietary counseling in obese subjects. *Sci. Rep.* **2014**, *4*, 6620. [CrossRef] [PubMed]
30. Stelmach-Mardas, M.; Mardas, M.; Walkowiak, J.; Boeing, H. Long-term weight status in regainers after weight loss by lifestyle intervention: Status and challenges. *Proc. Nutr. Soc.* **2014**, *73*, 509–518. [CrossRef]
31. Stelmach-Mardas, M.; Rodacki, T.; Dobrowolska-Iwanek, J.; Brzozowska, A.; Walkowiak, J.; Wojtanowska-Krosniak, A.; Zagrodzki, P.; Bechthold, A.; Mardas, M.; Boeing, H. Link between Food Energy Density and Body Weight Changes in Obese Adults. *Nutrients* **2016**, *8*, 229. [CrossRef]
32. De Melo, C.M.; Dos Santos Quaresma, M.V.L.; Del Re, M.P.; Ribeiro, S.M.L.; Moreira Antunes, H.K.; Togeiro, S.M.; Tufik, S.; de Mello, M.T. One-month of a low-energy diet, with no additional effect of high-protein, reduces Obstructive Sleep Apnea severity and improve metabolic parameters in obese males. *Clin. Nutr. ESPEN* **2021**, *42*, 82–89. [CrossRef]
33. Ng, S.S.; Chan, R.S.; Woo, J.; Chan, T.-O.; Cheung, B.H.; Sea, M.M.; To, K.-W.; Chan, K.K.; Ngai, J.; Yip, W.-H.; et al. A Randomized Controlled Study to Examine the Effect of a Lifestyle Modification Program in OSA. *Chest* **2015**, *148*, 1193–1203. [CrossRef]
34. Liu, A.; Cardell, J.; Ariel, D.; Lamendola, C.; Abbasi, F.; Kim, S.H.; Holmes, T.H.; Tomasso, V.; Mojaddidi, H.; Grove, K.; et al. Abnormalities of Lipoprotein Concentrations in Obstructive Sleep Apnea Are Related to Insulin Resistance. *Sleep* **2015**, *38*, 793–799. [CrossRef] [PubMed]
35. Dong, J.-Y.; Zhang, Y.-H.; Qin, L.-Q. Obstructive sleep apnea and cardiovascular risk: Meta-analysis of prospective cohort studies. *Atherosclerosis* **2013**, *229*, 489–495. [CrossRef]
36. García-Unciti, M.; Martinez, J.A.; Izquierdo, M.; Gorostiaga, E.M.; Grijalba, A.; Ibañez, J. Effect of resistance training and hypocaloric diets with different protein content on body composition and lipid profile in hypercholesterolemic obese women. *Nutr. Hosp.* **2013**, *27*, 1511–1520.
37. Snel, M.; Jonker, J.T.; Hammer, S.; Kerpershoek, G.; Lamb, H.J.; Meinders, A.E.; Pijl, H.; De Roos, A.; Romijn, J.A.; Smit, J.W.; et al. Long-Term Beneficial Effect of a 16-Week Very Low Calorie Diet on Pericardial Fat in Obese Type 2 Diabetes Mellitus Patients. *Obesity* **2012**, *20*, 1572–1576. [CrossRef]
38. Petersen, K.F.; Dufour, S.; Befroy, D.; Lehrke, M.; Hendler, R.E.; Shulman, G.I. Reversal of Nonalcoholic Hepatic Steatosis, Hepatic Insulin Resistance, and Hyperglycemia by Moderate Weight Reduction in Patients with Type 2 Diabetes. *Diabetes* **2005**, *54*, 603–608. [CrossRef]
39. Moss, J.; Tew, G.A.; Copeland, R.J.; Stout, M.; Billings, C.G.; Saxton, J.M.; Winter, E.M.; Bianchi, S.M. Effects of a Pragmatic Lifestyle Intervention for Reducing Body Mass in Obese Adults with Obstructive Sleep Apnoea: A Randomised Controlled Trial. *BioMed Res. Int.* **2014**, *2014*, 1–8. [CrossRef] [PubMed]
40. Gabryelska, A.; Białasiewicz, P. Association between excessive daytime sleepiness, REM phenotype and severity of obstructive sleep apnea. *Sci. Rep.* **2020**, *10*, 1–6. [CrossRef] [PubMed]
41. Mokros, Ł.; Kuczyński, W.; Gabryelska, A.; Franczak, Ł.; Spałka, J.; Białasiewicz, P. High Negative Predictive Value of Normal Body Mass Index for Obstructive Sleep Apnea in the Lateral Sleeping Position. *J. Clin. Sleep Med.* **2018**, *14*, 985–990. [CrossRef] [PubMed]
42. Chen, B.; Drager, L.F.; Peker, Y.; Vgontzas, A.N.; Phillips, C.L.; Hoyos, C.M.; Salles, G.F.; Guo, M.; Li, Y. Effect of CPAP on Weight and Local Adiposity in Adults with Obstructive Sleep Apnea: A Meta-Analysis. *Ann. Am. Thorac. Soc.* **2021**. [CrossRef] [PubMed]

MDPI
St. Alban-Anlage 66
4052 Basel
Switzerland
www.mdpi.com

Journal of Clinical Medicine Editorial Office
E-mail: jcm@mdpi.com
www.mdpi.com/journal/jcm

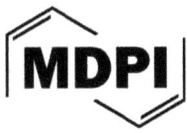

Disclaimer/Publisher's Note: The statements, opinions and data contained in all publications are solely those of the individual author(s) and contributor(s) and not of MDPI and/or the editor(s). MDPI and/or the editor(s) disclaim responsibility for any injury to people or property resulting from any ideas, methods, instructions or products referred to in the content.

www.ingramcontent.com/pod-product-compliance
Lightning Source LLC
LaVergne TN
LVHW070744100526
838202LV00013B/1302